MAXIMUM FOOD POWER
for Women

MAXIMUM FOOD POWER
for Women

HARNESS THE NATURAL POWER OF
FOOD, VITAMINS, AND HERBS
FOR TOTAL HEALTH AND WELL-BEING

BY JULIA VanTINE AND DEBRA L. GORDON

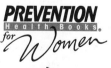

RODALE

Notice

This book is intended as a reference volume only, not as a medical manual. The information given here is designed to help you make informed decisions about your eating habits and health. It is not intended as a substitute for any treatment that may have been prescribed by your doctor. If you suspect that you have a medical problem, we urge you to seek competent medical help.

Library of Congress Cataloging-in-Publication Data

VanTine, Julia.
    Maximum food power for women : harness the natural power of food, vitamins, and herbs for total health and well-being / by Julia VanTine and Debra Gordon.
      p. cm.
    Includes index.
    ISBN 1–57954–246–8 hardcover
    ISBN 1-57954–411-8 paperback
    1. Women—Nutrition.   2. Women–Health and hygiene.   3. Food habits.
  I. Gordon, Debra, 1962–   II. Title.
  RA778 . V285   2001
  613.2'082—dc21   00–010990

Distributed to the book trade by St. Martin's Press

2 4 6 8 10 9 7 5 3 1   hardcover

2 4 6 8 10 9 7 5 3 1   paperback

Visit us on the Web at www.preventionbookshelf.com, or call us toll-free at (800) 848-4735.

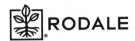

WE **INSPIRE** AND **ENABLE** PEOPLE TO IMPROVE
THEIR LIVES AND THE WORLD AROUND THEM

ABOUT *PREVENTION* HEALTH BOOKS

The editors of *Prevention* Health Books are dedicated to providing you with authoritative, trustworthy, and innovative advice for a healthy, active lifestyle. In all of our books, our goal is to keep you thoroughly informed about the latest breakthroughs in natural healing, medical research, alternative health, herbs, nutrition, fitness, and weight loss. We cut through the confusion of today's conflicting health reports to deliver clear, concise, and definitive health information that you can trust. And we explain in practical terms what each new breakthrough means to you, so you can take immediate, practical steps to improve your health and well-being.

Every recommendation in *Prevention* Health Books is based upon reliable sources, including interviews with qualified health authorities. In addition, we retain top-level health practitioners who serve on the Rodale Books Board of Advisors to ensure that all of the health information is safe, practical, and up-to-date. *Prevention* Health Books are thoroughly fact-checked for accuracy, and we make every effort to verify recommendations, dosages, and cautions.

The advice in this book will help keep you well-informed about your personal choices in health care—to help you lead a happier, healthier, and longer life.

MAXIMUM FOOD POWER FOR WOMEN STAFF

MANAGING EDITOR: Sharon Faelten

WRITERS: Julia VanTine, Debra L. Gordon

CONTRIBUTING WRITERS: Linda B. White, M.D.; Janis Jibrin, M.S., R.D.; Roberta Duyff, M.S., R.D.; Dayna Winter, M.S., R.D.; Kelly Garrett

RECIPE DEVELOPMENT: Susan McQuillan, R.D.

RECIPE EDITOR: Jean Rogers

ART DIRECTOR: Darlene Schneck

INTERIOR DESIGNER: Carol Angstadt

COVER DESIGNER: Christopher Rhoads

COVER PHOTOGRAPHER: Kurt Wilson

ASSOCIATE RESEARCH MANAGER: Shea Zukowski

PRIMARY RESEARCH EDITOR: Anita C. Small

RESEARCH EDITOR: Christine Dreisbach

EDITORIAL RESEARCHERS: Jennifer Bright, Carol J. Gilmore, Karen Jacob, Janice McLeod, Mary S. Mesaros, Deborah Pedron, Elizabeth B. Price, Sally A. Reith, Staci Ann Sander, Lucille Uhlman, Nancy Zelko

ASSOCIATE LIBRARIAN: Jennifer Keiser

SENIOR COPY EDITOR: Karen Neely

COPY EDITOR: Amy Morgan

TEST KITCHEN MANAGER: JoAnn Brader

FOOD RESEARCHERS: Lauri Centolanza, Renee Miller

EDITORIAL PRODUCTION MANAGER: Marilyn Hauptly

LAYOUT DESIGNER: Donna G. Rossi

MANUFACTURING COORDINATORS: Brenda Miller, Jodi Schaffer, Patrick Smith

Rodale Healthy Living Books

EXECUTIVE EDITOR: Tammerly Booth

EDITORIAL DIRECTOR: Michael Ward

VICE PRESIDENT AND MARKETING DIRECTOR: Karen Arbegast

PRODUCT MARKETING MANAGER: Stephanie Hamerstone

BOOK MANUFACTURING DIRECTOR: Helen Clogston

MANUFACTURING MANAGER: Eileen Bauder

RESEARCH DIRECTOR: Ann Gossy Yermish

COPY MANAGER: Lisa D. Andruscavage

PRODUCTION MANAGER: Robert V. Anderson Jr.

DIGITAL PROCESSING GROUP MANAGERS: Leslie M. Keefe, Thomas P. Aczel

OFFICE MANAGER: Jacqueline Dornblaser

OFFICE STAFF: Susan B. Dorschutz, Julie Kehs Minnix, Catherine E. Strouse

BOARD OF ADVISORS

ACKNOWLEDGMENTS

This book would not have been possible without the guidance and expertise of hundreds of experts in nutrition and health. In particular, the editor and writers would like to thank the following for their contributions to this book:

Roberta Duyff, M.S., R.D., a registered dietitian and food and nutrition consultant in St. Louis and author of *The American Dietetic Association's Complete Food and Nutrition Guide*, among other books.

Janis Jibrin, M.S., R.D., a registered dietitian and magazine writer living in Washington, D.C., and author of *The Unofficial Guide to Dieting Safely*.

Paul Lachance, Ph.D., professor of food science and nutrition in the food science department and executive director of the Nutraceutical Institute, both at Rutgers University in New Brunswick, New Jersey.

Shari Lieberman, Ph.D., a nutrition scientist in New York City, faculty member at the University of Bridgeport School of Human Nutrition in Connecticut, and author of *The Real Vitamin and Mineral Book*.

Susan McQuillan, M.S., R.D., a registered dietitian and food and nutrition writer. Her articles and recipes have appeared in *Prevention*, *Family Circle*, *Woman's Day*, *Cooking Light*, and *Country Living* magazines. She is also the coauthor of two low-fat cookbooks, *Simply Healthful Pizza* and *Simply Healthful Fish*.

Linda B. White, M.D., of Golden, Colorado, who writes widely on health issues, particularly natural health. She is the author of *Kids, Herbs, and Health* and other books and coauthor of *The Herbal Drugstore*.

Dayna Winter, M.S., R.D., a registered dietitian/nutritionist in New York City.

CONTENTS

NUTRITION FOR WOMEN
WHO LOVE FOOD—AND LIFE!

I love food. One balmy Saturday in autumn, I decided to make a pizza outdoors on our grill. I made a whole wheat crust and topped it with fresh grilled eggplant, tomatoes, onions, peppers, garlic, and olives, plus a sprinkle of sharp, freshly grated pecorino cheese. We ate dinner alfresco, on the deck, with a glass of vino rosso and the Stones serenading us on our outdoor stereo speakers. ("Thyme Is on My Side," as I recall.)

I got a boatload of healing nutrients in the bargain—lycopene from the tomatoes, lignans from the whole wheat crust, allicin from the garlic, and flavonoids from the wine, just to name a few. Vitamins never tasted so good!

Fast-forward to December. My husband, John, and I made our wish list for our millennium eve dinner. Steak. Lobster. Spinach salad with fresh mushrooms. Strawberries dipped in chocolate. Again, the nutrients flowed like bubbly: Beef supplies two essential minerals, iron (for concentration) and zinc (for strong immunity). Lobster is rich in DHA, a heart-protective fatty acid. Greens supply zeaxanthin, a plant substance that prevents a type of vision loss. Substances in shiitake mushrooms boost immunity, increasing resistance to infection. Ellagic acid, a component of strawberries, puts cancer cells out of commission. Even chocolate counts as a Power Food: Rich in phenols, chocolate offers the same antioxidants found in red wine that are known to lower the risk of heart disease and cancer. Chocolate boosts your body's overall antioxidant capacity to protect you against all kinds of age-related problems.

These are Power Foods—nature's blockbusters, packed with vitamin-like compounds that researchers never imagined existed back when women my age were in grade school learning about rickets and the four food groups.

At this point you're thinking, "That sounds great, Sharon. But if you typically eat that much food, you must weigh 250 pounds." *Au contraire.* I weigh 116 pounds, without my hiking boots. And my cholesterol? It's off the chart. *Below* the chart, that is. My risk of heart disease is so low that it doesn't show up in the lowest recommended range.

Why? Because I love the right foods, with the right nutrients. In the right amounts, Power Foods can even help you lose extra weight.

This book is written for you—a real woman who loves real food. A woman who wants to enjoy many, many more candlelight dinners, listening to her favorite music, maybe wearing clothes a size or two smaller, and possibly reducing her risk of diseases by as much as half.

Based on the latest research from pioneers in nutritional science, this book translates "what we know" into "what to do." Each chapter offers simple power-eating tips to help you apply these breakthrough discoveries to your life, starting today. You'll also find kitchen-tested Power Recipes that combine nature's top superfoods, along with tips for adding 101 Power Foods to your daily and weekly menus, no matter how busy you are. The 7-Day Food-Power Menu designed by a dietitian shows how. Plus, you'll find a customized supplement program for your body type. And you'll get straight answers on "nutriceuticals" that explain what exotic new supplements can and cannot do.

The benefits? This book shows you how to:

• Lose weight without obsessing over calories and "forbidden" foods

• Help yourself to isoflavones in soy and hundreds of other protective "phytonutrients" found naturally in other foods

• Head off heart disease, cancer, bone fractures, hot flashes, night sweats, wrinkles, and dozens of other threats to health

• Enjoy boundless energy from eating the right food

• Cut down on the frequency of colds and infections

• Free yourself from rigid diets based on strict "food rules" that don't work (and cause harm)

• Fine-tune your vitamin and mineral program to take into account individual differences

• Enjoy delicious food while building optimum health

• Look and feel fantastic

If you're tired of hearing what food can do *to* you, here is the book that will show you what food can do *for* you.

Sharon Faelten

Sharon Faelten
Managing Editor
Prevention Health Books for Women

WOMEN AND FOOD:
POWER ALLIES

Why Eat Right?
The Benefits Are B-I-G

Five nights out of seven, you'll find Sharon Keys Seal, a professional business coach, in her Baltimore kitchen, preparing dinner for herself and her two teenage sons.

"Last night, my younger son, Travis, had a wrestling match, which my older son, Carey, and I attended," says the 46-year-old mom. "We ate at 8:30, in the living room in front of the fireplace. We had pasta with meat sauce and," she laughs ruefully, "hot-fudge sundaes for dessert."

What? No vegetable?

"I usually do serve a veggie. We eat a lot of broccoli, steamed baby carrots, and snow peas," says Seal. "But since I didn't know what time Travis was coming home, I didn't make any. No one likes soggy broccoli."

For Seal, the lack of green in last night's meal is no big deal. Most nights—and days—Seal feeds herself and her sons in a way that would make a dietitian proud: lots of fresh fruits and veggies, oatmeal, whole grain bread, and low-fat yogurt. No soda, and very little junk. She studies food labels the way most of us study our supermarket receipts.

How does she eat healthfully, day after day? How does she exist without sour-cream-and-cheddar potato chips or Little Debbie snack cakes?

More important, *why* does she do it?

Because she wants to stick around to see her boys grow into men. Because she wants her middle and late years to be filled with zest and adventure, rather than medications and surgery.

Because she cares about herself, and that care extends to her body.

"I have this strong sense that I'm my body's caretaker," says Seal. "God gave me a strong body. It's like a gift. And when someone gives you a gift, you want to take care of it.

"I believe that how you treat your body today is going to impact it tomorrow," she adds. "And if you take the long view on your health, diet does make a difference."

The Nutrition Revolution

We all know that diet plays a pivotal role in our health—now. Yet it was only 30 years ago that the medical establishment snorted at the basic idea that too much dietary fat can lead to heart disease.

In the last decade, however, the breakthroughs in food science have accelerated. And the idea that diet can help prevent disease, once thought far-fetched, is fact rather than theory. Discovery follows discovery, with researchers putting together new pieces of the nutrition puzzle virtually every week.

"Nutrition is a dynamic area of research, and we're still at only the tip of the iceberg in terms of understanding the role food plays in promoting health and preventing disease," says Barbara Schneeman, Ph.D., assistant administrator for human nutrition at the USDA Agricultural Research Service in Washington, D.C.

But nutrition scientists find even the view from the tip of the iceberg exhilarating. And we, and most definitely our children, will be the beneficiaries of their ever-expanding knowledge. The blizzard of studies conducted in the past 5 years alone suggests that:

• A diet rich in whole grains can reduce a woman's risk of various cancers, including those of the colon, breast, endometrium (lining of the uterus), and ovary.

• Fibroids are linked to a diet high in red meat, while a diet high in green vegetables seems to have a protective effect.

• Calcium, long known to protect against the bone-thinning disease osteoporosis, also helps reduce blood pressure.

BUY GUM, BURN THOSE CALORIES

I n a study that is sure to be decried by etiquette experts nationwide, researchers have found that chewing a piece of gum fast hikes metabolism by 20 percent.

Researchers at the Mayo Clinic in Rochester, Minnesota, hooked seven men and women to a machine that calculates the amount of calories a person is burning at any given time. During a 30-minute rest period, the individuals burned, on average, 58 calories an hour. But when they chomped sugar-free gum at 100 chews per minute for 12 minutes, the rate shot up to 70 calories an hour. That's enough to burn off 11 pounds a year if you chew gum all the time you're awake.

The point of the study is not to tout chewing gum as a weight-loss tool, says study leader James Levine, M.D., an endocrinologist at the Mayo Clinic who also led the widely reported research on the calorie-burning power of fidgeting. "But the research does illustrate that small changes in daily activities, even something as trivial as chewing gum, can have a significant impact on weight loss."

- Substances in soy foods, called isoflavones, can slash "bad" LDL cholesterol, reducing the risk of heart disease. A soy-rich diet may also stave off osteoporosis.
- Regular consumption of leafy greens, such as spinach and kale, can help prevent cataracts and macular degeneration, two serious, age-related vision problems that can rob us of our precious eyesight.

Healing "Music" in Plant Foods

According to Phyllis Bowen, R.D., Ph.D., of the University of Illinois Functional Foods for Health Program in Chicago, one of the biggest breakthroughs of the past decade is the mounting certainty that free radicals promote disease, and the equally compelling evidence that substances in plant foods, called antioxidants and phytonutrients, help prevent them.

Free radicals are the price we pay for breathing. Generated by our own cells and by outside factors such as sunlight, smoking, and pollution, these "crippled" oxygen molecules damage healthy cells and are linked to the development of hardening of the arteries, cancer, and other chronic degenerative diseases.

The theory that free radicals contribute to disease has been around for decades. But researchers are just beginning to understand the havoc free-radical damage may wreak on our bodies. How it may trigger a chain of events that eventually chokes off the blood vessels of our hearts and brains, leading to heart attacks and stroke. How it may warp the structures of our cells and damage their DNA, which can lead to cancer. How the chemical reaction it unleashes, called oxidation, may be the trigger not just for age-related diseases but also for the aging process itself.

Equally as compelling is research that suggests that the antioxidants and phytonutrients in plant foods can slow free-radical damage and the resulting oxidation process. And file folders full of studies suggest a plant-based diet helps reduce the likelihood of developing cancer and heart disease, which tend to strike just as we're ready to cart the kids off to college, do some traveling, and savor the pleasures of our middle years.

"Plant foods speak to our bodies," says Keith Block, M.D., medical and scientific director of the Institute of Integrative Cancer Care and Block Medical Center in Evanston, Illinois, and clinical assistant professor at the University of Illinois College of Medicine in Chicago. "The antioxidants and phytonutrients they contain play piano chords on our genes." This chemical "music" helps stem free-radical damage to cells, shielding the DNA coiled within. Antioxidants and phytonutrients may also help block cancer-causing substances that damage DNA (which can lead to tumor formation) and may help prevent existing tumors from growing larger.

"Much like a plant, cancers thrive in certain environments and perish in others," says Dr. Block. "Nutrition is a potent strategy in changing this environment."

The Benefits Are Immediate

If you've ever tried to quit smoking (successfully, we hope), you've probably read that within hours of stubbing out your last butt, your lungs, along with the rest of you, reap significant health benefits.

GREAT MOMENTS IN NUTRITION

Like any science, nutrition evolves over time. This timeline highlights watershed events that have shaped women's nutrition over the years, going back to your great-great-grandmother's day.

1820–1830: Sylvester Graham travels the East Coast, extolling the health virtues of his fiber-rich cookie, the Graham cracker. Flouting the conventional medical wisdom of his time, Graham believed fiber was good for you.

1911: Russian researcher Nikolai Anitschkov feeds rabbits a diet of egg yolks. They die of hardening of the arteries. It's the first known research on the hazards of high blood cholesterol.

1912: American biochemist Casimir Funk coins the term "vitamine" for the unidentified substances in food that could prevent the deficiency diseases scurvy, beriberi, and pellagra.

1916: Caroline Hunt, a nutritionist in the Bureau of Home Economics of the USDA, creates the first USDA food guide.

1931: Lucy Wills, an early folic acid researcher, discovers that pregnant women with anemia become less anemic after they're given brewer's yeast, an excellent source of this B vitamin.

1941: The first loaf of Wonder bread is fortified with vitamins and minerals.

1943: The first set of Recommended Dietary Allowances, or RDAs, is published. The goal: to ensure that all Americans get the minimum amount of nutrients essential to good health.

1948: The Framingham Heart Study is launched. Over the years, this pioneering study of the residents of Framingham, Massachusetts, has defined key risk factors that increase the odds of developing heart disease, including obesity and a high-fat diet.

The benefits of switching over to a low-fat diet brimming with fruits, vegetables, and other plant foods are almost as instantaneous. That's a compelling reason to move toward a plant-based diet, especially if you have a family history of heart disease or cancer.

1954: Denham Harmon, M.D., introduces his free-radical theory of aging. His research suggests that compounds that fight free radicals, called antioxidants, might slow the aging process.

1976: Harvard Medical School and the Harvard-affiliated Brigham and Women's Hospital launch the Nurses' Health Study, the largest and longest-running women's health study in history. What the study has suggested so far: eating fruits and vegetables reduces the risk of breast cancer; moderate alcohol consumption reduces heart disease and stroke risk; and a high fiber intake reduces risk of type 2 diabetes.

1979: Dean Ornish, M.D., makes headlines with his first study, which finds that placing heart patients on an extremely low-fat diet and making stress-reducing changes to their lifestyles can actually reverse damage from heart disease.

1987: Noted fiber researcher James W. Anderson, M.D., shows that high-fiber diets help control blood sugar and reduce insulin needs.

1989: Research conducted at the University of Massachusetts Medical School in Worcester finds that a low-fat diet appears to increase resistance to some kinds of infection and disease and that a high-fat diet seems to depress immunity.

1991: The National Institutes of Health launches the Women's Health Initiative, a 15-year, 160,000-woman investigation of women and their health. One issue under study: whether consuming a low-fat, fruit- and vegetable-rich diet helps prevent breast and colorectal cancers and heart disease.

1992: A review of 156 scientific studies that analyzed the relationship between diet and cancer finds "extraordinarily consistent scientific evidence" supporting the protective effect of fruits and vegetables, among other foods.

1999: A study of 75,521 women, conducted by Harvard researchers, finds that eating more whole grains may protect against heart disease in women.

For example, "blood cholesterol drops within about 5 days of reducing your intake of dietary fat," says James W. Anderson, M.D., professor of medicine and clinical nutrition at the Veterans Affairs Medical Center in Lexington, Kentucky.

If you have high blood pressure, consuming less salt and more fruits, vegetables, and low-fat dairy products can significantly drop those numbers in as little as 2 weeks.

And within 3 weeks or so, your body will be able to mount a stronger defense against cancer, as the protective antioxidants and phytonutrients in plant foods are transported to your tissues and incorporated into your cells.

As if this instant gratification weren't reason enough to munch more stir-fried veggies, there are other, long-range benefits you can expect from eating right. In the pages that follow, you'll learn all about how focusing on well-researched Power Foods can deliver these benefits, which include increased energy; a slimmer, trimmer figure; a sharper memory; a strong, sturdy skeleton; and good digestive health.

In a way, eating smart is like investing in your 401(k). The more you "invest" now, the bigger the dividends in later life. These accrued benefits can help keep you healthy and active in your middle years and beyond.

Take Baby Steps

You don't need a book to tell you that eating an apple is better than eating a Twinkie or that you're better off ordering a salad instead of cheese fries.

Still, eating right isn't always that simple—or easy. The truth is, it can be hard, even painful, to choose grilled fish and brussels sprouts when you're quite happy with meat loaf and mashed potatoes.

This book will show you how to make dietary changes easier. The key? Start small. And spread the changes over time, says Dr. Schneeman. For example, if you tend to eat large portions of red meat every night, concentrate on eating smaller amounts 2 or 3 nights a week. Or if you can't remember the last time your lips touched a piece of fresh fruit or a salad, focus on adding one or two servings to your diet each day. Make the next healthy change when you've made the last one a habit.

Finally, be open to trying new foods or old favorites prepared in a healthful way, says Dr. Schneeman. Give soy burgers a whirl. Buy a vegetarian cookbook and rediscover the excitement of cooking. Prowl the produce aisle, pick the strangest-looking fruit or vegetable on display, and pop it into your cart.

REASON #1,289 TO LOVE CHOCOLATE

Low-fat double-fudge ice cream can't possibly taste as good as the real thing. Right? Wrong. A University of Missouri taste test found no significant difference in how much consumers like the flavor of low-fat chocolate ice cream compared to its full-fat counterpart.

It is chocolate's complex chemistry that makes the low-fat version just as yummy as the real thing, says study author Ingolf Gruen, Ph.D., of the university's food science and engineering unit. Chocolate contains some 500 flavor chemicals, which mask "off" flavors that can result from reducing the fat content. It's this chemical stew that helps chocolate retain its rich, creamy flavor, fat-free or not.

To conduct his study, Dr. Gruen used trained and untrained volunteers from the University of Missouri campus who weren't averse to getting ice cream for free. "People liked the nonfat chocolate ice cream, which contained less than 1 percent milk fat, just as much as the full-fat kind, which contained 9 percent milk fat," he says.

Alas, research shows that skimming the fat from other ice cream flavors significantly affects flavor. America's number one ice cream flavor, vanilla, has one dominant flavor chemical, vanillin. Research into the flavor chemistry of vanilla ice cream shows that people find the low-fat version tastes harsher and is less creamy than the regular kind. A similar study conducted in Finland reached the same conclusion in a taste test of fat-free versus regular strawberry ice cream.

In short, give your tastebuds a dose of adventure, instead of the same old thing.

"Research shows that children may taste a new food from six to eight times before they find it acceptable," says Dr. Schneeman. "So don't try a healthy food once and say, 'Never again.' Say, 'Well, this wasn't so tasty, but I'll try it again sometime, prepared a different way.' Keep trying and experimenting. It works. I never thought I'd come to like brussels sprouts."

Foods Women Eat, Foods Women Want

For Elizabeth Levi of Cedar Rapids, Iowa, breakfast is a cup of low-fat plain yogurt and fruit or an omelette made with egg substitute and tofu. But if the condition of her arteries or the circumference of her thighs were no object, she'd be digging into eggs Benedict.

Lunch for Theresa Krain of Eastpointe, Michigan? Most days, a Lean Cuisine or a Healthy Choice meal. But if she lived in a parallel universe where burgers and chocolate milkshakes were health food, that's what she would have.

And while Terri Minatra of Johnson City, Tennessee, often sits down to grilled chicken breast and salad for dinner, her very soul cries out for smoked salmon with decadent crème fraîche, followed by heartbreakingly delicious chocolate soufflé.

Choice versus Desire: The Great Divide

We may eat like angels, but we lust in our hearts. That's what *Prevention* magazine found when they ran a survey asking women what they typically eat—and what they really want to eat.

The short list of halo-over-our-heads fare includes high-fiber cereal, bagels, pasta, skinless chicken breast, and low-fat everything.

10

("I eat so much chicken and fish, I don't know whether to cluck or to swim," says Pat Perrier of Crest Hill, Illinois.)

But as you might imagine, the death-row wish list of forbidden foods evoked a flood of passion and longing.

"I'd have cheese lasagna and warm-from-the-oven chocolate chip cookies every day," says Tracey L. Dinneen of San Diego.

"I'm dreaming of breaded and fried fantail shrimp, eggplant parmigiana, and gooey chocolate chip cookies," says Luci Morrill of Rochester, New York.

"Cream-filled doughnuts—I haven't had one in years," sighs Trina M. Mallet of Topeka, Kansas.

Monica Shoemaker of Urbana–Champaign, Illinois, has actually created what she calls her deathbed list, which includes pecan pie and macaroni and cheese with bacon. "I will only eat from this list if I know that I have 24 hours to live," she says.

Time and again, survey respondents rhapsodized about "real" food. Real, as in real butter. Real cheese. Big, thick, calorie-laden cookies rather than low-fat substitutes. And the kind of deep-fried chicken that makes paper napkins stick to your fingers, rather than the oven-fried variety.

We also long for the food of our youth. One woman said that her fantasy foods include "anything my mom made in the 1960s before fat phobia, like meat loaf and mashed potatoes made with whole milk and real butter."

What's with the deprivation? There's good food to be eaten, and time's a-wastin'. We say: you want it, you eat it. And as you will see, nutrition and weight-loss experts heartily agree.

Waistline

Women's preoccupation with weight and body shape starts early. In one study of 548 girls in 5th through 12th grades, 69 percent said that pictures of models in magazines influenced their ideas of the "perfect" body. And 47 percent said the photos made them want to lose weight.

THE REAL WORLD:
20 FOODS WE EAT MOST OFTEN

If a survey of *Prevention* magazine readers is any indication, we're trying to eat nutritiously, and succeeding (barring the occasional Oreo gorgefest). Listed below are the top 20 foods the women who responded to the survey say they eat on an everyday basis.

1. Vegetables: 88%
2. Fruit: 77%
3. Chicken or turkey (prepared healthfully): 67%
4. Cereal: 52%
5. Fish: 48%
6. Bread: 44%
7. Milk: 36%
8. Lean meats: 35%
9. Cheese (all varieties): 33%
10. Snacks: 28%
11. Yogurt: 27%
12. Healthy fats, oils, or dressings: 25%
13. Pasta: 23%
14. Soy foods or beverages: 22%
15. Eggs or egg substitutes: 21%
16. Frozen yogurt or light ice cream: 20%
17. Rice: 20%
18. Juice: 18%
19. Soups and stews: 16%
20. Healthy baked goods: 16%

Why "Bad" Food Is Good

It may seem strange to encourage the enthusiastic noshing of so-called forbidden foods in a nutrition book. After all, scientific research is constantly unearthing new evidence of food's power to prevent and treat disease.

IN OUR DREAMS: TOP 20 FANTASY FOODS

If the mere thought of death-by-chocolate cake or fried mozzarella sticks sends your salivary glands into overdrive, you're not alone. Here are the savor-with-your-eyes-closed foods that women who responded to a *Prevention* magazine survey said they would eat if their health and the size of their jeans were no object.

1. Chocolate candy or dessert: 63%
2. Fried foods: 46%
3. Real cheese: 44%
4. Doughnuts: 39%
5. Full-fat ice cream: 39%
6. Red meat: 39%
7. Real butter, mayonnaise, or salad dressing: 38%
8. Pizza: 30%
9. Salty snack foods: 30%
10. Traditional breakfast foods (such as bacon and eggs): 29%
11. Nonchocolate desserts and baked goods: 28%
12. Cookies: 27%
13. Cream sauce or gravy: 24%
14. Cake: 23%
15. Mashed potatoes or baked potatoes loaded with toppings: 20%
16. Fruit pies, cobblers, or pastries: 17%
17. Cheesecake: 16%
18. Fast food: 13%
19. Chinese food: 9%
20. Barbecued chicken, ribs, or chicken wings: 5%

And, judging from the *Prevention* survey, health concerns, especially overweight, are our number one reason for healthy eating. Ruth Dutton of Ocqueoc, Michigan, started counting grams of fat when she learned that she had high blood pressure, while Perrier finds that healthy eating both relieves her hiatal hernia and reflux and gives her more energy. But we don't live in a laboratory. In the real world, food has an emotional impact on our lives as well as a physical one.

What's more, when you look at cold, hard statistics, denying ourselves the foods we love doesn't appear to be improving our health.

We diet constantly. At any one time, about 45 percent of all women are on a diet, compared to 28 percent of men.

Dieting doesn't seem to work. According to research from the Centers for Disease Control and Prevention, the number of us who are obese (defined as being 30 percent over ideal body weight) has jumped from 12 percent to nearly 18 percent in just 7 years. That's a startling 50 percent increase.

We're more aware of good nutrition, but we're getting sicker. We're fixated on eating by the numbers: counting calories, grams of fat, and milligrams of one nutrient or another, says Deborah Keston, professor of public health at the Institute for Health and Healing at the California Pacific Medical Center in San Francisco and author of *Feeding the Body, Nourishing the Soul.* "But this approach to food is obviously not working," she says. "We're the most overweight country in the world, and our risk of major diet-related diseases—diabetes, heart disease, some types of cancer, and high blood pressure—is rising."

So here's the big-money question: Is there a way to let the foods we love back into our lives? To eat for pleasure as well as for health?

You bet there is. But before we get to the solution, we need to see where we've been: how our feelings about food and eating developed, and how they influence our health—and our lives—today.

An All-Consuming Relationship

It's often said that women have a relationship with food, as we do with our mothers, our children, and our mates.

And as weird as it sounds, it's true. For what else but food—mashed potatoes with real butter, cream-filled doughnuts, chocolate chip cookies—can evoke such feelings of passion, love, guilt, and desperation?

There are a number of reasons food consumes us, says Susan J. Klebanoff, Ph.D., a clinical psychologist at the Eating Disorders Research Center in New York City.

We're still the "gatherers." While many of us hold down full-time jobs, we still do the bulk of the grocery shopping and cooking. These tra-

Waistline

When it comes to weight-loss books, our bookshelves are over-flowing. It all started in 1917, with *Diet and Health, with Key to Calories* **by Dr. Lulu Hunt Peters, the first diet book to achieve bestseller status.**

ditional responsibilities have given us a kind of intimacy with food, borne of countless years of thumping melons, devising unique ways to stretch a pound of ground beef or prepare pasta, and regularly conquering—or being defeated by—the temptations of the deli section.

We link food with nurturing. "To men, food is fuel. To women, it's emotional sustenance," says Gayle Reichler, R.D., president of Active Wellness in New York City and author of *Active Wellness: A Personalized 10-Step Program for a Healthy Body, Mind, and Spirit.*

Says Judy Strother of Fullerton, California, "Just the sight of cookies transports me back in time and links me to wonderful childhood memories."

Why isn't food emotional fuel for men, too? After all, we never think of a man curled up on the couch at 11:00 P.M. with a half-gallon of cookie-dough ice cream—and feeling guilty about it.

Generally speaking, we nurture, and men get nurtured, says Catrina Brown, author of *Consuming Passions: Feminist Approaches to Weight Preoccupation and Eating Disorders.* We've been raised to take care of others before we take care of ourselves, she says. But women need nurturing, too—which, for us, is harder to come by. And we've learned that food is the fastest, easiest, most time-efficient way to give ourselves the comfort we need.

We follow the rules. Many of us became aware of our bodies—and the enormous power that a shapely feminine form wields—in our early teens, says Reichler. Often, it's at this point that a woman's battle between deprivation and desire begins. One consequence of this never-ending battle? "Food rules"—what to eat, what not to eat, when to eat it, and how to eat it. "As we grow older, these rules stay with us and multiply," she says.

Waistline

Professional models are 23 percent lighter than today's average woman, making them an unrealistic benchmark for what's considered attractive.

Amen, says Perrier. "Most nights at around 10:30, my husband sits down with this huge cereal bowl full of chocolate or rocky road ice cream," she says. "He doesn't feel guilty about it. He just eats it. And I'm thinking, 'Why am I beating myself up because I had a few more grams of fat than I should have?'"

A Woman's Gotta Chew
What a Woman's Gotta Chew

There *is* a way to nourish your body while you nourish your soul. To balance what a woman's body needs (broccoli, skinless chicken breast, beans) with what it craves (Brie, brownies, KFC). To maintain or even lose weight without hallucinating cheese steaks or sticky buns.

In fact, more than a few survey respondents were proud to say that they occasionally fall off the wagon and eat their fantasy foods—and feel perfectly fine about it.

"It's all about balance," says Tess Johnson of Mesa, Arizona. "I don't eliminate foods or go crazy if I get a little off track for a day or two. I've managed to keep off 70 pounds for the last 2½ years without feeling deprived."

"If I don't permit the things I like once in a while, then I definitely overdo it when I do eat them," says Dinneen. "If I allow myself to have them once in a while, I can be more reasonable about portion size. I've lost about 65 pounds over 3 to 4 years, just by letting my body eat whatever it feels like eating."

Kathleen Stant of Richmond, Virginia, couldn't agree more. "Every once in a while you just have to indulge in a juicy steak, premium ice cream, or warm biscuits with lots of butter," she says. "About once a week, my husband and I go out and 'put on the feed bag' as a reward for being good the rest of the time."

These women have the right idea, says Brown. "Women have to move away from the idea that we eat only to fuel the body and to stay healthy," she says. "In my view, if we're going to achieve a more balanced approach to nutrition, we have to learn to make food choices that mesh with our emotional realities and social circumstances."

In other words, we need to get real about food.

Getting Your FAA License

To make peace with food, then, we have to balance our nutritional needs with our emotional needs. In short, we need to make what we're calling a Food Attitude Adjustment—FAA, for short.

The FAA is a new mindset that will enable you to eat for health while still eating for pleasure—without the side orders of deprivation and guilt. Once you have your FAA "license," you'll realize that your body's need for whole grain cereal and skinless chicken breast can coexist peacefully with your heart's desire for Twinkies and chocolate milk.

The word "adjustment" implies moving from one state to another. Here are some of the most important adjustments you can make to your thinking about food, according to experts.

From "good" and "bad" food to just "food." There's probably not one of us who hasn't said—or heard another woman say—"I've been bad (good) today—I ate (didn't eat) a piece of chocolate cake." Hold it right there. If you stop to think about it, cake is neither good nor bad. It's just, well, cake.

Waistline

Two-thirds of Americans say that it's important to eat fruits and vegetables, but consumption has increased only slightly since the late 1970s. And while more than 90 percent of adults say it's important to maintain a healthy weight, 40 percent say they eat too many calories.

"I don't think of food as bad anymore," adds Laurelee Roark, co-founder and director of Beyond Hunger in San Rafael, California, and coauthor of *It's Not About Food*. "It's just food—this is a sweet food, this is a green food. All around me, I hear women saying, 'I shouldn't be eating this' while they eat another of whatever it is. I just ask myself, 'Do you want it?' If the answer is yes, I have it. If the answer is no, I know that I don't have to eat it."

That said, some food choices are healthier than others, says Roark. But healthier doesn't necessarily mean better—especially if you feel chronically deprived.

From inflexibility to choices. Perhaps you know a woman who subsists on rice cakes, salads, and diet soda. Perhaps you even envy her sense of self-discipline. But let's get real: Is life without real cheese worth living?

The answer is no—but if you learn to balance healthy choices with not-so-healthy desires, there's no need to live without the foods you love. "The key is to be able to choose satisfying alternatives instead of feeling deprived," says Reichler. "Choices come from having more knowledge. And you want to have enough knowledge to eat healthfully 90 percent of the time."

Making a conscious choice to eat or not eat a so-called forbidden food can be incredibly freeing, says Brown, because you have put the power in *your* hands, rather than relinquishing it to the food in question. "You're making a deliberate choice to eat the ice cream, as opposed to feeling that whether or not you eat it is out of your control."

From eating "for the heart" to eating "from the heart." "We've been trained to eat for health," says Keston. "But for other societies, eating is a pleasure. We seem to have forgotten that."

To make your peace with food, you need to blend your desire for good health with a genuine appreciation for food, she says. "Food is as life-giving and as life-containing as we are," says Keston. "The key to physical, emotional, and spiritual health is to eat fresh whole foods—fruits, vegetables, beans, whole grains—as often as possible. And when you want a doughnut, have it—and enjoy every single bite."

Food Fantasies
and Attitudes:
Getting Your FAA License

There's no such thing as a "bad" food. You can enjoy your personal fantasy foods as long as you also consume your fair share of Power Foods—whole grains, extra fiber, and five to nine fruits and vegetables a day. (After all, they even served corn dogs at the American Dietetic Association's national conference.) You just have to get your FAA—that's female Food Attitude Adjustment—license.

Fantasies, according to Webster's dictionary, are "unrealistic or improbable mental images." Images like comfortable yet sexy high heels. A husband who doesn't snore. Or spending your 50th birthday in Fiji partying with Mick Jagger.

When *Prevention* magazine surveyed readers about the fantasy foods they ate—or wanted to eat but didn't—women listed mixed nuts, brownies, chocolate milkshakes, doughnuts, and pizza among the things that they felt they couldn't or shouldn't have. Yet there's no real reason that you can't get just as excited about strawberries, blueberries, whole grain rolls, or hearty minestrone soup.

It's all about adjusting your attitude.

So put on your studying caps, ladies. Here are the 10 steps to getting your FAA license. (As for your other fantasies—well, you're on your own.)

I. Stop Dieting

Envy women who never diet? Their lives don't revolve around obsessing over good and bad foods. You can be one of them.

"We need to get back to eating normally," says Tammy Baker, R.D., a Phoenix-based spokesperson for the American Dietetic Association. When we diet, we frequently stop depending upon our bodies' own signals of hunger and fullness, she says, leading to potential bingeing on fantasy foods.

Consider the classic milkshake study. Researchers at Northwestern University in Evanston, Illinois, divided dieters and nondieters into three groups. The first group drank two milkshakes before eating some ice cream; the second drank one milkshake before the ice cream; and the third got no milkshake.

While the nondieters in each group responded in logical ways—eating less ice cream when they'd had a milkshake first, for example—the dieters reacted exactly the opposite. Those who had no milkshake ate just a little ice cream, while those who had two milkshakes lost control entirely and ate the most ice cream of all.

Self-imposed limits, or "forbidden" foods, can be a problem, says Baker. "When you have a bad day, the first thing you'll do is go to the foods you think you're not supposed to have. If all foods are okay in moderation, then it's much easier to practice portion control and lose weight over the long haul."

At the same time, be realistic about your weight, and take into account your genetic makeup and family history, says Susan Adams, R.D., a spokesperson for the American Dietetic Association who is based in Seattle. "Some of us come from ethnic groups where people just tend to be more stout and have heavier body weights."

"Being content with a somewhat higher weight goal will enable you to enjoy food more, eat more realistically, and still be healthy," Baker says.

2. Look Back and Ahead

Stop focusing just on what you ate today. Instead, think about what you ate in the past 2 weeks, says Adams. If you're making even a minimal effort to choose Power Foods, chances are that they will more than compensate for the fantasy foods you consume.

"You have to think about how you can eat in a way that is healthy over

LOW-FAT CHOCOLATE ICE CREAM GETS HIGH MARKS

To many, low-fat vanilla ice cream just doesn't measure up to its full-fat counterpart. But low-fat chocolate is more convincing. Researchers at the University of Missouri gave chocolate ice cream with differing fat levels to 100 people and asked them to rate them. The low-fat versions scored just the same as the high-fat ones: delicious.

The reason may be because the process of formulating low-fat ice cream affects the taste of vanillin, the dominant flavor chemical in vanilla ice cream. But chocolate ice cream's mix of more than 500 flavor chemicals, none of which is dominant, makes it easier to mask any off flavors that may result from tinkering with the fat content.

your lifetime," she says. That means you can enjoy special occasions and holidays, complete with the extra fat and calories that come along with them. "Put it in perspective: Maybe you do overeat, but then you go back to your regular eating habits afterward."

When you do choose an item on your most-wanted list, don't beat yourself up, says Suzanne Havala, R.D., a nutrition consultant for the Vegetarian Resource Group in Baltimore and author of *Good Foods, Bad Foods: What's Left to Eat?* Having a fast-food outlet on nearly every street corner and a bakery in every supermarket makes it impossible to pretend that those foods don't exist. "Just being aware that it's not you, it's the system, can help prevent you from throwing up your hands altogether and giving up any attempt to eat healthfully," Havala says.

3. Make Bad Choices Better

What's a turkey sandwich without the side of crisp, salty potato chips? Or watching *Ally McBeal* without a bowl of rich chocolate mocha ice cream? Indulge. Just find the best "bad" choice you can make. Here's how.

• Choose baked chips instead of fried. Try some of the baked tortilla products available in grocery stores. Or for your own baked tortilla chips, cut corn tortillas in half, then into 1-inch strips, spray with cooking spray, season with salt, garlic powder, and cumin and toss in a bowl or plastic bag to coat evenly. Then bake on a baking sheet at 475°F for 5 minutes.

- Make your French toast with fat-free milk instead of whole milk. Bake it using cooking spray instead of frying, saving 152 calories and 12 grams of fat.
- Replace 1 cup of premium ice cream with 1 cup of premium sorbet, saving 360 calories.
- Order your pizza with anchovies and spinach—getting valuable omega-3 fatty acids and phytonutrients like beta-carotene that may protect against cancer and heart disease. Choose oatmeal cookies for their fruit and fiber content, or make the Power Cookies on page 156.
- Grate full-flavor cheeses on foods to satisfy your cheese urges. Feta and Parmesan are both good choices because they add texture and interest to meals and are slightly lower in fat than other cheeses.
- Grab a turkey hot dog instead of beef or pork franks. You'll only cut 32 calories per dog, but you will be down 5 grams of fat.

4. Bank Your Calories

If you simply must have a cream-filled doughnut, find caloric room for it by giving up something you really don't care about, says Havala. For instance, replacing your morning cup of granola with a cup of Life cereal banks 343 calories, more than the doughnut's 270.

Or substitute two glasses of water, flavored seltzer, or diet soda for the two glasses of cola you drink every day, saving 304 calories.

Can you live without the pat of butter in your mashed potatoes and the splash of cream in your coffee? You've just rescued 65 calories, enough for a chocolate chip cookie.

5. Limit, Don't Eliminate

If you deny yourself that slice of cake in favor of some fresh fruit, chances that are you're going to eat your sweet later—maybe even a double portion. So ditch denial.

Instead, make fantasy foods the postscript to your regular diet, the little somethings that fill in the cracks, instead of the mortar that holds up the entire structure. Limiting will be easier if Power Foods—whole grains, lean meats, lots of fruits and vegetables, and mega amounts of fiber—make up the bulk of your diet.

If that still doesn't work for you, try portion control. Here are some ideas that may be helpful, says Havala.

- Shake a small handful of mixed nuts into a dessert dish and put the container away.
- Share a luscious dessert with a friend (or two).
- Buy individually wrapped ice cream treats. Pass up half-gallon containers of ice cream for pint-size ones.
- Buy one small candy bar instead of an entire bag.
- Slice off a piece of cake and wrap up the rest of it so you aren't tempted to chisel away at it.
- Eating out? Eat half of your chocolate cake (or pie or mousse) and ask the waiter to wrap the other half to go.
- Split an order of fries with at least one friend (preferably two).

6. Savor, Don't Scarf

Appetizers are a marketers' ploy. They give you something to keep your hands busy while you wait for your entrée, but you don't really need the extra food.

If you truly love the tangy spiciness of Buffalo wings offset by the cool creaminess of blue cheese dressing, go ahead and order them. But if you just need something to do, ask for a steamed vegetable platter as an appetizer.

"Either way, eat deliberately, with full intent, being conscious the whole time of taste, texture, and body responses," says Baker. "This minimizes haphazard, casual, and indiscriminate eating and helps you feel satisfied."

If you were mindful of how you were feeling while gulping half a chocolate cake, she says, you'd realize that it didn't feel very good in your stomach. And take time to smell your food. Studies show that once you start eating, smelling your food can make you stop eating sooner by satisfying you faster.

Like many dietitians, Baker recommends keeping a food diary. Write

YET ANOTHER REASON TO CHOOSE OLIVE OIL

As the benefits of olive oil have become known, more restaurants are making it their preferred spread. But does dipping your bread in olive oil land you the same number of calories as buttering it? Here's what researchers at the University of Illinois Food and Brand Lab found out.

After observing 307 diners at two Italian restaurants over 3 nights, weighing their bread, butter, and olive oil before and after their meals, the verdict came in. Although diners did use more olive oil than butter per piece of bread, they ate less bread, for an overall calorie savings of 52 calories.

Ask for extra-virgin olive oil when dining out, and also use it at home. A small study at the University of Granada in Spain showed that LDL oxidation (the process that makes "bad" artery-clogging cholesterol), was significantly slower in people who used extra-virgin oil than in those using more refined olive oil, suggesting that refining oil robs it of certain beneficial antioxidants.

down what you eat and when, and note any strong emotions you may have been feeling at the time. "Then you'll see when you're most vulnerable." If you find a pattern emerging, consider why you are eating the way you do. For instance, most of us eat the bulk of our calories after 4:00 P.M., she says. If your log shows that you're heading to the fridge as soon as you get home, look for ways to change that behavior, such as going for a walk or taking a bubble bath instead of eating.

So before you open that bag of chips or slice off a piece of cheesecake, Baker suggests that you stop and ask yourself these questions.

• Am I hungry—or am I bored, angry, frustrated, or sad? Unless you're hungry, close the refrigerator and focus on the emotion, not the food.

• Do I crave this food or its taste sensation? For instance, if you simply need something salty and crunchy, will air-popped popcorn do instead of potato chips? If it's creamy you're after, does it need to be the cheesecake or will cheesecake-flavored yogurt satisfy you?

• Where am I going to eat this food? If it's standing up in the kitchen, then you're eating for the wrong reason. If you plan to sit down at the table and slowly take small bites, closing your eyes after each bite to savor the richness, saltiness, crunchiness, sweetness (or even greasiness) of whatever delicacy you've chosen, then give yourself the green light for that food.

7. Get Over Your Fat Phobia

When green creatures from outer space sort through the remnants of our civilization centuries from now, here's one question they'll undoubtedly ask: If so many Earth foods were low-fat or fat-free, then why were so many Earthlings so fat?

If we were still around, we could answer them: "When was the last time *you* ate only two fat-free cookies?"

The problem with our glut of low-fat and fat-free foods is that in most cases, they have the same number of calories as regular versions. Excess calories of any kind eventually turn into fat. Also, we've deceived ourselves into thinking that it's okay to eat more of these foods since they're low in fat.

To test how low-fat and fat-free labels affected eating, researcher Barbara Rolls, Ph.D., professor of nutrition at Pennsylvania State University in University Park, gave 48 women three raspberry-flavored yogurts— high-fat/high-calorie, low-fat/high-calorie, and low-fat/low-calorie— that were otherwise indistinguishable. When the women ate the yogurts labeled low-fat, they ate significantly more calories during the lunch and dinner that followed than after eating the yogurt labeled high-fat.

"One of the things that happen when people try to eat a lot less fat is that they're hungry all the time," says Adams. Fat slows down the emptying of our stomachs, helping us feel fuller longer. Even just a tiny bit—a pat of butter on your toast in the morning—can make a difference, she says.

8. Forget the Food Myths

Anyone who has been reading about nutrition for years knows that it's a constantly moving field. It seems that nearly everything that used to be bad for us now has some redeeming quality.

Yet many of us still place items like shrimp and eggs (too much cholesterol), steak sandwiches and cheeseburgers (too much fat), and chocolate (too much of everything) on our verboten lists.

Consider the following:

• Most shellfish contains no more cholesterol than many cuts of meat and poultry—and some contain less. But it's not dietary cholesterol that's the instigator in heart disease, it's saturated fat, which in shellfish is relatively low. In fact, a study performed at Rockefeller University in New York City found that healthy adults eating 10½ ounces of shrimp a day maintained healthy cholesterol levels and even lowered overall blood levels of fatty triglycerides. The researchers concluded that eating 10½ ounces of shrimp a day had less impact on cholesterol levels than eating two eggs a day. The reason? Heart-healthy omega-3 fatty acids, found in shrimp and many other types of seafood.

• Yes, red meat contains saturated fat. But a study of 191 men and women with mild to moderately high cholesterol levels showed that eating lean red meat (like beef, veal, or pork) was no more likely to boost their cholesterol levels (and heart disease risk) than eating lean white poultry or fish.

• Eggs contain cholesterol—about 212 milligrams per egg. But they also provide a good low-calorie source of protein, unsaturated fats, essential amino acids, and B vitamins. Still worried about the cholesterol? Try one whole egg mixed with two egg whites for your omelette or scrambled eggs.

• Chocolate isn't all bad. Not only is chocolate good for you emotionally, it's good for you physically. Chocolate contains substantial amounts of phenylethylamine, a compound that raises levels of serotonin and dopamine, brain chemicals associated with mood. But chocolate also contains catechin, a type of antioxidant that may protect against heart disease and possibly cancer. Animal studies suggest it may even be beneficial to the immune system.

9. Go Ahead and Cheat

Nutritionists call it the what-the-hell effect: "What the hell, I ate a piece of cake, I may as well eat the entire cake." "What the hell, I scarfed a french fry from my husband's plate, so I may as well order my own basket."

Stop right there. Allowing yourself a treat doesn't mean you've lost

Waistline

According to the Calorie Control Council, which tracks food and beverage consumption:

- 44 percent of Americans drink diet soft drinks
- 40 percent of Americans drink sugar-free or light noncarbonated soft drinks
- 32 percent of Americans use sugar substitutes
- 30 percent of Americans chew sugar-free gum
- 30 percent of Americans eat sugar-free frozen desserts, ice cream, or frozen yogurt

Still, 54 percent of Americans are overweight. So all those foods don't seem to be helping us stay fat-free.

control, and denying yourself doesn't mean you're in control. All it proves is that the very thing you most want is controlling you. And you're a grown woman. Just how does it feel to be controlled by a pepperoni pizza?

"I think the slippery slope is a problem that stems from goals being too great a leap," says Havala. It also goes back to the denial, or forbidden foods, issue. Instead, take the time to build your dietary goals gradually. For instance, if you customarily eat fast food for lunch every day, don't switch to Power Foods entirely. Cut out a fast-food lunch each week until you're down to one, then switch what you're eating at McDonald's from a Big Mac to a plain hamburger.

And don't be too hard on yourself.

"There should be room for cheating in any program," says Jose Antonio, Ph.D., assistant professor of exercise science at the University of Nebraska in Kearney and author of *Diets Drive Me Nuts*.

10. Get Off the Couch and Exercise

So you've followed our advice, and you're allowing yourself a handful of guilt-free chocolate-covered peanut butter candies, a wedge of baked Brie, or a grilled cheese sandwich made with real cheese.

Then, with a contented sigh, you go lie on the couch in front of the fire.

Not so fast. Not denying yourself is one thing; putting on the pounds is another. So get off the couch and start exercising. "There's simply no better way to be able to eat what you want without gaining weight than to incorporate some kind of regular exercise into your life," says Dr. Antonio.

That doesn't mean taking a 30-minute jog to try to make up for the pint of Häagen-Dazs you ate. It means balancing your exercise with your food intake over the course of the week, says Dr. Antonio. He recommends some sort of aerobic activity three times a week (you can walk, right?) and 2 days of weight training. Don't have a gym? You can do pullups or pushups at home, or fill water bottles with water and use them for arm curls.

If you're really starved for time, incorporate extra movements into your daily routine, suggests Baker. "Take things upstairs one at a time, or walk your paperwork down the hall. Even little things like holding in your stomach muscles while driving can make a difference."

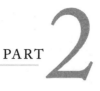

POWER-MAKER FOODS

Beans: Core Ingredients of a Healthy Diet

Power Maker #1: Eat ½ cup of beans at least four times a week—even more (1 cup a day) if you need to lower your blood cholesterol.

Not so long ago, beans got little more culinary respect than pigs' knuckles.

"Folks definitely looked down on beans," says legume guru James W. Anderson, M.D., professor of medicine and clinical nutrition at the Veterans Affairs Medical Center in Lexington, Kentucky, who has spent more than a decade investigating and touting the health benefits of beans.

Now, beans are the crown jewels of a healthy diet. Low in fat, high in both complex carbohydrates and protein, beans are stuffed with the woman-friendly nutrients folate and iron. Beans are also loaded with fiber, which research suggests can help lower cholesterol, help manage diabetes, and may reduce the risk of cancer.

But although vegetarianism is popular and we do love our Mexican food, most of us still eat a paltry amount of legumes—8 pounds a year, less than ½ ounce per day. Compared to the 128 pounds of meat women eat annually, that's a pretty small hill of beans.

Magic Bullets for Cholesterol Control

In one of the earliest studies on the link between diet and blood cholesterol levels, researchers found that Trappist monks, who typically follow a vegetarian diet, ate significantly less fat and had lower cholesterol levels than their Benedictine brothers, who typically consume Western-style diets.

One of the staples of the Trappist menu? Beans. And what's good for monks is good for the rest of us, too.

Beans are loaded with soluble fiber, long known to lower both total and "bad" low-density lipoprotein (LDL) cholesterol. You'd have to eat seven slices of whole wheat bread to get the amount of soluble fiber in just ½ cup of navy beans.

"Eating a cup of any type of beans a day—particularly kidney, navy, pinto, black, garbanzo (chickpea), or butter beans—can lower cholesterol about 10 percent in 6 weeks," says Dr. Anderson. That 10 percent gives you a big advantage: For every 1 percent you reduce your cholesterol, you reduce your heart disease risk by 2 to 3 percent. Experts aren't sure how soluble fiber sends cholesterol south. Among the most accepted theories, says Dr. Anderson, is that it increases the amount of bile acid—a substance produced by the liver that helps you digest fats—that is excreted in bowel movements. Because your body uses cholesterol to make bile, reducing the amount of bile in your system also reduces your cholesterol.

Another theory is that beans may create a mini-microbrewery in your

FIVE-STAR PERFORMERS

While virtually all beans are excellent sources of fiber, some varieties achieve superstar status. You can get a lot of fiber in just 1 cup of beans. Here are five top performers.

- Black beans: 15 grams
- Lima beans: 13 grams
- Kidney beans: 11 grams
- Chickpeas: 10.5 grams
- Black-eyed peas: 8 grams

POWER
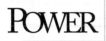

D I P

HUMMUS PLATTER

You can feel virtuous eating this creamy dip. It's loaded with the complex carbs, protein, fiber, folate, and iron that beans are famous for. And the garlic multiplies the cholesterol-reducing power of the beans. Even the garnishes (onions and parsley) and the vegetable dippers add a variety of health-building nutrients, like beta-carotene, cancer-zapping quercetin, and bone-strengthening vitamin K.

4	whole wheat pitas
1	can (19 ounces) chickpeas, rinsed and drained
1/3	cup tahini
1/3	cup lemon juice
3	cloves garlic, chopped
1/2	teaspoon salt
1/2	cup finely chopped red onion
2	tablespoons chopped fresh parsley
2	sweet red peppers, thinly sliced
1	cucumber, thinly sliced

colon. As they bubble-bubble away in your colon, they produce substances called short-chain fatty acids (SCFAs) such as acetate, propionate, and butyrate. "SCFAs work almost like the statin drugs used to lower cholesterol. They hinder the production of cholesterol by blocking an enzyme," says Dr. Anderson.

Conquer the Blood-Sugar Roller Coaster

Diabetes is a hydra-headed monster of a disease. Left uncontrolled, it can wreak havoc on a woman's eyes, liver, and kidneys and leave her from two to four times more vulnerable to suffering heart disease or stroke.

Preheat the oven to 425°F. Cut each pita into eight triangles and separate each triangle into two pieces. Spread the triangles, rough side up, on two large baking sheets.

Bake for 8 to 10 minutes, or until crisp. (This can be done ahead of time. Cool the triangles completely and store them in a covered container for up to 3 days.)

In a food processor, combine the chickpeas, tahini, lemon juice, garlic, and salt. Pulse for 30 seconds to mix. Process for 2 minutes, or until very smooth, scraping down the sides of the container as necessary.

Transfer to a serving dish. Sprinkle with the onion and parsley. Serve with the pitas, peppers, and cucumber.

Makes 8 servings

Per serving: 207 calories, 7 g protein, 29 g carbohydrates, 8 g fat, 0 mg cholesterol, 6 g dietary fiber, 439 mg sodium

Note: To jazz up hummus and give it more beta-carotene, add a roasted red pepper to the basic recipe and puree along with the other ingredients.

The good news: Eating right can do much to head off these serious complications. And that's where the humble bean comes in.

"The soluble fiber in beans can help regulate blood sugar levels," says David M. Klurfeld, Ph.D., professor and chairman of the department of nutrition and food science at Wayne State University in Detroit. Unlike refined carbohydrates (sugars), such as table sugar and honey, which flood the bloodstream with glucose within minutes, complex carbohydrates (starches) combined with soluble fiber found in beans take hours to digest, he explains. So glucose enters your blood gradually, keeping blood sugar on an even keel.

You don't have to eat heaping helpings of beans to reap their beneficial effects. Research on men and women with diabetes has shown that eating small quantities of beans—approximately ½ cup a day—helps to manage their blood sugar levels.

Thwart Cancer with Legumes

Low in total and saturated fat and high in fiber, beans may be some of the best cancer-preventive foods we can eat. But beans also contain specific plant chemicals, called phytochemicals, or phytonutrients, that have been found to wage war against cancer cells themselves.

"The phytochemicals in beans, such as isoflavones, saponins, sterols, phytates, and protease inhibitors, have been shown in test tubes and some animal studies to hinder cancer-cell growth," says Leonard Cohen, Ph.D., section head of the nutrition and endocrinology program at the American Health Foundation in Valhalla, New York. In some cases, they also appear to keep normal cells from turning cancerous.

In one study, Dr. Cohen and other researchers from the American Health Foundation and New York Medical College, also in Valhalla, analyzed the diets of 214 White, Black, and Latina college-age women. They found that the Latina women ate significantly more beans—7.4 servings per week, compared to 4.6 servings per week for Black women and less than 3 servings per week for White women.

"There's no doubt that Latina women as well as female vegetarians eat more beans and that both groups tend to have lower incidence rates of breast cancer than the general population," says Dr. Cohen. "It remains to be seen whether the chemicals present in beans afford protection against breast cancer, or whether protection can be attributed to other lifestyle or dietary factors that are associated with high levels of bean consumption."

Beans also contain proteins called lectins. Research suggests that some of the lectins found in beans may help prevent colorectal cancer, which kills about 15 out of every 100,000 women in this country each year.

Fava beans, a staple of Italian, French, Spanish, Greek, and Middle Eastern kitchens, seem to have cancer-blasting potential. Researchers at the Imperial College of Science, Technology, and Medicine at Hammersmith Hospital in London found that adding a specific type of lectin—*Vicia faba* agglutinin—found in favas to cancerous cells in test tubes made the cells act more like healthy cells and stopped the cancerous cells from multiplying.

POWER

TACOS

SOFT PINTO BEAN TACOS

Mexican food, sometimes criticized for being high in fat, can be super healthy if you're smart about how you prepare it. When making tacos, use soft tortillas instead of fried ones, and stuff them with a lean, fiber-filled bean mixture. As for toppings, pile on plenty of shredded dark green lettuce (romaine has seven times the cancer-fighting carotenoids of iceberg) and chopped tomatoes (with lots of lycopene for further cancer protection).

1	tablespoon canola oil
1	large onion, finely chopped
1	can (15½ ounces) pinto beans, rinsed and drained
⅓	cup salsa
4	large flour tortillas
1	cup shredded reduced-fat Cheddar cheese
1½	cups finely shredded romaine lettuce
1	tomato, finely chopped

In a medium saucepan, warm the oil over medium heat. Add the onion and cook, stirring, for 5 minutes. Stir in the beans and salsa. Cook for 5 more minutes.

Remove half of the bean mixture. With a potato masher, mash half of the mixture to a paste. Return the mashed mixture to the saucepan.

Wrap the tortillas in a paper towel and microwave on high power for 1 minute.

Divide the bean mixture evenly among the tortillas, spooning it into the centers. Sprinkle evenly with half of the cheese. Top with the lettuce, tomato, and remaining cheese. Roll to enclose the filling.

Makes 4 servings

Per serving: 304 calories, 14 g protein, 35 g carbohydrates, 12 g fat, 20 mg cholesterol, 5 g dietary fiber, 629 mg sodium

The lectins in favas may interact with specific molecules on the surface of the cells that line the colon, says lead study author Mark Jordinson, M.D., Ph.D., research fellow in the department of gastroenterology. Those molecules—called cell surface adhesion molecules—may function as a kind of on/off switch for cell growth, thereby influencing the development of cancer.

There's no telling how many fava beans you have to eat to get "the lectin effect," says Dr. Jordinson. But since many legumes contain cancer-crippling compounds, he says it's wise to make all varieties a part of your healthy, low-fat diet.

MASKED DISASTER

Refried Beans

If you're dining out on Mexican cuisine, skip the refried beans. Many restaurants start with otherwise healthy, low-fat beans and add lots of fat (including lard), bacon, and cheese. One survey of restaurant offerings found refried beans that supplied one third of an entire day's allowance of saturated fat in a ¾-cup serving. For meals at home, choose canned refried beans marked fat-free or made with an oil that isn't labeled "hydrogenated." Hydrogenation is a process that increases the saturated fat levels of oils, making them less heart-healthy.

Little Package, Big Nutrients

Every bean is like a tiny jewelry box, aglitter with woman-friendly nutrients that our diets often lack.

Take folate. In the Nurses' Health Study, a large, ongoing study of 80,082 women, Harvard researchers found that those who consumed high amounts of this B vitamin (the naturally occurring form of folic acid) cut their risk of developing heart disease nearly in half. In another study of 386 women at the University of Washington in Seattle, women with the highest blood levels of homocysteine, an amino acid that research has linked to an increased risk of heart disease, had double the heart attack risk of those with the lowest levels. Interestingly, they also had the lowest levels of folate.

Too much homocysteine may damage arterial walls, allowing fatty deposits to clog arteries and cause blood clots. It's thought that folate breaks down homocysteine, sending it packing before it can damage your arteries.

CANNED BEANS ARE PERFECTLY OKAY

Few of us have the time or the inclination to soak and cook dried beans. The solution? Reach for your can opener. Canned beans are just as good for you as dried, says James W. Anderson, M.D., professor of medicine and clinical nutrition at the Veterans Affairs Medical Center in Lexington, Kentucky. They do contain more sodium, so drain and rinse canned beans before using them.

Beans are excellent sources of folate. One cup of black beans, for example, contains 256 micrograms of folate, 64 percent of the recommended 400 micrograms a day. The same amount of kidney beans contains 229 milligrams of folate, while large lima beans contain 156 milligrams.

Beans are also an excellent source of iron, a mineral that, if you're premenopausal, is especially vital to your health. If you don't get enough, you're at risk for becoming one of the 8 million girls and premenopausal women with iron deficiency, the most common nutritional deficiency among American women. Left untreated, iron deficiency can lead to the more serious iron-deficiency anemia and leave a woman's body cells starving for oxygen.

One cup of kidney beans contains 5.2 milligrams of iron, about one-third of the 15 to 18 milligrams recommended for premenopausal women. A cup of lima beans contains 4.5 milligrams of iron, while a cup of black beans packs 3.6 milligrams.

Preparing Your Hill of Beans

You already know to add beans to soups, stews, chili, and casseroles. But you probably haven't even considered the unique serving suggestions below. Give them a whirl.

• Whip up a savory Southwestern omelette, suggests Jay Solomon, chef and owner of Emily's Gourmet-to-Go in Denver and author of *Lean Bean Cuisine*. Combine ¼ cup of canned or cooked black beans, 2 tablespoons each of corn kernels, minced red or green pepper, diced

POWER

SOUP

BLACK BEAN SOUP

Eating a cup of beans a day can help lower cholesterol. With dishes like this savory Tex-Mex soup to choose from, you'll have no trouble meeting that quota. Feel free to spike it with hot-pepper sauce. The capsaicin it contains is also good for your heart.

1   tablespoon olive oil
1   large onion, finely chopped
1   small carrot, finely chopped
1   teaspoon ground cumin
2   cans (15 ounces each) black beans, rinsed and drained
3   cups water
1   bay leaf
    Juice of 1 lime
¾   cup fat-free plain yogurt
½   cup finely chopped fresh cilantro

In a medium saucepan, warm the oil over medium heat. Add the onion and cook, stirring, for 3 minutes. Add the carrot and cumin. Cook, stirring, for 2 minutes longer. Stir in the beans, water, and bay leaf. Simmer for 15 minutes. Remove and discard the bay leaf.

Remove about one-third of the bean and vegetable mixture. Using a potato masher, mash the mixture to a paste. Return the mashed mixture to the saucepan. Stir in the lime juice. Serve topped with the yogurt and cilantro.

Makes 4 cups

Per cup: 187 calories, 10 g protein, 29 g carbohydrates, 5 g fat, 0 mg cholesterol, 10 g dietary fiber, 706 mg sodium

tomato, and minced scallions, 1 tablespoon of diced jalapeño pepper, 1 tablespoon of dried cilantro, and ¼ teaspoon of ground cumin. This is enough to stuff an omelette made with three eggs or 1½ cups of egg substitute.

• To give homemade rice pudding a Hawaiian-inspired touch, add sweet adzuki beans to your next batch, suggests Solomon. Add 1 cup of cooked or canned adzukis to 3 cups of cooked rice. You might also add two mashed bananas. Adzukis can be found at health food stores and some grocery stores.

• "Pizza is a canvas, a way to express your culinary creativity," says Solomon. He likes topping his homemade pizzas with ½ cup of cooked kidney or black beans, 1 cup of shredded spinach, and four to six sliced mushrooms.

• While most of us think of hummus as a dip for pita bread or baby carrots, it also makes a wonderful salad dressing, says Greg Hottinger, R.D., a registered dietitian with the Duke University Diet and Fitness Center in Durham, North Carolina. To thin it down, dilute it with a bit of water or lemon juice.

• For a savory bean salad, combine 1 cup each of navy beans, chickpeas, and red kidney beans with ½ cup of coarsely chopped fresh mint leaves, two chopped tomatoes, one diced cucumber, two or three minced scallions (or ¼ cup of minced red onion), two minced cloves of garlic, and 4 ounces of crumbled feta cheese. Dress with 2 tablespoons each of olive oil and vinegar, 2 tablespoons of minced fresh parsley (or 1 tablespoon of dried), and salt and pepper to taste.

• The next time you make potato salad, use sweet potatoes instead of white and add 1½ cups of navy or great Northern beans, suggests Solomon. (He also adds 1 cup of shredded mustard or dandelion greens and ½ cup each of slivered red onion and chopped celery.) For the dressing, use ½ to ¾ cup of olive or canola oil, ⅓ cup of red wine vinegar, 1 teaspoon of dried thyme, 1 teaspoon of sugar (optional), and salt and pepper to taste.

Soy: A Natural Hormone Balancer—And More

Power Maker #2: Shop around for a soy food or beverage you like, then pick it up every time you buy groceries and make it a routine part of your weekly menu.

Y ou know soy has gone mainstream when Starbucks sells soy milk latte and the articles in the *New York Times* report on its health virtues. Food companies are allowed to tout the benefits of soy on product labels, and you can buy soy burgers, soy ice cream, soy flour, and soy foods like tofu and tempeh in most supermarkets.

There's a reason for the soy mania: A growing body of evidence shows that the humble legume may lower our cholesterol levels, reduce our risk of breast and colon cancers, and possibly protect against osteoporosis and memory problems after menopause.

In fact, some experts say it's only a matter of time before doctors routinely recommend soy for many women past menopause.

What Makes Soy Special?

Researchers started to take notice of soy years ago. Here's what they observed about the connection between soy and health.

1. Nearly all of the soybeans grown in this country (about half the world's soy) are either exported or fed to animals, whereas people eat nearly all of the soy grown in Asia.

2. The Japanese eat an average of 23 pounds of soy per person per year, compared to the 2 pounds per person eaten in the United States.

3. The Japanese have a longer life expectancy than ours, breast cancer and heart disease rates one-fourth as high as ours, and colon cancer rates one-third as high as ours.

4. When the Japanese move to our country and begin eating our food, their rates of cancer shoot up.

"People in Asian countries have existed on a soy-based diet for literally centuries, apparently with little or no detriment and, in fact, with great benefit," says Helen Kim, Ph.D., research associate professor in the department of pharmacology and toxicology at the University of Alabama at Birmingham.

Studies on individuals suggest that the benefits are more than a coincidence. Soy is loaded with substances collectively known as phytochemicals, or phytonutrients, which promote health in several ways. Soy contains at least five classes of anticarcinogenic compounds, including isoflavones, saponins, phytates, protease inhibitors, and phytosterols. Many of these are also found in a variety of fruits, vegetables, and whole grains. But isoflavones, a kind of plant-based compound that shares some properties with the female hormone estrogen, are nearly exclusive to soy.

In the body, three types of isoflavones—daidzein, genistein, and

SOY BONUS: LONGER MENSTRUAL CYCLES

Don't be surprised if your period arrives a little later than usual after you start eating soy. Women in China and Japan, who eat more soy, have menstrual cycles nearly 4 days longer than ours. They also experience one-fourth as much breast cancer as we do.

Scientists believe that a longer time between periods—equating to fewer menstrual cycles in your lifetime—may be a protectant against breast cancer. So fewer periods are better.

POWER

STEW

SAVORY SOYBEAN STEW

Soybeans have great healing potential—everything from blocking heart disease and cancer to strengthening bones and easing the effects of menopause. If you think you don't like soybeans, you'll be pleasantly surprised by this savory stew. It's delicious, hearty, and ready in a cool half-hour, thanks to canned beans.

1	tablespoon olive oil
1	large onion, finely chopped
½	cup finely chopped green bell pepper
1	tablespoon finely chopped garlic
1½	teaspoons ground cumin
1½	teaspoons ground coriander
¾	teaspoon ground ginger
1	small butternut squash, peeled, seeded, and cut into ½" cubes
2	cups water
2	cans (15 ounces each) soybeans, rinsed and drained
1	can (8 ounces) tomato sauce
1½	teaspoon salt

In a large saucepan, warm the oil over medium heat. Add the onion and cook, stirring constantly, for 3 minutes. Add the pepper, garlic, cumin, coriander, and ginger. Cook, stirring constantly, for 2 minutes. Stir in the squash and 1 cup of the water. Bring to a boil. Reduce the heat to medium-low, cover, and simmer for 5 minutes.

Stir in the soybeans, tomato sauce, salt, and the remaining 1 cup water. Simmer for 20 minutes, or until thickened.

Makes 6 cups

Per cup: 192 calories, 12 g protein, 21 g carbohydrates, 8.2 g fat, 0 mg cholesterol, 4 g dietary fiber, 543 mg sodium

glycitein—act like kinder, gentler versions of our own natural estrogen. Most researchers believe that these isoflavones are what make soy beneficial—at least as food. In some cases, supplements don't have the same effect.

More Soy, Fewer Heart Attacks?

Soy gets a lot of credit for protecting against heart disease, and for good reason, says Kenneth D. R. Setchell, Ph.D., director of clinical mass spectrometry and professor of pediatrics at Children's Hospital Medical Center in Cincinnati. It appears to play an important role in a complex chain of events that leads to artery disease. You know about the "good" cholesterol, HDL, and about the "bad" cholesterol, LDL. Now say hello to the really bad cholesterol: oxidized LDL. This is LDL cholesterol that's been attacked by free radicals, rampaging scavenger cells that steal molecules from other cells, damaging them in the process. Oxidized LDL is like a kid on a lollipop binge: it sticks to everything, particularly the arteries leading to and from your heart. This could block blood flowing to your heart, leading to heart disease and heart attacks.

Soy, however, appears to prevent LDL from being oxidized, explains Dr. Setchell. He and his colleagues saw this happen in a study of 47 postmenopausal women. Even though they had normal cholesterol levels to begin with, just 12 weeks of drinking three 8-ounce glasses of soy milk a day reduced their oxidized LDL levels about 10 percent. Each glass of soy milk contained 22 to 24 milligrams of isoflavones.

In another study of 51 perimenopausal women—women who missed at least three menstrual periods in the past 12 months—adding one or two doses per day of 20 grams of soy protein containing 34 milligrams of isoflavones lowered their overall cholesterol and LDL, which would be expected to reduce their heart disease risk 12 percent. This dosage is as much soy protein as in about 1 cup of cooked soybeans.

That's considered a substantial drop in cholesterol, especially since the women had normal levels to begin with. Other studies suggest that soy may also increase levels of the good cholesterol, HDL, in women.

In another study, monkeys who were fed a high-cholesterol diet containing soy isoflavones dropped their risk of stroke just as much as monkeys who were given Premarin, a widely used hormone-replacement drug prescribed for its cardio-protective effects in menopausal women. Unlike

POWER

QUICHE

ASPARAGUS QUICHE
WITH BROWN RICE CRUST

The problem with most quiches is their heavy-cream filling. This one uses tofu to achieve a silky smooth texture without excess fat. And, of course, the tofu has cancer-preventing benefits that the cream could never rival. As a bonus, the high-fiber rice crust is a healthy alternative to a standard butter-based pie shell.

CRUST

2½   cups cold cooked brown rice

⅓   cup grated Parmesan cheese

2   egg whites, lightly beaten, or ¼ cup liquid egg substitute

FILLING

12   ounces low-fat silken tofu

4   eggs, lightly beaten, or 1 cup liquid egg substitute

1   tablespoon cornstarch

½   teaspoon salt

⅛   teaspoon ground nutmeg

1   pound asparagus, trimmed, cut into 1" pieces, and steamed

hormone-replacement therapy (HRT), soy doesn't increase women's triglyceride levels, which are yet another risk factor for heart disease.

Isoflavones may be the active ingredient, but in isolation they give little, if any, protection. "You need both soy protein and isoflavones," says Thomas Clarkson, D.V.M., professor of comparative medicine at Wake Forest University in Winston-Salem, North Carolina, who has studied postmenopausal monkeys, who are reproductively similar to humans. Evidently, the isoflavones send cholesterol to your gut, where it binds to the soy protein and eventually passes through your body.

3   ounces reduced-fat Swiss cheese, shredded

2   ounces ham-flavored soy deli slices, finely chopped

2   scallions, finely chopped

Preheat the oven to 350°F. Lightly coat a 10" deep-dish pie plate with cooking spray.

To make the crust: In a large bowl, mix the rice, cheese, and egg whites or egg substitute. Press evenly in the bottom and up the sides of the pie plate. Bake for 15 minutes.

To make the filling: In a food processor, combine the tofu, eggs or egg substitute, cornstarch, salt, and nutmeg. Process until smooth, scraping down the sides of the container as necessary.

Sprinkle the asparagus, cheese, soy slices, and scallions over the baked crust. Pour in the tofu mixture, stirring gently to blend slightly.

Bake for 45 minutes, or until firm in the center. Let stand for 5 minutes before slicing.

Makes 6 servings

Per serving: 261 calories, 27 g protein, 25 g carbohydrates, 8.3 g fat, 151 mg cholesterol, 2 g dietary fiber, 524 mg sodium

Can Tofu Guard against Colon Cancer?

If protecting your heart isn't enough reason to eat more soy foods, evidence strongly suggests it can also protect you against colon cancer.

Maurice R. Bennink, Ph.D., professor of food science and human nutrition at Michigan State University in East Lansing, added 39 grams a day of either soy protein or a soyless protein to the diets of 29 men and 10 women who either had previous colon cancer or had polyps that tend to develop into cancer. One year later, changes in the cells lining the colons of the men and women eating soy protein indicated that their risk of colon cancer had been cut in half.

Soy's protective effects didn't surprise Dr. Bennink; he'd seen similar results in years of animal studies. What really excited him was that all he did was to add soy to the men's and women's diets, not change the entire way in which they ate.

"So you don't have to make radical changes in your diet to get the benefit of soy," he says (although there are plenty of good reasons to add other protective foods to your diet).

Subtle Benefits for Breasts

In population studies, scientists have found that compared to women who don't eat soy foods, women who do get less breast cancer. Laboratory and animal studies show that certain compounds in soy can destroy breast cancer cells or reduce animals' risk of developing the cancer.

What worries some doctors is the estrogen-like action of soy. In our bodies, estrogen seems to stimulate the division of breast cells—healthy as well as cancerous—and in some women it increases the risk of breast cancer. Theoretically, adding the phytoestrogens found in soy might increase the risk even more.

A variety of studies in humans have not shown that soy acts like estrogen, says Mindy Kurzer, Ph.D., associate professor of food science and nutrition at the University of Minnesota in St. Paul. Though there are few, studies in women that suggest that eating soy foods may reduce the risk of breast cancer are encouraging. At the University of South Carolina, researchers compared the levels of isoflavones in the urine of 60 women with breast cancer with that of an equal number of women who did not have the disease. Those with the highest levels of isoflavones had about half the cancer risk of those with the lowest levels—a good sign, since the levels correspond with soy food consumption.

And intriguing studies by Wake Forest researchers suggest that soy phytoestrogens may be the "magic" ingredients that might counteract the higher rate of breast cancer that hormone-replacement therapy causes.

In other reassuring research at Wake Forest, J. Mark Cline, D.V.M., Ph.D., associate professor of comparative medicine, studied the combined effects of soy protein and estrogen on postmenopausal monkeys, whose breast and uterine tissues are very similar to those in humans. Cell divi-

POWER

PARFAITS

BERRY VANILLA PUDDING PARFAITS

Soy milk is an excellent substitute for regular milk in loads of recipes. Here we use the vanilla-flavored variety to make classic homemade pudding that's not just comfort food but also a good source of disease-preventing isoflavones.

3	cups vanilla soy milk
⅓	cup sugar
3	tablespoons cornstarch
¼	teaspoon almond extract
1	cup thinly sliced strawberries
1	cup blueberries
½	cup low-fat granola

In a medium saucepan, whisk together the milk, sugar, and cornstarch. Bring to a boil over medium heat, whisking constantly. Reduce the heat to medium-low. Whisking constantly, simmer for about 15 minutes, or until the mixture is very thick. Remove from the heat and stir in the almond extract.

Divide half of the pudding among individual dessert dishes. Sprinkle with the strawberries and blueberries. Top with the remaining pudding and sprinkle with the granola. Loosely cover and refrigerate for at least 1 hour. (The pudding will set further as it cools.)

Makes 6 servings

Per serving: 154 calories, 3 g protein, 33 g carbohydrates, 2 g fat, 0 mg cholesterol, 2 g dietary fiber, 70 mg sodium

sion in the monkeys' breasts and uteruses—a cancer marker—declined. This was the first study to show this effect.

While scientists have several theories, they don't yet know precisely how soy might affect breast cancer.

Yet Another Way to Build Bone

Some studies suggest that soy may also help protect a woman's bones, even if she's not getting quite enough calcium.

Bone is formed by cells called osteoblasts and destroyed by cells called osteoclasts. Estrogen acts like handcuffs on the osteoclasts, preventing them from breaking down much bone, says Dr. Setchell. But after menopause, when the levels of estrogen in our bodies drop dramatically, the handcuffs come off, and the bone-consuming osteoclasts step up their activity. Dr. Setchell thinks that soy may be one key to reining them in.

He gave 43 postmenopausal women three glasses of soy milk a day containing between 60 and 70 milligrams of isoflavones. At the end of 12 weeks, he found the levels of bone-eating osteoclasts decreased while the levels of bone-producing osteoblasts increased significantly. To make sure calcium wasn't a factor, they consumed no calcium during the study. Normally, that would increase bone loss. But soy milk prevented that, says Dr. Setchell.

Food for the Female Brain

Preliminary studies in monkeys suggest that soy protein may help lower a postmenopausal woman's risk for Alzheimer's disease. It certainly couldn't hurt.

Dr. Kim studied the brains of postmenopausal monkeys who ate an isoflavone-containing diet, looking for changes indicative of Alzheimer's disease. Instead she found changes indicating protection from Alzheimer's. When she compared the brains to those of monkeys who ate either soy protein without isoflavones or who were given Premarin, she found no protection. "It appears that eating the whole soy protein protected the brains of the postmenopausal monkeys from at least some of the bio-chemical changes that appear in brains with Alzheimer's," she says.

She's encouraged by another study, this one on rats, conducted by Wake Forest researchers that showed that postmenopausal rats who received either soy phytoestrogens or estrogen replacement performed better on maze tests than those receiving no treatment.

"On balance, our studies suggest that soy isoflavones provide a beneficial effect on brain function, protecting against dementia," says Dr. Clarkson.

SOY MAY RELIEVE PAIN NATURALLY

Doctors have stumbled on a hidden benefit of soy: It may relieve pain. In one instance, two similar studies of pain sensitivity in rats produced different results. The chow fed to one group contained a lot of soy protein, and the chow fed to the others did not. The group fed soy chow tolerated pain better.

In another study, French researchers gave 75 men and women with osteoarthritis in their knees or hips a pill containing soybean and avocado oil. Another 69 received a placebo. At 6 months, nearly half of the 75 people taking the oil capsules used less pain medication, compared to just a third of those given the placebos. And more than half of those taking the oil capsules rated their treatment as "very good" or "good" compared with just 30 percent of those given the placebos.

A Hormone Helper

Despite the potential benefits of soy, some menopausal women may still need to take hormone-replacement therapy.

But by adding soy protein with isoflavones to their diets, Dr. Clarkson says, women may eventually be able to take estrogen only, not progesterone. Added to the estrogen to counteract increased cancer risk, progesterone causes many of the side effects, such as breakthrough bleeding and headaches, that many women experience on HRT. Soy has no such side effects.

Taste the "New" Soy

If you ever tried soy only to find it bitter, bland, or mushy, consider giving soy foods a second chance.

Thanks to technology, soy foods taste pretty normal. Today, you can get your soy meat Cajun-, Asian-, or Mexican-style. Soy cream cheese actually tastes like cream cheese. Soy milk is found in the dairy case next to the cow juice in luscious flavors like vanilla, chocolate, and strawberry. Technology has enabled food manufacturers to develop more realistic flavors for soy foods as well as to remove some of the not-so-pleasant ef-

GOING FOR SOY? SHOP AROUND

Soy foods vary widely. Some contain far more isoflavones (considered to be the active ingredient for health) than others. As a bonus, some offer a fair amount of calcium or fiber.

Here's a quick guide to some widely available soy foods.

SOY FOOD	SERVING SIZE	CALORIES
Soy cereal (sold under the brand name Nutlettes)	¼ cup	70
Soy shakes, dry mix (follow package directions)	1 oz	100
Soy protein bars	1 bar	210
Textured vegetable protein (TVP)	¼ cup	56
Soybeans, roasted	3 Tbsp	152
Soybeans, canned	½ cup	140
Tempeh	½ cup	160
Soy flour, defatted	¼ cup	82
Soy milk	1 cup	80
Soy pudding	½ cup	150
Soy protein isolate	3 Tbsp	96
Tofu, raw, firm	½ cup	140
Soy hot dogs	1	60
Miso	2 Tbsp	70
Green soybeans, boiled	½ cup	127
Soy burgers	1 patty	137
Soy cheese	1 oz	70
Low-fat soy nondairy frozen dessert	½ cup	120
Premium soy nondairy frozen dessert	½ cup	190

fects of soy from the bean itself, explains Nancy Chapman, executive director of the Soyfoods Association of North America. For instance, some beans are higher in simple carbohydrates, so they're sweeter. Other beans are lower in indigestible carbohydrates that cause some gas when eaten in their raw form.

You can find everything from soy biscotti to soy protein bars to soy

"Don't get overly concerned with isoflavone content, though," says Gregory Burke, M.D., professor in the department of public health sciences at Wake Forest University in Winston-Salem, North Carolina. "Just pick something you like, and enjoy it regularly."

FAT (g)	FIBER (g)	CALCIUM (mg)	ISOFLAVONES (approx. mg)
0.7	4.5	80	61
1	0	700	55
0	2	250	49
0.2	1.8	41	47
8	5.7	4	41
6	3	100	38–41
9	2	92	36
0.3	4.3	60	33
2.5	0	300	30
4	1	47	30
0.9	1.6	50	28
8	1.7	532	24
2.5	0	40	16
2	1.8	22	15
6	4	130.5	11
4	5.7	102	9
5	0	0	4
2	0	0	3–4
11	0	0	3–4

pizza and ice cream at your supermarket, health food store, or by mail order, so there's no need to get your soy in pills. They won't protect your heart, and the effects of taking supplements that contain a concentrated form of soy are unknown. If you eat the recommended amount of soy-based foods, you'll get soy's specific benefits along with fiber and other nutrients, says Dr. Kim.

"I suggest eating soy at the same levels that people in Asia do: one serving a day," says Dr. Kurzer. One serving equals ½ cup of tempeh, 1 cup of soy milk, 3 tablespoons of roasted soybeans, or a soy protein bar. All of these will provide 30 to 50 milligrams of isoflavones, an amount experts say is a sensible goal for most Americans. And make sure that whatever you're eating contains isoflavones. Alcohol extraction of soy protein concentrates and isolates used in some products can remove as much as 90 percent of the isoflavones.

Sneak In More Soy

Adding soy to your diet isn't complicated. Here are some ideas to get you started.

Fill your flour jar. You can substitute soy flour for one-third of the wheat flour in recipes.

Snack on it. Dry-roasted soy nuts make a wonderful snack, saving you 23 calories and 3 grams of fat compared to potato chips.

"IS IT SAFE FOR MY HUSBAND TO EAT SOY?"

It's one of the most common questions soy researcher and gynecologist John A. Eden, M.D., hears from women. "They've heard that soy acts like a natural source of estrogen, and they want to know if soy is going to feminize their husbands," says the associate professor of reproductive endocrinology at the University of New South Wales in Australia.

To put their minds at rest (and answer some scientific questions of his own), Dr. Eden gave 27 men 28 grams of soy protein containing 65 milligrams of isoflavones. After taking the soy protein daily for 12 weeks, the men's HDL cholesterol levels had increased 9.5 percent with no effect on their levels of the male hormone testosterone. HDL cholesterol is the so-called good cholesterol—the higher the level of HDL, the lower the risk of heart disease, explains Dr. Eden.

In other words, there really is no good reason for him not to eat soy burgers, too.

Toss it. Sprinkle lightly steamed, young, green soybeans, called edamame, in your salad.

Splash it. Pour soy milk on your cereal.

Combine it. Use half soy meat crumbles and half ground turkey or lean ground beef when making spaghetti sauce, tacos, or any other ground-meat recipe.

Marinate it. Marinate tofu and use it for stir-fries and grilling.

Add it. Add soy isolate or concentrate to other foods such as milk-shakes or smoothies.

Grill it. Soy burgers, even without the ketchup, can be a hit with your teenagers.

Puree it. Puree soft tofu and flavor it with onion soup mix for dip.

Garlic: This Bulb Could Save Your Life

You might say garlic (*Allium sativum*) is like a woman: full of sweetness and character when handled properly, and powerful enough to influence everything that comes near.

Garlic especially influences our health. After all, when a vegetable is mentioned in the Bible, you have to figure it's more than a great way to flavor a leg of lamb. Yet it wasn't until after nearly 1,300 studies that scientists and doctors realized what ancient Romans and Greeks had always known: Garlic is powerful.

"I'm incredibly impressed with the diversity of positive effects that garlic has on health," says John Milner, Ph.D., head of the nutrition department at Pennsylvania State University in University Park, who is known in scientific circles as Dr. Garlic.

More Than Meets the Nose

Crush, cut, or chop it, and you'll likely smell it on your hands all day, thanks to a substance called alliin, a sulfur-containing version of an amino acid. Alliin has no taste or smell, but if you damage the garlic, it sets off a chemical reaction that turns alliin into another sulfur compound called allicin, giving garlic its pungent scent and taste. Once released, allicin transforms into dozens of other compounds, some so ephemeral that they can't even be captured for study, others with medicinal properties that rival some antibiotics or heart disease drugs. The compounds created and the benefits that garlic yields depend on how you prepare it.

"If you crush garlic and let it sit for 15 minutes, 20 different compounds form," says John Pinto, Ph.D., director of the nutrition research laboratory at Memorial Sloan-Kettering Cancer Center and associate professor of biochemistry at Weill Medical College of Cornell University, both in New York City. "Then, when you eat the garlic, these compounds, called phytonutrients, are transformed into other compounds that either by themselves or in any combination may have beneficial effects."

A Natural Prescription for Your Heart

When it comes to benchmarks of heart health like blood pressure and cholesterol levels, "I don't know of any other natural substance that can produce the kind of results garlic does," says Manfred Steiner, M.D., Ph.D., a hematologist retired from East Carolina University in

EXTRACTS ARE CONVENIENT AND EFFECTIVE

If you're looking for a way to get your garlic without offending your friends, try using supplements.

Look for aged garlic extracts, says Earl Mindell, R.Ph., Ph.D., professor of nutrition at Pacific Western University in Los Angeles. These products contain a variety of garlic's beneficial compounds but are odorless, so they won't leave you with bad breath. They're available in tablet, capsule, and liquid forms. Follow dosage instructions on the label.

Do not use garlic supplements if you are on anticoagulants (blood thinners) or before undergoing surgery, because garlic thins the blood and may increase bleeding. Avoid supplements if you're taking drugs to lower your blood sugar.

Greenville, North Carolina, who has studied garlic's effects on various aspects of heart disease.

He supplemented 41 volunteers' diets with 7.2 grams of aged garlic extract a day for 6 months—the equivalent of a clove of garlic daily. At the end of the study, volunteers' blood pressure levels had dropped 5 to 6 percent and their total cholesterol and LDL levels had dropped 7 to 8 percent. Additionally, their blood platelets were less sticky, even when exposed to adrenaline, a hormone that typically makes platelets clump together, setting off a chain reaction that can lead to stroke or heart attack.

"None of these effects by itself was huge, but the combined effect was beneficial," Dr. Steiner says. To get similar effects with drugs would take at least three different medications. The results bode well for women with slightly elevated cholesterol or blood pressure levels, or even those who simply have a family history of heart disease.

Other studies found that garlic compounds prevent LDL oxidation, the process some doctors think leads to sticky, fatty cholesterol accumulations on blood vessel walls. In Germany, researchers actually reversed the effects of plaque buildup in arteries by supplementing the diets of 61 men and women with ⅓ teaspoon of garlic powder a day.

Garlic also appears to keep arteries elastic, delaying or possibly preventing a common occurrence in old age that may result in heart attacks or strokes. Lifelong exposure to fats clogs arteries and makes them stiff and brittle. Hardened arteries can no longer stretch to absorb the blood pumping through them. Each heartbeat sends a wave of pressure through the body, causing a form of hypertension that is implicated in strokes and other cardiovascular problems. When German researchers compared 101 healthy adults who used supplements (averaging about half a clove of garlic a day for 7 years) with those who used no supplements, they found that the arteries of the garlic-using subjects—even those who already had high blood pressure—weren't nearly as stiff as the arteries of those who didn't take supplements.

Not a Magic Bullet—But Powerful

Dozens of studies show that various forms of garlic can reduce cholesterol levels by an average of 9 to 12 percent. Yet in two studies, neither garlic oil nor garlic powder tablets had any effect on cholesterol. How could the results be so different?

COOKED OR RAW? MINCED OR SLICED?

So what's the best way to use your garlic in food? Garlic researcher John Milner, Ph.D., head of the nutrition department at Pennsylvania State University in University Park, offers these tips.

- Peel the garlic before heating. Keeping the peel on prevents various disease-preventing compounds from forming.

- Let garlic rest for 10 to 15 minutes after it's cut or crushed. Letting garlic "breathe" allows time for the important sulfurous compounds to form.

- Garlic compounds appear to stay in your body for several days, so eating garlic once a week should suffice. Since garlic thins the blood, don't exceed two cloves per day prior to surgery or if you are taking anticoagulants.

How does "Dr. Garlic" get his regular dose of this magical vegetable? "I married an Italian," he says.

Perhaps the studies didn't account for the participants' diets and exercise habits. Evidence shows that the benefits from garlic improve as fat content in the diet increases, says Dr. Milner. He thinks that it has something to do with the individual fatty acids we ingest. "This doesn't mean you should eat a high-fat diet, but since many Americans do, they would likely benefit from the addition of garlic to their diets."

"Garlic isn't the sole remedy for high cholesterol, but combined with an overall program that includes a low-fat diet and regular exercise, garlic can reduce cholesterol levels even further," says Yu-Yan Yeh, Ph.D., professor of nutrition at Pennsylvania State University, which houses one of the country's premier garlic research centers.

Detoxify with Garlic

Our bodies are constantly bombarded with cancer-causing toxins. In turn, our bodies fight back with powerful detoxification enzymes that convert the cancer-causing chemicals into benign substances that we can shake off like a bad day. If our bodies produce too few of these enzymes, the cancer gets a foothold, which is where garlic comes in.

POWER

PESTO

BASIL PESTO

Here is a versatile recipe using that disease-fighting giant, garlic. Pesto perks up just about everything—from pasta, broiled chicken, and steamed vegetables to soup, rice, and baked potatoes. You can literally eat it every day and not run out of delicious ways to use it. For variety, replace some or all of the basil with other fresh herbs, like marjoram or parsley.

$\frac{1}{3}$ cup chopped walnuts

2   cups packed fresh basil leaves

$\frac{1}{2}$ cup grated Parmesan cheese

$\frac{1}{3}$ cup extra-virgin olive oil

1–2   cloves garlic, halved

$\frac{1}{8}$ teaspoon ground black pepper

In a small skillet, stir the walnuts over low heat for 2 minutes, or until golden and fragrant. Let cool, then transfer to a blender or small food processor. Add the basil, cheese, oil, garlic, and pepper. Pulse until smooth, scraping down the sides of the container as necessary.

Makes 1 cup (enough for 1 pound of pasta)

Per tablespoon: 73 calories, 2 g protein, 1 g carbohydrates, 7 g fat, 2 mg cholesterol, 0 g dietary fiber, 59 mg sodium

Note: Store the pesto in a covered container for up to 5 days in the refrigerator or up to 1 month in the freezer.

When scientists in New Zealand fed rats a garlic extract called diallyl disulfide, an allicin daughter, production of one protective enzyme increased up to 60 percent. "The dose was the equivalent of half a clove of raw garlic, showing that even relatively small intakes of garlic could be useful in protecting against certain types of cancer," say study authors Rex Munday, Ph.D., and his wife, Christine, of the Ruakura Agricultural Research Centre in Hamilton, New Zealand.

In laboratory experiments, various garlic compounds have been found to slow the growth of cancers of the breast, colon, lung, rectum, esophagus, skin, and stomach. Certain garlic compounds seem to have an anti-angiogenesis effect, halting the growth of blood vessels that feed tumors.

In studies of populations in China, Italy, and the United States (including a study of 42,000 women in Iowa), those who regularly ate raw or cooked garlic had lower rates of stomach and colon cancers.

"The scientific evidence appears to be convincing," says Aaron Fleischauer, a Ph.D. candidate at the University of North Carolina in Chapel Hill, who completed a metanalysis of 20 different studies on the effects of garlic on cancer incidence, especially colon and stomach cancers.

Nature's Antibiotic

Garlic is such a strong antimicrobial that you could practically clean your kitchen with it.

"Garlic is a natural killer of cells, but it's selective, destroying tumor cells, virus-infected cells, and foreign invaders but not normal cells," says Earl Mindell, R.Ph., Ph.D., professor of nutrition at Pacific Western University in Los Angeles.

In some circles, garlic is referred to as Russian field dressing. During World War II, the Soviet army relied on garlic to treat the wounded when penicillin and sulfa drugs weren't available. In more recent years, doctors have found that garlic stops the growth of a fungus that causes meningitis, fights off a flu-causing virus (in tests with mice), and kills the fungi that cause athlete's foot and ringworm.

Garlic doesn't produce the side effects of typical antibiotics, like those used to treat yeast infections, diarrhea, and other stomach upsets. And bacteria don't seem to develop a resistance to garlic, unlike medicinal antibiotics.

That's not to say that you should give up antibiotics. Garlic's actions are slower and weaker than many of the potent prescriptions we have today, says Stephen Fulder, Ph.D., in his book, *The Garlic Book: Nature's Powerful Healer*. It is best used to treat chronic and less dangerous infections like sinusitis, sore throats, bronchitis, and skin infections rather than pneumonia or infected wounds.

Dr. Mindell recommends using garlic to treat ear infections also. "You don't have to take a lot of it for any of these conditions—just a clove a day for an anti-infective action."

Power Steps: For a sore throat, take a glass of water and keep adding salt while stirring until the salt no longer dissolves. Then add 10 drops of liquid aged garlic extract, which is the equivalent of one clove, and gargle two or three times a day, says Dr. Mindell. Repeat for 2 to 3 days, or until the symptoms are relieved. See your doctor if the condition persists.

For ear infections, warm a bottle of aged garlic extract by holding it in your hands or under a warm tap. Then put several drops into the affected ear. Plug your ear with a cotton ball for 20 minutes. Do this two or three times a day for 2 to 3 days. If your symptoms aren't relieved, seek medical attention.

Bad Breath, Good Memory?

It sneaks up on you inexorably. One day you can't remember someone's name, the next day you forget where you parked your car. You don't need a mnemonic, you need some garlic. Believe it or not, it works on rats.

STOP FAMILY BICKERING WITH GARLIC BREAD

Studies show that unpleasant odors generate aggression and hostility, and pleasant odors improve people's moods. Where does garlic fit in?

To find out, scent researcher Alan R. Hirsch, M.D., neurologic director at the Smell and Taste Treatment and Research Foundation in Chicago, manipulated the smells during what, in many families, has become the daily battleground: the dinner hour.

He fed 50 families spaghetti dinners, bringing garlic bread to the table 1 minute after they were seated, and observed their interactions. Those family members who like the aroma and taste of the fragrant bread fought less.

"Maybe garlic bread, like baked goods, induces a nostalgic feeling in people," suggests Dr. Hirsch. The effect was the same even if family members didn't eat the bread. So, for stressed-out working moms, serving garlic bread at dinner could have physical *and* emotional benefits.

Japanese researchers fed rats that were specially bred for fast memory loss a diet containing 2 percent aged garlic extract. Not only did the rats do better on mazes but their brains actually shrank less. This result surprised the researchers, since brain matter normally deteriorates with aging.

The researchers claim that their results raise the possibility that aged garlic extract prevents physiological aging and may be beneficial for age-related cognitive disorders in humans.

Help Yourself to Garlic

Here's how to reap a heap of garlicky benefits.

- Thread three or four peeled garlic cloves on pointed toothpicks and lightly brush with oil. Grill until soft, about 5 to 8 minutes per side.

- To add garlic flavor, lightly rub a salad bowl with a cut fresh clove before adding greens and dressing. Lightly rub toast or grilled bread slices with garlic before serving. A few swipes imparts a nice mellow flavor, minus the bite.

- Put a few cloves of peeled, crushed garlic in a bottle of vinegar and refrigerate it for 2 to 3 days before using.

- Make a series of ½-inch-deep slits in an eggplant or in roast beef, lamb, or pork. Insert large slivers of peeled garlic in each slit, then roast or grill as you normally would.

- Add garlic flavor without garlic chunks to sauces and sautéed dishes. Put cloves on toothpicks and cook them with the other ingredients. Then simply pluck out the skewered garlic before serving.

- Sauté garlic only until it turns a pale golden color. It may turn bitter if cooked longer.

- Bake one whole head of unpeeled garlic per person in a baking pan in a 350°F oven until soft, about 40 minutes. Cut in half widthwise and spread on toast, or mix into mashed potatoes, rice, sauces, or pasta. Although some of the beneficial effects may be lost by this cooking method, you can still enjoy the flavor and aroma of roasted garlic.

To get rid of garlic breath, chew on fresh parsley, mint, or citrus peel. Get garlic odor off your hands by rubbing them with lemon juice or vinegar.

Grains: Powerhouses of Nutrition

Power Maker #4: Eat at least three servings of whole grain foods a day in place of foods made with white flour. One serving equals one slice of whole grain bread, ½ to 1 cup of cold cereal (check labels for the amount that will provide 70 to 90 calories), ½ cup of hot cereal, or ½ cup of whole grain pasta.

Are you a white-bread-and-minute-rice kind of gal? You have plenty of company. Of the three to five servings of bread, pasta, and grains most of us eat each day, less than one serving is whole grain.

Most of these foods are made from refined grains. That's white flour, the nutritional equivalent of cardboard. Bad move. "The amount of whole grains a woman eats—or doesn't eat—can have a profound impact on her health," says Shari Lieberman, Ph.D., a clinical nutritionist in New York City. The evidence is overwhelming.

• In a study of 34,492 postmenopausal women, researchers at the University of Minnesota in Minneapolis found that those who ate three or more servings of whole grains a day were 30 percent less likely to die of heart disease than those who ate only three servings or fewer a week.

- Another study by the same researchers found that women who ate just one serving of whole grains a day had a 15 percent lower risk of dying *of all causes* than those who didn't eat any.

- Studies of women who regularly eat whole grains suggest that they have lower rates of breast cancer. Conversely, researchers in Italy found that women with breast cancer ate more refined grains in the form of bread, cereal, and cake than women without breast cancer.

- In a 6-year study of 65,173 nurses, researchers at the Harvard School of Public Health found that those who ate the fewest whole grain foods and the most refined grains were 2½ times more likely to develop diabetes.

The healthiest women in these studies weren't scarfing platefuls of grains with unpronounceable names. They simply ate two to three servings of whole grain foods a day, mostly breads, cereal, and popcorn.

Milled Grain Falls Short

What's the difference between whole grains and refined ones? Simple.

Mother Nature clothed all grains in a thin, flaky shell known as bran and tucked in a nugget of germ, the tiny bud from which a new plant will sprout. But when whole grains are milled into white flour, as most are, they're stripped of these good-for-you "garments."

It's a nutritional travesty. "Removing a grain's bran and germ removes more than 80 percent of the minerals, trace minerals, and many vitamins, essentially leaving you with starch, which has little nutritive value. So manufacturers add back a handful of nutrients and call it enriched. It's a joke," says Dr. Lieberman.

A Package Deal

"When Mother Nature created whole grains, she put together an excellent nutritional package," says David R. Lineback, Ph.D., director of the Joint Institute for Food Safety and Applied Nutrition at the University of Maryland in College Park. Unwrap the package, and you'll find several potent disease fighters.

Antioxidants. Found in fruits and vegetables, antioxidants wage war on free radicals, cell-damaging forces that can contribute to your risk of age-related illnesses, including heart disease and cancer.

Whole grains are one of the few food sources of vitamin E, the mother of all antioxidants. And most of it is concentrated in the germ. There's strong evidence that vitamin E protects women's hearts, possibly by preventing undesirable LDL cholesterol from sticking to artery walls. In a multicenter study of 21,809 postmenopausal women, those who got more than 10 IU of vitamin E a day from food, not supplements, had 62 percent less risk of heart disease.

Unfortunately, the average woman gets only about 11.3 IU of vitamin E a day—about one-third the Daily Value of 30 IU. Whole grains such as wheat germ and brown rice can help make up the shortfall.

Phytonutrients. These plant-derived compounds appear to act as disease repellents. Oats contain tocotrienols (a form of vitamin E), ferulic acid, and caffeic acid, all of which act as powerful antioxidants. Brown rice contains oryzanol, shown to reduce cholesterol production. And each particle of wheat germ is a tiny anti-cancer grenade, packed with vitamin E, folate (the naturally occurring form of folic acid), and selenium.

When grains get stripped, it's bye-bye phytonutrients. Refining wheat, for example, reduces its phytonutrient content two- to three-hundredfold.

Trace minerals. Whole grains are excellent sources of trace minerals that most of our diets lack: zinc, an immunity-boosting antioxidant; magnesium, which protects against heart disease and high blood pressure; and iron, which acts as the body's oxygen-transport system.

The Fiber Factor

The last goodie in the whole grain package is fiber, and lots of it. Stacks of studies suggest that this tough, stringy, indigestible part of plant foods helps protect against diseases that disproportionately strike women: heart disease, breast cancer, colon cancer, and, possibly, diabetes. It also promotes regularity and fights constipation.

Fiber comes in two forms, soluble and insoluble. Soluble fiber forms good-for-you goo in the intestines that engulfs cholesterol and whisks it out of your body. Barley and oats are especially rich in soluble fiber. Insoluble fiber prevents constipation and seems to protect against colon cancer; wheat bran is a stellar source. Ideally, you should consume both soluble and insoluble fibers, says Dr. Lieberman.

But soluble and insoluble fibers also work as a team. A multicenter

NEW GRAINS TO TRY

Sorting through the wide variety of whole grains at upscale supermarkets and health food stores may seem daunting. This primer can help.

Most whole grains have a nutlike flavor and a pleasant, chewy texture. A timesaving tip is to make big batches of whole grain dishes and refrigerate them in airtight containers for up to 4 days.

GRAIN	COOKING TIPS	SERVING SUGGESTIONS
Barley (whole or pearled)	Soak overnight in enough water to cover, then drain. Cook 1 part barley in 3 parts boiling water for 50 minutes, or until tender.	Add to strong-flavored, hearty dishes such as lamb stew and mushroom soup
Brown rice	Simmer 1 part rice in 2 parts water for 30–40 minutes	Use in place of white rice in rice pudding, homemade chicken-and-rice soup, and stuffed peppers or grape leaves
Buckwheat groats (kasha)	Simmer 1 part groats in 2 parts water for 15 minutes	Add ½ cup cooked kasha per pound of ground meat for meatballs or meat loaf
Bulgur	Pour 1½ cups boiling water over 1 cup bulgur and let stand for 30 minutes	Add cooked bulgur to your favorite coleslaw recipe
Kashi (combination of whole wheat, rye, buckwheat, and bulgur)	Simmer 1 part Kashi in 2 parts water for 25 minutes	Cover with your favorite vegetables sautéed with olive oil, garlic, and onions, or mix ½ cup cold cooked Kashi into low-fat frozen yogurt
Oats (rolled)	Simmer 1 part oats in 2 parts water for 10 minutes	Stir low-fat fruit yogurt into cooked oatmeal, then add raisins or fresh or frozen fruit; use uncooked oats in baked goods such as muffins, cookies, and breads
Quinoa	Rinse, then simmer 1 part quinoa in 2 parts water for 15–20 minutes	Mix cold quinoa with cucumbers, tomatoes, garlic, mint, and parsley; add olive oil and lemon juice

study of 68,782 nurses co-led by Harvard Medical School found that women who ate an average of 23 grams of fiber a day from whole grains had 23 percent lower risk of heart attack compared with women who averaged only 11.5 grams a day.

POWER

FRUIT AND NUT OATMEAL

Imagine a hot, hearty breakfast in 5 minutes—and we're not talking just plain old oatmeal. Mix a batch of this dry cereal base and keep it on hand for near-instant morning meals. We started with basic oats but gave them a power boost of fruit, wheat germ, and other superfoods. The result? A cereal packed with fiber, protein, calcium, B vitamins, vitamin E, and even omega-3's.

2	cups rolled oats
1½	cups nonfat dry milk
1	cup oat bran
1	cup chopped mixed dried fruit
½	cup chopped walnuts
½	cup toasted wheat germ

In a large bowl, mix the oats, milk, oat bran, fruit, nuts, and wheat germ.

To make the hot cereal: add ½ cup of the dry mix to 1 cup of boiling water in a saucepan. Simmer, stirring occasionally, for 5 minutes. Let stand a few minutes to thicken. If desired, sweeten to taste or serve with milk, fruit-flavored yogurt, or fresh fruit.

Makes 6 cups

Per ½ cup: 186 calories, 9 g protein, 31 g carbohydrates, 5 g fat, 2 mg cholesterol, 4 g dietary fiber, 67 mg sodium

Note: Store the dry mix in a covered container in the refrigerator for up to 1 month.

Further, low-fiber, highly processed carbohydrate foods cause blood sugar and insulin levels to alternately spike and plummet, which may increase the risk of diabetes, heart disease, and weight gain. Whole grains and other high-fiber foods are digested slowly, so blood sugar rises gradually and insulin levels stay steady, all of which may help to control diabetes or in some cases prevent it.

What to Look For

Sneaking more whole grains into your diet is easier than you may think. Here's how to zero in on whole grain products and prepare them in speedy, tasty ways.

Check your loaf's label. If the first ingredient is whole wheat flour (or another whole grain), buy it. If the first word is "enriched," "unbleached," or "unbromated," leave it on the shelf; it's made with refined flour.

Don't be fooled by dark breads. That healthy-looking hue may be food coloring. Be wary of multigrain breads, too: They're frequently made with refined flour.

Switch to whole grain cereals. The first ingredient should be described as whole or whole grain, as in whole grain oats, wheat, rice, corn, or barley. Among the easiest to find are Kellogg's All-Bran, General Mills' Fiber One and Multi-Bran Chex, Post Raisin Bran and Shredded Wheat 'N Bran, and Kashi Seven Whole Grains and Sesame.

For variety, mix ½ to 1 cup of a fiber-rich cereal (approximately 70 to 90 calories' worth) with ½ cup of low-fat fruit yogurt. The yogurt is a delicious alternative to fat-free milk, and it will soften up those spiky nuggets.

Select whole grain pastas. Your local supermarket is bound to stock at least whole wheat pasta. Look for more exotic varieties, made with amaranth, quinoa, or buckwheat (including Japanese buckwheat noodles more commonly known as soba noodles), at upscale grocery or health food stores. You'll enjoy their denser texture and sweet, almost nutty flavor. Here are three serving suggestions.

- Mix with steamed vegetables and 1 to 2 tablespoons of olive oil. Top with a small amount of grated cheese.

- Whip up a no-cook sauce of chopped fresh tomatoes, basil, jarred roasted red peppers, and a little reduced-fat mozzarella cheese.

- Toss soba noodles with sautéed onions, mushrooms, and peppers. Season with sesame oil, soy sauce, and cilantro.

Try these other painless ways to get whole grains into your diet, suggests Marlene Bumgarner, author of *The New Book of Whole Grains.*

- Snack on popcorn. (How hard is that?) If you buy the microwaveable kind, opt for low-fat varieties.

- Make oat pancakes. Mix 1 cup of oat flour, 1 teaspoon of baking powder, ½ teaspoon of baking soda, ½ teaspoon of salt, one egg, ½ cup of plain yogurt, and ½ cup of fat-free milk.

- When making baked goods, replace all or most of the white flour with whole grain flour such as oat or spelt. (Spelt is a grain related to wheat; look for it in health food stores.) Oat flour makes delicious muffins and cookies, while spelt flour's lighter texture is well-suited for breads, cakes, and biscuits.

- Look for cornmeal that is labeled "water-ground" or "stone-ground." It has more of the bran and germ than regular. Use it for cornbread and muffins.

- Stir wheat germ into low-fat yogurt. Or sprinkle it over salads.

- Buy tortillas made with whole wheat or corn flour.

- Stuff peppers with a mixture of cooked bulgur, beans, mushrooms, celery, and basil.

- For a hearty, healthier meat loaf, mix 1 cup of cooked whole millet into each pound of ground meat.

- For a tasty cold salad, toss cooked quinoa with chopped parsley, cucumbers, tomatoes, and minced garlic. Dress with olive oil and lemon juice.

- Combine cold cooked brown rice with black or green olives, celery, tomatoes, and your favorite creamy salad dressing.

MASKED DISASTER

Granola

"Granola" has such a wholesome ring. Too bad so few brands are whole grain, and that most are a veritable bomb of calories and sugar. Just ½ cup of low-fat granola packs 213 calories, 13.4 grams of sugar (almost 3 teaspoons), and a mere 3 grams of fiber.

Stick to unsweetened whole grain cereals, such as Kellogg's All-Bran. A ½-cup serving contains 79 calories, 6 grams of sugar, and 10 grams of fiber.

Greens: Meganutrients in Every Bite

Power Maker #5: Eat at least one ½-cup serving of cooked greens (such as kale, bok choy, or collards) or one 1- to 2-cup serving of raw greens (like radicchio or arugula) a day, preferably more. Iceberg lettuce doesn't count.

Greens look so gorgeous in the produce aisle. That handsomely beruffled kale nestled against the broad, crinkled leaves of Swiss chard. Those bunches of slender, emerald-hued mustard and turnip greens. And the spinach! Velvety smooth, yet temptingly springy, the kind poor Popeye never got to experience.

Yet many of us breeze right by all this beauty and reach for anemic-looking iceberg lettuce. If you're like many women, you're confounded by anything less familiar than spinach or romaine. Most likely, you don't know how to cook them, assuming that collards are relegated to the South and bok choy to Asian cooking.

But if you don't know greens, it's time to make their acquaintance, because they're a nutritional bonanza. From arugula to watercress, a serving of greens can pack up to a dozen nutrients, including folate, calcium, and iron—a power trio of nutrients vital to a woman's health—as well as vitamins A and C, depending on the type of greens. In general, the darker the color, the more nutrient-rich they are. Greens are also excellent sources of phytonutrients, plant compounds shown to decrease the risk for developing cancer and other chronic diseases. Here's why you should make these green giants a part of your Power-Eating Plan, and how to prepare them in a snap.

Give Your Heart the Green Light

Greens do more than please your palate. They also help protect your heart.

Lynn Bailey, Ph.D., loves her greens. "My personal favorite is raw spinach salad with mushrooms and tomatoes," says Dr. Bailey, professor in the department of food science and human nutrition at the University of Florida in Gainesville. "And as a Southerner, I grew up on turnip greens."

But Dr. Bailey is also a nutritionist, which makes her appreciate greens even more.

Greens are significant sources of folate. This B vitamin (the naturally occurring form of folic acid) lowers blood levels of homocysteine, an amino acid research links with an increased risk of heart disease. Greens also contain vitamin B_6, which works in tandem with folate and vitamin B_{12} to reduce blood levels of homocysteine.

In itself, homocysteine (formed when your body breaks down other amino acids in your blood) is perfectly innocent. But evidence is mounting that abnormally high levels of homocysteine cause the tissues lining your arteries to thicken and scar. Cholesterol lodges in these damaged arteries, which can lead to clogs and blood clots.

Folate converts homocysteine into a harmless substance called methionine, preventing a toxic buildup of homocysteine in the blood. In a Harvard study of 80,000 nurses, those with the highest intake of folate (about 696 micrograms a day) had a 31 percent lower risk of heart disease than those with the lowest intake.

As a source of folate, cooked spinach reigns supreme: One cup packs 262 micrograms of folate, two-thirds of the Daily Value of 400 micrograms. Other greens that are good sources of folate include turnip greens, which deliver 170 micrograms per cup, and mustard greens, which contain about 103 micrograms per cup.

A FLAVOR GUIDE TO UNFAMILIAR GREENS

New and unusual greens are a gold mine of nutrition, but they cost more than run-of-the-mill romaine lettuce and spinach. You may want some idea of what broccoli raab or arugula or kale tastes like before you plunk down your hard-earned food dollars. This handy flavor guide will give you an idea of which greens will most appeal to your palate.

- **Arugula: Powerfully peppery**
- **Beet greens: Mild, somewhat earthy flavor**
- **Bok choy: Slightly more pronounced than regular green cabbage**
- **Broccoli raab: Pungent, somewhat bitter when plain; milder when sautéed Mediterranean-style in garlic and olive oil**
- **Collard greens: A cross between spinach and watercress**
- **Dandelion greens: Young leaves are pleasantly bitter; older leaves are very bitter**
- **Kale: Mild, cabbagelike**
- **Mustard greens: Tangy, mustardlike flavor**
- **Radicchio: Sweet with bitter undertones**
- **Spinach: Musky yet mild**
- **Swiss chard: Sweet, earthy, with a slightly bitter undertone**
- **Turnip greens: Young greens are slightly sweet; older greens are strongly flavored**
- **Watercress: Spicy, peppery taste**

Battle Armor against Cancer

"I come from a Mediterranean family and actually grew up eating dandelion and other wild greens. Our mother picked them in the early spring and served them with lemon and a little olive oil," says Maria G. Boosalis, Ph.D., associate professor of clinical nutrition at the University of Kentucky in Lexington.

Smart woman—studies of large groups of people have found that those who eat the most leafy greens develop less cancer than those who eat the least.

Greens boast an arsenal of phytonutrients—substances in plant foods found to lower the risk of cancer and other chronic diseases, says John Pinto, Ph.D., director of the nutrition research laboratory at Memorial Sloan-Kettering Cancer Center and associate professor of biochemistry at Weill Medical College of Cornell University, both in New York City. These include:

- Dithiolthiones and isothiocyanates, found to stimulate the body's cancer-battling phase-I and phase-II enzymes. These enzymes help detoxify a number of cancer-causing chemicals, including those found in cleaners and pesticides, environmental toxins such as PCBs (polychlorinated biphenyls), and heterocyclic amines, which are formed when meats are cooked at high temperatures during frying, broiling, or grilling.

- Indole-3-carbinol. This phytonutrient chemically alters estradiol—the form of estrogen believed to fuel the development of breast cancer—into a less reactive form, thereby helping to protect against breast cancer in premenopausal women.

- Lutein, alpha-carotene, and beta-carotene, members of the carotenoid family of phytonutrients. As antioxidants, carotenoids help neutralize the destructive force of free radicals, harmful molecules generated by both our own bodies and the environment that damage cellular DNA and lead to an increased risk of developing cancer.

The findings of the test tube and animal studies seem to extend to people, too. In one study, Harvard researchers who tracked the eating habits of 47,909 middle-aged men for 10 years found that those who ate more than five servings a week of cruciferous vegetables—broccoli, cabbage, collards, watercress, kale, and mustard and turnip greens—were half as likely to develop bladder cancer as those who ate one serving a week or less, no matter how many other vegetables they ate. Broccoli and cabbage were the most protective. Experts say the results also apply to women.

In another study, researchers in Chile compared 61 men with lung cancer with 61 men of similar age and smoking habits who were cancer-free. The one difference? The men with cancer ate significantly fewer carotenoid-rich foods, especially Swiss chard, spinach, and cabbage, than those without the disease. Again, the results apply to women as well.

POWER
G R E E N S

BOK CHOY WITH OYSTER SAUCE

Like other cabbage-family vegetables, bok choy is full of disease-preventing antioxidants. And it's a good source of folate, which guards
against heart disease and cancer. If you're at a loss to know how to cook
it, try this Asian recipe, which lightly glazes the slender white stalks and
green leaves with a savory soy mixture.

1	large head bok choy
2	cloves garlic, finely chopped
1	cup water
2	tablespoons oyster sauce
1	tablespoon soy sauce
2	teaspoons cornstarch

Cut the bok choy into quarters lengthwise. Cut each quarter in half cross-
wise. Place in a large skillet and add the garlic and ½ cup of the water.
Bring to a simmer over medium heat. Cover and cook for 3 minutes. Drain
and return to the skillet.

In a small bowl, whisk together the oyster sauce, soy sauce, cornstarch, and the remaining ½ cup water. Pour over the bok choy. Cover and
simmer for 5 minutes, or until the bok choy is tender and glazed.

Makes 4 servings

Per serving: 45 calories, 4 g protein, 8 g carbohydrates, 0.4 g fat, 0 mg cholesterol,
4 g dietary fiber, 807 mg sodium

Sight-Saving Greens

For reading, driving, or gazing at our loved ones, our eyesight is precious. But it's also vulnerable, especially as we grow older.

That's where greens come in.

Two of the same phytonutrients in greens that help battle cancer, lutein and zeaxanthin, may also help save your sight. Research shows that they may help prevent cataracts—which occur when the eyes' normally clear lenses become clouded—and age-related macular degeneration, the leading cause of irreversible vision loss in women age 65 and older.

In a 12-year study of almost 78,000 nurses, researchers found that those who ate the most lutein and zeaxanthin were 22 percent less likely to develop cataracts than those who ate the least. Spinach appeared to be the most protective.

In a study of 876 people with and without macular degeneration, those who ate the most carotenoid-rich foods, including spinach, collards, carrots, and broccoli, reduced their risk of the disease by 43 percent

FOOLPROOF TIPS FOR COOKING GREENS

On impulse, you throw a bunch of kale or beet greens or collard greens into your shopping cart. You bring the bunch home. You think, "How do I cook this stuff?" Not to worry. This how-to guide makes cooking greens a no-brainer. (Chopping helps speed cooking time.)

Don't be intimidated by greens bundled in humongous bunches. Greens cook down considerably—to one-quarter or less of their original volume. For example, a pound of raw kale will yield about 2½ cups cooked.

WILTING. Wash the greens and leave them wet. Set them in a colander. For every 3 cups of chopped greens, add 1 teaspoon olive oil to a large nonstick skillet. When the oil is hot, add some chopped garlic, to taste, and sauté until golden brown. Add the wet greens. Cook, covered, over medium-high heat until the greens are wilted and bright green.

BRAISING. Cooking greens a bit longer in a small amount of water or stock after they are wilted softens tougher greens and makes a delicious sauce that Southerners call pot liquor. (Sop it up with a hunk of crusty bread.) To braise, follow the directions above for wilting the greens. After they have wilted, add liquid until the greens are partially submerged. Cover and cook on medium-low heat for 5 minutes, or until the greens are soft.

compared with those who ate the least. What's more, those who ate lutein- and zeaxanthin-rich spinach or collard greens two to four times a week were almost half as likely to develop the disease as those who ate them less than once a month. Kale, mustard, and turnip greens also contain substantial amounts of these two carotenoids.

Lutein and zeaxanthin concentrate in the retina, the part of the eye that "photographs" visual images, similar to the way the film in a camera works. These two phytonutrients are the major components of the central yellow pigment in the retina. It's thought that they serve as filters by absorbing blue light, which is particularly damaging to the photoreceptors in the retina. Studies have shown that a more dense pigment may protect against this damage. They may also act as antioxidants, and so stem free-radical damage to the eyes.

BLANCHING. This method, in which greens are "flash boiled," also softens tough greens. Although more "assertive" greens, like collards, will lose some of their strong taste and become more tender if they're cooked in large amounts of water, some of their nutrients will leach into the water. To minimize this loss, follow this method for "shallow blanching." In a large skillet, bring 2 cups of water to a boil. Add greens. Cover with a tight-fitting lid and boil from 3 to 10 minutes, or until tender. The time depends on the type of greens; the more tender ones, like spinach, will take less time. Drain and enjoy. You can also save the cooking water and use it to add nutrients and flavor to your soups and stews.

MICROWAVING. Toss greens into a glass dish. Splash with water or stock. Cover with vented plastic wrap. Microwave on high until just tender, about 2 minutes for 2 cups of greens. Let stand for 2 minutes, then drain. Enjoy them alone or add them to casseroles, stir-fries, or pasta or rice dishes.

STEAMING. You can steam greens, but some cooks advise against it. Steaming greens, especially strongly flavored ones, can turn them an unpalatable shade of grayish green and turn strong greens bitter. For similar reasons, do not cook greens in aluminum cookware.

CAN IT, LADY

Don't have time to wash and chop greens? Grab your can opener. Canned kale and turnip or mustard greens contain about as much folate, calcium, and iron as fresh greens. (You'll lose out on some vitamin C, however, which is partially destroyed during the heat processing.)

Iron without Meat, Calcium without a Milk Mustache

Getting enough calcium and iron in your diet? Chances are, you may not be, says Dr. Boosalis. The price you pay is greater odds of developing the bone-thinning disease osteoporosis or iron-deficiency anemia, a blood condition that can leave you physically weak and fatigued, pale, and with lower endurance and shortened attention span.

You can help reduce those risks by heaping your plate with greens.

Some greens are good sources of iron, which you use to transport oxygen from your lungs to the rest of your body. One-half cup of cooked spinach contains 3.2 milligrams of iron, a good chunk of the daily 15 to 18 milligrams recommended for premenopausal women, while the same amount of cooked Swiss chard contains 2 milligrams of iron.

Your body doesn't absorb the iron found in plants, called nonheme iron, as efficiently as the heme iron found in meats, unless it's teamed at the same meal with vitamin C. Greens are two-for-one veggies: Along with their substantial amounts of iron, some are also rich sources of vitamin C, which significantly improves your absorption of the iron in greens. While most greens contain ample amounts of C, kale, bok choy, and mustard greens pack the most.

Certain greens also supply some calcium. For example, 1 cup of cooked shredded bok choy contains 158 milligrams of calcium—about half of the 300 milligrams in a glass of fat-free milk. The same amount of cooked chopped kale contains 93 milligrams—not enough on which to rely heavily, but it certainly contributes to your total. "What's more, the calcium in some greens, such as broccoli, kale, bok choy, and Chinese cabbage is more readily absorbed by the body than that in milk," says

Connie M. Weaver, Ph.D., professor and director of the department of foods and nutrition at Purdue University in West Lafayette, Indiana.

Just don't depend on spinach, Swiss chard, collards, and beet greens to help meet your calcium quota. All contain oxalates—compounds that block calcium absorption from these greens and other sources, making them poor calcium choices.

Going Green

Once you learn the basics of greenery, you'll find dozens of unique and delicious ways to enjoy them. These quick fixes will get you started.

- In 1 teaspoon of peanut oil, stir-fry two sliced leeks and two julienned carrots for 1 to 2 minutes. Add 4 cups of chopped mustard greens, 4 cups of chopped kale, and 3 tablespoons of chicken broth. Cover and cook for 3 minutes. Serve over rice.

- Add tomato sauce to canned kale or other canned greens. (Use ½ cup of sauce to each can of greens.) Heat and enjoy.

- Sauté one large chopped red onion in 1 tablespoon of olive oil. Stir in ¼ cup of tomato paste and 1 teaspoon of honey. Cook 1 minute, then add 4 cups of cooked or canned chickpeas and 1 cup of water. Bring to a simmer. Add 1½ pounds of trimmed, shredded Swiss chard. Cover and simmer for 20 minutes, or until the greens are wilted and tender. Serve hot as a main course or cold as a salad.

- In a large bowl, combine 3 cups each of watercress leaves and arugula leaves, torn into small pieces, or you can use 6 cups of spinach leaves. Add 3 cups of sliced strawberries. Dress with ¼ cup of orange juice, 2 teaspoons each of olive oil and poppy seeds, and ½ teaspoon of grated orange rind. Or replace the watercress and arugula with 6 cups of torn spinach leaves. To add crunch, toss in ⅓ cup of sliced toasted almonds.

- Slice the stalks and leaves of one head of bok choy, keeping the stalks and leaves separate. Stir-fry the stalks with two sliced red peppers in 2 teaspoons of olive or canola oil with 1 tablespoon of minced fresh ginger and three minced garlic cloves. Add the leaves and 3 table-spoons of water. Cover and cook until the leaves are wilted and the stalks are crisp-tender. If you like, stir in ½ teaspoon of sesame oil and sprinkle with 1 tablespoon of toasted sesame seeds.

Fruit: Pick a Peck
of Disease Protection

Power Maker #6: Eat at least two, and preferably three, servings of fruit a day, including nutrient-dense tropical fruits such as kiwifruit, mango, and papaya.

The way some women pass up fruit, it might as well be chopped liver. Two-thirds of us don't eat the recommended two servings a day. We're twice as likely to start the day with coffee as with OJ. And for every 10 snacks, we rarely choose one packaged in a peel.

So help yourself to a piece of fruit, already. Each time you slice a banana over your cereal, stir strawberries into your yogurt, or munch a bunch of red grapes, you help protect yourself against a slew of illnesses, from heart disease and stroke to cancer and infections.

The following are among fruit's disease-fighting substances.

- Phytonutrients. These are the plant pigments that give fruits and vegetables their Crayola-bright hues. "Every apple, blueberry, and grape contains a chemical stew that can block or retard carcinogens, lower cholesterol, reduce fatty deposits in your arteries, and fight the effects of aging," says Stephanie Beling, M.D., a physician at Canyon Ranch, a health and fitness resort in Lenox, Massachusetts, and author of *Power Foods*.

- Antioxidants, especially vitamin C and beta-carotene. These compounds act as a kind of body-wide security system, protecting your cells from disease-promoting molecules called free radicals.
- Fiber. It has been found to lower cholesterol levels, is linked to a reduced risk of colon and rectal cancers, and may possibly reduce the risk of breast cancer.
- Potassium. This mineral supports heart health and may also protect against stroke.

The best part is that all fruits offer at least some of these benefits. Here are details on some of the most common ones. Let the fruitfest begin!

Apples: Skin-Deep Benefits

Crunch into a McIntosh or a Red Delicious, and you do your heart good, thanks to quercetin, a phytonutrient in apple skin that's been linked to healthy heart function. In a study of 34,492 postmenopausal women, those who consumed the most quercetin—equivalent to the amount in half an apple a day—were afforded the most heart disease protection. Other studies have shown similar results. Remember that much of an apple's quercetin content is found in the skin.

Apples are also rich in the soluble fiber pectin. Like a sponge soaks up spills, pectin mops up excess cholesterol in your intestine before it can enter your blood and gunk up your arteries. Then the pectin is excreted, taking fat and cholesterol along with it.

Bananas: A Bunch of Protection

A monkey's favorite fruit is one of the top sources of potassium, a mineral linked to lower blood pressure and a reduced risk of stroke.

Researchers at the Harvard School of Public Health followed 43,738 men for 8 years and found that those who ate the most potassium from food lowered their risk of stroke by 38 percent. A banana a day plus other fruits and vegetables will get you well on your way toward a hefty amount of potassium.

Potassium's ability to lower blood pressure may play a small role in stroke protection, says Alberto Ascherio, M.D., Dr.P.H., assistant pro-

FIBER UP WITH FRUIT

Trying to get the recommended 20 to 35 grams of fiber a day? Reach for fruit. Here is the fiber content of some popular varieties.

FRUIT	SERVING SIZE	FIBER (g)
Red raspberries	1 cup	11.0
Guava	1 cup	9.0
Papaya	1 med	5.5
Blueberries	1 cup	3.9
Apple	1 med	3.7
Strawberries (whole)	1 cup	3.3
Orange	1 med	3.1
Mango	1 cup	3.0
Banana	1 med	2.8
Kiwifruit	1 med	2.6
Red grapes	1 cup	1.5
Pink grapefruit	½ med	1.4

fessor of nutrition and epidemiology at the Harvard School of Public Health. In addition, he says, potassium might also prevent undesirable LDL cholesterol from sticking to artery walls and, ultimately, blocking bloodflow to the brain.

Blueberries: High-Octane Power

These tangy-sweet berries kick free-radical butt. In fact, in a study of more than three dozen fruits and vegetables, blueberries emerged as the number one source of antioxidants.

"A half-cup of blueberries provides as much antioxidant power as five servings of other fresh fruits and vegetables," says study leader Ronald Prior, Ph.D., chief of the phytochemical lab at the Jean Mayer USDA Human Nutrition Research Center on Aging at Tufts University in Boston.

Besides helping our cells withstand free-radical damage, blueberries may keep us mentally sharp as we age or even reverse age-related memory decline. And they may also stave off the bane of many a woman's existence, urinary tract infections (UTIs).

"Like cranberries, blueberries contain condensed tannins, compounds found to prevent the bacteria responsible for UTIs from sticking to the walls of the bladder," says Amy Howell, Ph.D., a research scientist at the Rutgers University Blueberry and Cranberry Research and Extension Center in Chatsworth, New Jersey. "Our research suggests that it would take about a cup of blueberries a day to prevent recurrent UTIs. You could even get your quota in blueberry pie, as long as you are getting your full cup's worth," she says.

Citrus Fruits: A Juicy Trio of Benefits

Want cancer protection, a healthier baby, or a strong heartbeat? Start peeling. Besides being excellent sources of the antioxidant superstar vitamin C, oranges and grapefruit provide hesperetin and naringin, phytonutrients shown to halt the growth of some kinds of breast cancer cells.

After injecting rats with breast cancer cells, researchers at the University of Western Ontario supplemented their diets with orange juice, grapefruit juice, naringin, naringenin (a form of naringin), or water. After 4 months, the OJ-guzzling mice had developed 50 percent fewer tumors than the other groups; those that got naringin, 37 percent fewer.

Orange juice and oranges are also sources of the B vitamin folate (the naturally occurring form of folic acid), which helps prevent brain and spinal cord birth defects. Folate also guards our hearts by breaking down an artery-damaging amino acid before it can do harm. Grapefruit is also packed with cholesterol-lowering pectin.

Waistline

Amount the National Cancer Institute spends each year to promote eating fresh fruits and vegetables: $1 million.

Amount a major candy manufacturer spent in 1 year on advertising just one type of candy: $64 million.

Women of all ages should get at least 400 micrograms of folate a day. Oranges can help you meet that quota, as can other citrus fruits, dark leafy greens such as spinach, and enriched breads and cereals. But if you're thinking of getting pregnant, or are at high risk of heart disease, ask your doctor about supplements.

Grapes: Purple Globes of Power

Wine drinkers rejoiced when research suggested that their favorite Chianti could help protect their hearts. There's more good news on the grape. Regular munching of red or purple grapes is being studied for its promising potential to stave off breast and other cancers.

Red and purple grapes (but not green grapes) contain resveratrol, a phytonutrient found in their skins and seeds. Test tube studies have shown that resveratrol stops normal cells from turning cancerous, prevents precancerous cells from turning malignant, and prevents tumors from growing bigger.

Resveratrol also holds promise in fighting breast cancer, says Ginette Serrero, Ph.D., associate professor in the department of pharmaceutical sciences at the University of Maryland School of Pharmacy in Baltimore. It may be that, like the phytoestrogens found in soy foods, resveratrol helps reduce the overall amount of estrogen in a woman's body. "And women with high blood estrogen levels in breast tissues appear to have a higher incidence of hormone-fueled cancers such as breast cancer," she says.

Strawberries and Red Raspberries: Crimson Cancer Fighters

One cup of plump, ruby red strawberries contains more vitamin C than an orange, and an equal amount of red raspberries contains more folate. But strawberries and red raspberries also contain ellagic acid, yet another phytonutrient that may put cancer cells out of commission.

Ellagic acid might fight cancer by causing apoptosis, or programmed cell death, says Daniel W. Nixon, M.D., president of the American Health Foundation in New York City. Unlike normal cells, which are "programmed" to die at a certain point, cancer cells just keep multiplying and may eventually form tumors, he explains. In laboratory studies, ellagic acid appears to quash this out-of-control growth.

POWER

FRUIT TOPPING

RASPBERRY-MELON MÉLANGE

Get your day going in the best way possible, with a colorful, antioxidant-rich compote. The fruit, almonds, and even the ginger help keep cholesterol under control. Serve with low-fat granola and vanilla yogurt or use to top pancakes and waffles in place of butter and syrup. This is also a great way to add low-fat pizzazz to desserts like angel food cake, baked apples, and poached pears.

$\frac{1}{4}$ cup honey or sugar

2   tablespoons orange juice

2   tablespoons finely chopped crystallized ginger

$\frac{1}{4}$ teaspoon ground ginger

1   cantaloupe, cut into $\frac{1}{2}$" cubes

1   cup raspberries

$\frac{1}{4}$ cup toasted sliced almonds

In a large bowl, combine the honey or sugar, orange juice, crystallized ginger, and ground ginger. Add the cantaloupe and toss to coat. Refrigerate for at least 2 hours, stirring occasionally. Just before serving, gently stir in the raspberries and almonds.

Makes 3 cups

Per $\frac{1}{2}$ cup: 120 calories, 2 g protein, 23 g carbohydrates, 3.5 g fat, 0 mg cholesterol, 2 g dietary fiber, 10 mg sodium

Tomatoes: Sauce Reigns Supreme

Yes, tomatoes qualify as fruit—and as powerful cancer fighters, thanks to lycopene, a phytonutrient and potent antioxidant.

In a review of 72 studies by researchers at the Harvard School of Public Health, 57 linked high tomato consumption or high blood levels

TRY THE TROPICS

Fruits like mango, kiwifruit, and papaya are among the most nutrient-dense foods that can pass our lips.

Researchers at Rutgers University in New Brunswick, New Jersey, analyzed 33 common fruits to determine which were the best sources of critical nutrients such as vitamin C, vitamin E, folate, and fiber. The hands-down winner? The little-known guava. A 1-cup serving of the fruit contains the vitamin C of almost four oranges and ample amounts of fiber and potassium. The runner-up: kiwifruit, high in C and a low-fat source of vitamin E. Third place went to vitamin C–rich lychee, a Chinese fruit now grown in California, Florida, and Hawaii. Papaya and cantaloupe (the only nontropical fruit in the bunch) came in fourth and fifth. Both are brimming with C and are good sources of the B vitamin folate.

Here's how to use these island all-stars.

GUAVA. The pink flesh of these pink or yellow lemon-size fruits tastes like a cross between strawberry and pineapple. Add slices to salads. For a tropical slush, puree one or two guavas, mix with fat-free plain yogurt, and freeze until firm; run through a food processor until slushy.

KIWIFRUIT. This fuzzy, egg-shaped fruit tastes much like guava but is more commonly available. Peel, dice, and add to chicken salad, coleslaw, and other salads. Or just cut them in half and spoon out the succulent flesh.

PAPAYA. It looks like a yellow or orange avocado. The inside is orange-pink with edible black seeds. Add the flesh to salads and salsas; use the seeds to give spicy crunch to a salad.

of lycopene with reduced risk of lung and stomach cancers. Lycopene also seems to thwart the growth of breast cancer cells. In an Israeli study, animals injected with lycopene had fewer breast cancer tumors than those given either beta-carotene or nothing at all.

Tomato sauce seems to provide more protection than tomatoes alone, says Dr. Ascherio, possibly because it's a concentrated source of lycopene. In a landmark study of 48,000 men, those who consumed 2 cups of tomato sauce a week had a 34 percent lower risk of prostate cancer. That amount should help protect women from other forms of cancer, he adds.

10 Fast Fruit Fixes

By all means, drop berries on your cereal or crunch an apple on the run. But don't stop there. These simple but unique serving ideas can help you sneak fruit into your diet deliciously.

- Add diced red apples (with skins) to your favorite coleslaw recipe.

- For a snack or dessert, simmer a banana and some raisins in ¼ cup of apple juice, ¼ teaspoon of vanilla, and a dash of cinnamon for 10 minutes. Remove the banana and blend a few tablespoons of fat-free vanilla yogurt into the juice. Spoon over the banana.

- Top desserts with a quick fruit sauce: Whir 2 cups of fresh blueberries, strawberries, or raspberries; ½ cup of sugar; and ⅓ cup of water in a blender until thick. Serve over low-fat frozen yogurt, angel food cake, or sliced fruit.

- For a smooth and fruity shake, puree in a blender 2 cups of frozen blueberries; 1 cup of frozen mixed fruit; your choice of 1 cup of fat-free, rice, or soy milk; 1 tablespoon of sugar; and 2 teaspoons of vanilla extract.

- Blend ¾ cup of orange juice with ¼ cup each of vinegar, olive oil, and water. Pour over a mixed green salad studded with chunks of pink grapefruit and orange.

- Add quartered red grapes to tuna or chicken salad.

- Marinate five or six sliced tomatoes in 3 tablespoons of olive oil and 1 tablespoon of balsamic vinegar for 1 hour. Arrange on a pizza shell, sprinkle with minced garlic and crumbled goat cheese, then bake.

- Add bananas, strawberries, or blueberries to pancake or waffle batter. Serve topped with more fruit.

- Cook whole wheat couscous or bulgur in diluted orange juice instead of water. To turn it into a salad, add diced papayas, mangoes, kiwifruit, strawberries, orange segments, and a dash of honey. Chill. If desired, stir in a little apple juice and chopped mint.

- Add chopped oranges, papayas, mangoes, or pineapple to store-bought salsa.

Fatty Acids: The Multitasking Ingredient in Fish

Power Maker #7: To eat more omega-3 fatty acids and balance omega-6 fatty acids, replace corn, sunflower, and safflower oils and margarine with olive, canola, and flaxseed oils. And while you're at it, eat tuna three times a week for lunch and salmon once a week for dinner.

What if we told you that there was something you could do just two or three times a week to reduce your risk of heart disease, cut your chances of dying from a heart attack in half, improve your mood, treat arthritis, possibly protect against osteoporosis as well as breast and other cancers, and even reduce menstrual cramps and PMS?

The best part is that it doesn't involve sweating.

Two words, ladies: Eat fish. But not just any fish. Go for fattier, cold-water fish like tuna, salmon, and mackerel.

From humble tuna-noodle casserole to grilled salmon, cold-water-fish dishes are just dripping with a number of polyunsaturated fats collectively known as omega-3 fatty acids. Omega-3's enable fish to function in the chilly waters of the North Atlantic, Pacific Northwest, or Arctic oceans. If you balance your omega-3's with another type of fatty acid—omega-6's (found in vegetable oils like corn, safflower, and sunflower, and in meat), you will find yourself sharing characteristics of some of the healthiest people in the world, like the Inuit Eskimos and the Greeks on the island of Crete.

Cold Fish, Healthy Hearts

Eskimos thrive on one of the highest-fat diets in the world—heavy on roasted whale blubber and light on fresh fruit, vegetables, and fiber. Plus, they smoke. You'd expect them to keel over from heart attacks even as you read this. Yet a key discovery was made in the 1970s: When researchers looked at 10 years of health records for a hospital in Greenland that served 2,000 people, they found nary a death caused by a heart attack.

The reason is that their diets are high in omega-3's. These Eskimos get 5 to 7 grams per day of eicosapentaenoic acid (EPA) and docosahexaenoic acid (DHA), two critical types of omega-3's, in their diets.

Omega-6's, in contrast, cancel out many of the good things that omega-3's do.

"Cancer, heart disease, asthma, and autoimmune disorders occur less and less frequently in populations who eat fewer omega-6's and more omega-3's," says Artemis P. Simopoulos, M.D., president of the Center for Genetics, Nutrition, and Health in Washington, D.C., and author of *The Omega Diet*.

These are some of the benefits of omega-3's.

Lower blood pressure. Reducing saturated fat in your diet also does this, but if you reduce the saturated fat in your diet to about 25 percent

Waistline

If you followed the National Institutes of Health recommendation to eat about 13½ ounces of fish a week, you would be reeling in nearly 44 pounds of fish a year. Currently, Americans eat about 14 pounds a year. You've got a long way to go, baby.

and aim for up to three fish meals per week, you'll lower your blood pressure even more than by just cutting down on total fat.

Smoother cell membranes. They are less likely to clump and cause blood clots that can lead to heart attacks. While omega-3's may reduce the risk of blood clots, omega-6's may encourage them.

Lower incidence of irregular heartbeats (arrhythmias). These are a major cause of death from coronary heart disease.

How much fish should you eat for better cardiovascular health? It depends. If your blood pressure tends to run high, you need to eat cold-water fish about five times a week. But just one palm-size piece of salmon weekly can cut your risk of cardiac arrest from arrhythmias in half. And a healthy diet of fish two or three times a week can make a difference in blood clots.

Anti-Cancer Potential for Fish Lovers

Contemporary medical wisdom links high levels of dietary fat to breast tumors. Yet Inuit Eskimos don't worry much about breast cancer. Could whale blubber have something to do with it?

Cancer researcher Ronald S. Pardini, Ph.D., professor of biochemistry and associate director of the University of Nevada agricultural experimental station in Reno, wanted to know. So he implanted human breast cancer cells in mice and fed the mice one of three diets: a low-fat diet with just 5 percent corn oil rich in omega-6 fatty acids; a high-fat diet with 25 percent of fat coming from omega-6's; and a high-fat diet composed of 20 percent omega-3's and 5 percent omega-6's. The more omega-3's, the slower the tumors grew in the mice. The more omega-6's, the faster the growth.

"So you begin to wonder if saying that going on a low-fat diet is enough," says Dr. Pardini. "What might really matter is the *kind* of fat people eat." He tested his theory with four different cancers—breast, pancreatic, prostate, and ovarian—and found similar results.

On a side note, fish-oil supplements seem to enhance some chemotherapies, making them more toxic to the tumor but less toxic to the rest of the body, thus producing fewer side effects in those undergoing cancer treatment. If he had cancer, Dr. Pardini says, "I'd be slamming this stuff down. No question about it."

SUSHI SAFETY

So you like your salmon raw, with a dab of wasabi, wrapped in seaweed, rice, and ginger. No problem. Just don't do it at home. Most cases of illness related to sushi come from that made at home, says the FDA.

That's because in order to kill bacteria, viruses, and parasites that could make you sick, the fish must be frozen to −31°F for 15 hours or −10°F for 7 days. Home freezers just don't get that cold.

If you purchase sushi, make sure that the retailer and supplier have high standards. Not all take-out sources or grocery stores do. Experienced sushi chefs (if they've ever worked in Japan, you can count on them having at least 7 years of training) and reputable restaurants tend to be the safest. And always ask if the sushi fish, including salmon, shrimp, and tuna, has been frozen.

Other signs of freshness include a fishy taste, not smell, and smooth fish flesh. Tiny bumps are another sign of parasites.

If you are pregnant or have any kind of compromised immune system, you shouldn't have raw fish of any kind.

Experts at the FDA say that your chance of getting sick from fish, cooked or raw, is actually much less than getting sick from chicken or meat. One kind of sushi, blowfish, contains a powerful nerve poison that can leave you paralyzed or dead. It's very rarely served in the United States, but avoid it while traveling.

But Wait—There's More

Not only do Eskimos have unbelievably healthy hearts and a lower incidence of breast cancer, they also show amazingly low rates of diabetes, asthma, arthritis, Crohn's disease, multiple sclerosis, and psoriasis, most of which result from overreactive immune systems. With autoimmune disease, your body wages war with itself, with white blood cells attacking parts of your body as invaders, leading to inflammation, swelling, and pain.

But omega-3's can quell the runaway train of inflammation by limiting the number of white blood cells speeding to affected parts of the body. With rheumatoid arthritis, for instance, a disease three times more

POWER

TUNA SALAD

ALBACORE TUNA SLAW WITH CREAMY LEMON-DILL DRESSING

Is tuna salad one of your lunch staples? Smart you! Albacore or bluefin tuna is one of the richest suppliers of omega-3 fatty acids. There's only one way you can improve on this universal favorite: Add crunchy coleslaw mix to the fish. You'll reap cancer-preventing indoles from the cabbage and beta-carotene from the carrots. For even more meganutrients, serve the salad over baby spinach leaves (or add them to your sandwich—and be sure to use whole grain bread).

¼	cup reduced-fat mayonnaise
1	tablespoon lemon juice
1	teaspoon dried dillweed
1	teaspoon Dijon mustard
2	cups packaged coleslaw mix (see note)
2	cans (6½ ounces each) water-packed albacore tuna, drained and flaked

In a medium bowl, mix the mayonnaise, lemon juice, dillweed, and mustard. Add the coleslaw mix and toss to coat. Gently stir in the tuna.

Makes 4 servings

Per serving: 135 calories, 19 g protein, 7 g carbohydrates, 3 g fat, 30 mg cholesterol, 1 g dietary fiber, 449 mg sodium

Note: Buy a coleslaw mix that contains carrots and other vegetables, or add a shredded carrot.

common in women than in men, between 3 and 5 grams a day of EPA and DHA—at least 7 ounces of a fish like salmon—may provide enough relief to reduce the amount of ibuprofen and other nonsteroidal anti-inflammatory drugs that you need to take.

Even women with kidney disease may benefit. James V. Donadio, M.D., professor emeritus at the Mayo Clinic in Rochester, Minnesota, has used fish-oil supplements to treat men and women with a common form of kidney disease—IgA nephropathy—since 1987, with excellent results. Just 3 to 4 grams of DHA and EPA supplements daily reduced the inflammation that leads to permanent scarring in the kidney—and ultimately kidney failure. "They're still taking it," he says, "because their conditions improved or remained stable"—unusual in this disease for which there is no other treatment.

Increasing omega-3's in the diet may also improve symptoms of Crohn's disease, ulcerative colitis, and lupus. In most cases, the addition of fish-oil supplements enabled patients to reduce, if not discontinue, their traditional medications. However, if you are under medical care for the management of a chronic disease, you should never change your medications without first consulting your doctor.

Depressed? Feed Your Brain

More and more researchers are taking a look at how fish oil affects our mental well-being (although actual dosages have yet to be determined). Some population studies show that, on the average, the more fish that people consume, the lower the prevalence of major depression. Coincidence? Maybe not.

Brain serotonin is a neurotransmitter important to the biochemistry of depression. A growing amount of data suggests an association between omega-3's and serotonin. Down in the dumps? Low levels of omega-3's may be leaving you short-tempered or irritable. When researchers gave one group of students placebos and another group fish-oil supplements in the midst of their most stressful time—university exams—those taking fish oil were significantly calmer.

Other studies show that omega-3's may be effective in treating bipolar disorder (manic-depressive disorder). And it may help prevent Alzheimer's. Researchers found that those people with high levels of omega-3 DHA in their blood were more than 40 percent less likely to develop dementia, including Alzheimer's, during the next 9 years than people with low DHA levels. But if you are taking a prescription antidepressant, don't stop taking your medication without talking to your doctor.

PMS? THINK TUNA

When he gave teenage girls fish-oil supplements, Zeev Harel, M.D., assistant professor of pediatrics at Brown University in Providence, Rhode Island, found a 30 to 40 percent decrease in 18 different problems associated with menstruation, including cramps, headaches, diarrhea, and acne. Similar results have been shown in older women in Denmark.

The good news is that you don't need massive amounts of DHA and EPA for relief: just 1.8 grams of the fatty acids a day—or about 4 ounces of fish.

Strike a Balance

Nearly a century ago—when we ate more leafy vegetables, more wild game and poultry that fed on these vegetables, and more fish—we had nearly a 1-to-1 ratio between omega-3's and omega-6's. Today, most of us get way more omega-6's than omega-3's in our diets—close to a 25-to-1 ratio. We should be at about 4 to 1 or less.

While omega-3's slow the growth of certain cancers, omega-6's make them grow faster. "Not only that," says Dr. Simopoulos, "but high ratios of omega-6's increase inflammation, have little effect on triglycerides, and lower our 'good' cholesterol, HDL."

So how did our diets get so out of whack?

By focusing on reducing overall fat as a way to lower cholesterol and prevent heart disease—and forgetting about essential fatty acids like omega-3's. Dr. Simopoulos and other experts recommend between 4.5 and 7 grams of EPA and DHA a week, preferably from fish. If you don't like the taste of fish, you can take supplements.

With about 1.2 grams of DHA and EPA in a typical 3-ounce serving of fish, you'll need between four and six servings of fish a week. And if you suffer from some of the physical problems for which omega-3's are recommended, like depression, heart disease, or autoimmune diseases, you'll need more.

We're not talking about some exotic fish you can't pronounce or afford (although caviar is a pretty good source), we're talking about the glassy-eyed mackerel staring at you from behind the glass case, the slabs of Atlantic salmon sold in every grocery store, and the cans of albacore tuna sitting on your cupboard shelves.

On the East Coast? You're lucky. You can get bluefish, which has 1 gram per serving. Midwest? You have cold-water lake trout—1.2 grams per serving. And everyone can find sardines, herring, and anchovies. They each contain at least 1 gram of omega-3's per 3-ounce serving, and most have more.

Don't forget shellfish. Although they don't have as many omega-3's per serving, they still pack a wallop. One-half cup of shrimp or mussels, for instance, gives you 0.5 gram of EPA and DHA. A half-cup of squid or Pacific oysters gives slightly more. Buy shellfish in the shell, toss them in the boiling water when you cook pasta, drain, peel, add a bit of olive oil and Parmesan cheese and voilà!—a hefty helping of omega-3's in less than 10 minutes.

But forget fish sticks. When Dr. Simopoulos analyzed the fatty acids in a commercial fish patty, she found no trace of omega-3 fatty acids.

Right about now you're thinking, "Fatty fish? I'm trying to reduce fat in my diet." No problem. A 3-ounce serving of omega-3-rich coho salmon gives you 157 calories; the same amount of skinless chicken breast has about 142. Even though some fish do pack more calories, like the Atlantic mackerel with 223 calories (61 percent of them from fat), you shouldn't worry, says Joyce Nettleton, R.D., D.Sc., a dietitian in Amherst, Illinois, and author of *Omega-3 Fatty Acids and Health*. "We should be eating more of this kind of fat, not less."

MASKED DISASTER

Restaurant Tuna Salad

Scanning the lunch menu looking for something low-fat and healthy? Like a tuna sandwich, maybe?

Not so fast. Tuna salad served in a typical restaurant is likely to weigh 11 ounces with 720 calories—twice the calories of homemade. Even a tuna sub from Subway packs 540 calories, 6 percent of them from fat.

And you're not necessarily getting the maximum omega-3's, since restaurant tuna is mostly yellowfin, not a high omega-3 fish. A better bet is to order the salmon. A piece the size of a deck of cards packs nearly 2 grams of DHA and EPA.

ARE FARM-RAISED FISH BETTER?

While plenty of fishermen still troll the ocean for their catches, more and more of the fish you eat is farm-raised, but it varies from state to state.

Chances are, you won't notice a difference in taste. And while fish raised in captivity is safe to eat, so is ocean fish, says Dan Herman, director of food technical affairs for the National Fisheries Institute in Arlington, Virginia. That's because when fish hits our shores, it's subject to tough inspection standards at the processing plant by FDA investigators.

"Some people say that fish raised on fish meal have less intense flavor than fish caught in the wild," says Herman.

As for omega-3's, farm-raised fish may have the same levels per ounce, since some aquaculture farmers add extra dollops of omega-3's to their traditional feed.

Sneaky Ways to Eat More Fish

Three to five servings a week may sound like a lot of a fish. The key is to find clever ways to add fish to your regular menu. Experts offer these suggestions.

- Chop up a few sardines or other types of fatty fish like canned albacore tuna or mackerel and throw them into the tomato sauce for pasta.
- Try sardines sautéed in a bit of olive oil with lemon and capers on pasta.
- For a tasty, healthy appetizer, spread sardines canned in mustard sauce on low-fat crackers or pita bread.
- Use fish, instead of chicken or meat, in casseroles and stews. Try fish tacos, salmon lasagna, or pasta primavera made with fish as well as vegetables. Sprinkle some shrimp on your pizza or order pizza with anchovies.
- Instead of chicken soup, try fish soup, using bottled clam juice as a base stock.

Flaxseed: An Onshore Alternative

So you hate fish. And there's no way your husband or kids will eat it.

Don't despair. There's a form of omega-3 fatty acid called alpha-linoleic acid, or ALA, that comes from plants.

You get it from flaxseed oil or, better yet, flaxseed meal, which is not only high in omega-3's but also a great source of fiber. Sprinkle it over yogurt or cottage cheese, use it in place of about ¼ cup of flour in baking, or just mix it up in water and drink it. Buy whole flaxseed, keep it refrigerated, and grind only what you'll use at one time.

Other good sources of ALA include walnut and canola oils, dried seaweed, and raw and mature soybeans. Canola oil, in particular, has been shown to have heart-benefiting effects, cutting the risk of a second heart attack by 70 percent.

Still, when it comes to the health benefits of omega-3's, plant sources pale compared to fish, says C. Leigh Broadhurst, Ph.D., a nutrition chemist with a government human nutrition research lab. It takes about 10 times as much ALA to equal 1 gram of EPA. And most of the research on the health effects of omega-3's were done with fish-oil supplements, not ALA.

Where Supplements Come In

If you can't seem to get fish on the menu more than a couple of times a month, fish-oil supplements may be another way to get omega-3's. "You'll get the same benefits within 95 percent of what you get from fish," says Dr. Broadhurst.

But read the labels. Check how much EPA and DHA are in each recommended dose, then do the math to ensure that you're getting the amount you need. For instance, if the capsule is 1,000 milligrams, with 200 milligrams of EPA and 300 milligrams of DHA, to get 1 gram of these fatty acids, you need to swallow two capsules. Don't turn to cod-liver oil, though, because it could result in toxic amounts of vitamins D and A. And when you open a new bottle of supplements, cut one or two open. If they smell really bad (unlike regular fish smell), throw them away or ask the store for your money back. Try to stick with name-brand supplements, rather than generic.

If you have asthma, diabetes, or clotting disorders, talk to your doctor before taking any supplements.

Meat: Best Choices for Nutrition-Savvy Women

Power Maker #8: To benefit from what meat has to offer, eat at least 3 ounces of lean meat two or three times a week.

To some women, eating a small piece of meat is akin to running up their credit card bill at a factory outlet—a pleasure that will come back to haunt them.

Too much fat. Too many calories. A shortcut to heart disease and cancer. Women have been saying no to meat with very good intentions. Even women who do eat meat consume far smaller amounts than men do. The average woman eats about 128 pounds of meat a year, compared with the average man, who eats 183 pounds.

"Some women don't simply tell me that they eat red meat—they confess it," says Susan Nitzke, Ph.D., professor of nutritional sciences at the University of Wisconsin in Madison. "They think a nutritionist is going to scold them."

Dr. Nitzke and other nutritionists sigh over this red-meat phobia. Lean meat—not just beef but also pork, lamb, and game meats such as venison—is an excellent source of zinc and iron, essential minerals that are frequently lacking in the diets of premenopausal women.

An iron-poor diet puts you at risk of becoming one of the millions of adolescent girls and premenopausal women who have iron deficiency, the most common nutritional deficiency among American women of child-bearing age. Once your iron stores are drained, you are vulnerable to the more serious stages of iron-deficiency anemia, which can sap your physical and mental energy. If untreated, it can lead to dire health problems. (Of course, you don't have to eat meat to fill your iron quota. Research shows that vegetarians on well-planned diets are no more likely to develop anemia than meat eaters.)

DE-MYTHIFYING MEAT

True or false? Eating meat equals an increased risk of cancer and heart disease.

The fact is that the data are very inconsistent, at least for cancer, according to Martha Slattery, Ph.D., professor of epidemiology at the University of Utah in Salt Lake City. "Most of the scientific literature does not show that eating meat is a risk factor for cancer, especially for breast cancer."

In a study of 4,402 people with and without colon cancer, coauthored by Dr. Slattery, eating red meat was not shown to raise the risk of colon cancer. In another study, research conducted at the National Center for Toxicological Research in Jefferson, Arkansas, found no association between meat consumption and breast cancer.

Most likely, it's the overall American diet—high in fat, sugar, and refined flour and low in fiber—that increases cancer risk, says Dr. Slattery. "Meat is just one part of this Western dietary pattern."

Her advice? Eat meat in moderation. And use your grill in moderation. High-temperature cooking, such as grilling, converts substances in meat to potential cancer-causing chemicals called heterocyclicamines, which have been shown to increase cancer risk.

What about heart disease? There's no question that a high-fat diet leads to clogged arteries, says Dr. Slattery. But if you choose the leanest meats and eat in moderation, your risk of heart disease—from eating meat, at least—is likely to be reduced.

And if you still think meat is a fatfest, think again. More than 40 percent of all beef cuts have no external fat, a 3-ounce serving of pork tenderloin contains just 4 grams of fat, and a skinless chicken thigh contains more fat than a 3-ounce portion of lean lamb.

Welcome to the Iron Gap

Like a lust for shoes, iron deficiency is primarily a woman thing. One in five women of childbearing age has low iron stores, compared with 1 in 60 men.

Men's sheer physical size allows them to store more iron than women. A man's body contains from 1 to 1.4 grams of stored iron; a woman's, well below 0.5 gram.

MEAT ADDITIVES: WHAT YOU SHOULD KNOW

That succulent steak, pork chop, or chicken breast on your plate delivers more than good taste. It also contains antibiotics, growth hormones, or both, given to protect livestock from disease and to fatten them. Should you eat with gusto—or misgivings? Here's the lowdown on these substances.

ANTIBIOTICS. Virtually all pigs and poultry (less often, beef cattle) receive low doses of antibiotics, most commonly penicillin or tetracyclines. Given in water or feed or by pill or shot, antibiotics promote animals' growth and prevent the spread of disease among animals in close quarters. But there's growing concern that giving livestock antibiotics may eventually make the drugs less able to kill bacteria, both in the animals and the people who eat them. This means that if you get sick from food contaminated by *Escherichia coli*, salmonella, or campylobacter, the antibiotics typically given to destroy these bacteria may not work.

There's no conclusive evidence that giving animals antibiotics leads to bacterial resistance in people. So it's too early to steer women away from meat. Nevertheless, the government isn't taking any chances. In 1996, it established the National Antimicrobial Resistance Monitoring System to track antibiotic resistance in animals and humans. "We take this issue seriously," says Stephen F. Sundlof, D.V.M., Ph.D., director of the Center for Veterinary Medicine at the

Moreover, if you think of stored iron as savings, men are misers, while women are spendthrifts. "Men have more iron in the bank because they don't make as many withdrawals as women," says Dr. Nitzke.

Blood loss is one of the main causes of iron deficiency. Women's biggest and most frequent withdrawal from their iron account is menstruation. Depending on the flow, you lose from 1 to 2 milligrams of iron each day of your period, with heavy bleeders losing the most. That's on top of the 1 milligram of iron both sexes normally lose each day via bowel movements. Pregnancy and childbirth also strain a woman's iron reserves.

Finally, most women don't make adequate deposits to their iron stores through diet, because they eat less food than men and because they don't eat enough iron-rich foods, says Dr. Nitzke. If you're of childbearing age,

FDA in Washington, D.C. "Our intent is to preserve the effectiveness of these drugs, both for animals and humans." Smart consumers will continue to monitor this issue for new developments.

HORMONES. Up to 90 percent of all U.S. beef cattle (but not pigs or poultry) receive low doses of hormones injected under their skins. The hormones in question are estradiol, testosterone, and progesterone, which are produced naturally in both animals and people, and the synthetic hormones trenbolone acetate, zeranol, and melengestrol acetate.

Hormone-treated cattle gain weight more rapidly, producing more tender and flavorful meat. And the sooner cattle reach market weight, the cheaper it is to process them into steaks and roasts, a savings that is passed on to us. But some consumer groups fear that hormone-treated beef may fuel the development of hormone-related cancers, such as breast and prostate cancers.

Experts deem this practice to be safe. The FDA has researched the effects of growth hormones for decades and has consistently found that they pose no risk to people at all, says Dr. Sundlof. The amounts used are very low, he adds. For example, a 1-pound portion of beef given estradiol contains about nine million times less of this hormone than the amount produced by a pregnant woman.

LOWER IRON, SLOWER BRAINS?

Feel dumber when you diet? Evidence suggests that low-calorie diets, particularly those under 1,200 calories a day, can lower your iron reserves and your ability to concentrate.

Going on that evidence as well as on the knowledge that children who don't get enough iron may fall behind in their mental development and have attention problems, Molly Kretsch, Ph.D., a research nutrition scientist at the USDA Western Human Nutrition Research Center in Davis, California, wanted to find out how dieting might affect a woman's iron stores and her powers of concentration.

In Dr. Kretsch's study, 14 overweight premenopausal women consumed diets of 1,000 to 1,200 calories a day, half their usual amount. By the end of the 4½-month study, iron levels had dropped significantly in 8 of the women. This was despite the fact that they were consuming a total of twice the 18 milligram Daily Value for iron in the form of food and a supplement.

"For reasons we don't understand, it appears that their bodies didn't utilize the dietary iron. It may be that iron isn't used as effectively when we restrict calories," says Dr. Kretsch.

Further, these eight women scored 50 percent lower on a computer test that measured their ability to focus and sustain attention. Did they also report losing their train of thought or other symptoms of mental murkiness? "Our study didn't gather that kind of information," says Dr. Kretsch. "But clearly, women on low-calorie diets talk about losing their ability to concentrate."

It's smart to get a blood test that checks your levels of iron, hemoglobin, and ferritin (stored iron) before starting a reduced-calorie diet. "If your doctor informs you that you are anemic or that your iron stores are low, then it would be prudent to improve your body's iron status by eating iron-rich foods before beginning a low-calorie diet," says Dr. Kretsch. Recommended sources of iron include: lean meat, legumes, breads, and cereals. It will probably take 3 to 4 months to improve your iron status. A repeat blood test will let you know if you have been successful.

there's a strong chance that you're not getting the recommended 18 milligrams of iron a day. Fully 75 percent of us don't.

Menstrual iron losses combined with an iron-poor diet can push you into iron-deficiency anemia, which affects more than three million adolescent girls and premenopausal women. "This condition has serious consequences for a woman's physical health, mood, and mental performance," says Gayle Reichler, R.D., president of Active Wellness in New York City and author of *Active Wellness: A Personalized 10-Step Program for a Healthy Body, Mind, and Spirit.*

Iron Helps Cells "Breathe"

Iron is vital because it helps your body utilize a substance that's essential to life: oxygen.

Most of the scant amount of iron normally found in a woman's body—0.2 to 0.4 gram—can be found in hemoglobin, the protein in red blood cells that delivers oxygen from your lungs to the rest of your body. Iron enables red blood cells to carry oxygen to every part of your body: the brain, muscles, nervous system, and organs.

If you don't eat enough iron-rich foods, or if your iron stores dip too low, you are in danger of developing iron deficiency. That is, your red blood cells can't carry as much oxygen to where it's needed, which is everywhere.

Iron deficiency is sneaky—you can't "feel" yourself running on empty. But if you develop iron-deficiency anemia, you may know your health has taken a turn for the worse. This condition is a nutritional endgame: the final and most debilitating stage of iron deficiency.

The body of a woman with this condition is literally starving for oxygen. So she's tired—very tired. She's also physically weak, pale, cold, and irritable. What she's not: productive. Iron-deficiency anemia also saps a woman's ability to think and concentrate.

Absorption Is the Key

Of course, iron-deficiency anemia is usually preventable if you take in enough iron through your diet. And lean meat can help you meet your iron quota. "Lean meat may be especially important to women of childbearing age as a source of iron," says Janet Hunt, Ph.D., a research nutritionist at the USDA Human Nutrition Research Center in Grand Forks, North Dakota.

But what's so special about beef or pork, when you can also get iron from iron-fortified breads and cereals and iron-rich fruits, vegetables, and legumes?

Iron comes in two forms: heme and nonheme. Heme iron is found only in meats, poultry, and fish. Nonheme iron is found in both plant and animal foods, and it's the kind of iron in fortified foods. Your body is able to use heme iron better than the nonheme variety. In fact, heme iron is absorbed two to three times more effectively than the nonheme iron in plant and iron-fortified foods.

Heme iron-rich animal foods such as meat, fish, and poultry also contain a kind of "nonheme helper," allowing your body to absorb the nonheme iron of foods eaten with them. "So eating a small portion of meat at lunch or dinner helps your body absorb the iron in the rest of your meal," says Dr. Nitzke.

Chicken contains significantly less total iron than beef and other meats. Three ounces of chicken breast contains a bit over half a milligram of iron, compared with almost 3 milligrams found in 3 ounces of beef loin, so beef weighs in with almost five times more total iron than chicken. Poultry also falls short on heme iron. One study conducted at Utah State University in Logan found that from 55 to 80 percent of the iron in beef is the heme variety, depending upon the cut. That's about double the 29 to 40 percent in chicken.

The upshot? If skinless chicken breast is the primary source of meat in your diet and you're not eating enough iron-rich foods, you may not be getting the iron your body needs, says Molly Kretsch, Ph.D., a research nutrition scientist at the USDA Western Human Nutrition Research Center in Davis, California.

Beef Up on Zinc and B$_{12}$

Meat is packed with the trace mineral zinc, another nutrient that the average woman doesn't get enough of in her diet.

Zinc strengthens the immune system, which protects you from colds and other infections. It also may help keep your bones thick and strong; in women of all ages, as zinc intake increases, bone loss decreases. The

ALL OF THE FLAVOR, NONE OF THE GUILT

Stop feeling guilty when you sink your teeth into a nice piece of sirloin. In fact, here are seven cuts of beef that contain between 4 and 9 grams of fat per 3-ounce serving—about the amount in a skinless chicken breast or thigh. And virtually all of them contain more iron, zinc, and B_{12} than the chicken. A 3-ounce serving of meat is about the size of a deck of cards or a bar of soap.

CUT (3 oz)	FAT (g)	IRON (mg)	ZINC (mg)	VITAMIN B_{12} (mcg)
Eye round	4.2	1.7	4.0	1.8
Top round	4.2	2.4	4.7	2.1
Tip round	5.9	2.5	6.0	2.5
Top sirloin	6.1	2.9	5.5	2.4
Bottom round	6.4	2.9	4.6	2.1
Top loin	8.2	2.1	4.4	1.7
Tenderloin	8.6	3.0	4.8	2.2
Chicken breast	3.1	0.9	0.9	0.3
Chicken thigh	9.2	1.1	2.2	0.3

Daily Value (DV) is 15 milligrams, and you can easily get one-third that amount from 3 ounces of lean beef.

Most meat is also a good source of B vitamins, particularly B_6 (needed for strong immunity), niacin (crucial for healthy skin, nerves, and digestion), and thiamin (which helps convert blood sugar into energy).

It's also one of the few sources of vitamin B_{12}, which you need to keep your red blood cells healthy and maintain myelin, the fatty sheath that covers nerve cells. What's more, not getting enough B_{12} can raise blood levels of homocysteine, a substance research suggests may raise the risk of heart disease.

Since the best sources of B_{12} are meat, eggs, milk, and cheese, total vegetarians may not get enough of this crucial vitamin, which is why nutritionists urge them to eat fortified soy beverages and meat replacers or to take B_{12} supplements. Lean meat can make a significant deposit to your B_{12} account. One 3-ounce portion of tip round steak, for example, contains 2.5 micrograms of B_{12}—41 percent of the DV.

POWER

BURGERS

SALSA BEEF PATTIES

How do you make a burger healthier? Add some spicy pepper and tomato salsa. It'll give you a hefty shot of vitamin C to help your body absorb iron from the meat, plus cancer-fighting lycopene and beta-carotene. Meanwhile, the whole wheat bun supplies fiber, and the dark green romaine lettuce adds even more beta-carotene.

1	pound ground eye round
¼	teaspoon ground black pepper
3	plum tomatoes, finely chopped
1	jarred or freshly roasted red bell pepper, finely chopped (see note)
2	tablespoons finely chopped red onion
1	tablespoon finely chopped fresh cilantro
1–2	teaspoons finely chopped jalapeño pepper (wear plastic gloves when handling)
4	whole wheat buns, split
	Romaine lettuce leaves

Preheat the oven to 450°F. Form the eye round into 4 patties ½" thick. Season with the black pepper. Place on a broiler pan. Bake for 8 minutes. Turn and bake for 8 to 10 minutes longer, or until no longer pink in the center.

To make the salsa, mix the tomatoes, bell pepper, onion, and cilantro in a small bowl. Stir in jalapeño pepper to taste.

Line the bun bottoms with lettuce leaves and spoon on half of the salsa. Place the burgers on the salsa. Add the remaining salsa and the bun tops.

Makes 4

Per burger: 356 calories, 26 g protein, 22 g carbohydrates, 18 g fat, 68 mg cholesterol, 3 g dietary fiber, 323 mg sodium

Note: Blacken a red bell pepper on all sides under the broiler. Wrap it in foil and set aside until cool enough to handle. Remove and discard the charred skin, seeds, and inner membranes. Chop the flesh.

Maximum Iron, Minimum Fat

We can just hear you now, saying, "What about the fat?"

Today's meats are leaner than ever. If you consume sensible portions, you can get the nutrients you need without the extra fat and calories you don't need, says Dr. Nitzke. Here's how.

Make the grade. When possible, choose "select," the leanest grade of beef, says Richard J. Epley, Ph.D., professor of meat science in the department of food science and nutrition at the University of Minnesota in St. Paul. Ask your supermarket what grade of meat it carries. "Choice" and "prime" are the other options, with prime having the most fat.

Stick to round steak. Whatever the grade, you'll get the least amount of fat from beef cuts that include "round" in the name. Shop for eye round, followed by top, tip, and bottom, says Dr. Epley. Choosing carefully can make a big difference in your fat "budget." In fact, 3 ounces of broiled top round contains half the fat of the same amount of roasted dark-meat chicken without the skin. Other lean cuts of beef include sirloin and tenderloin.

Know the ground rules. The leanest varieties of ground beef are also marked "loin" or "round." Also, choose ground beef by color: Generally speaking, the redder the meat, the less fat it contains.

MASKED DISASTER

Liver

Did you ever force yourself to eat liver because "it's good for you"? Well, you can stop. Although beef liver is an excellent source of iron, a 3-ounce serving contains 331 milligrams of cholesterol—more than the recommended daily limit of 300 milligrams. Chicken livers are even worse, with 536 milligrams. By contrast, a luscious 3-ounce portion of lean beef tenderloin weighs in at 71 milligrams cholesterol—a fraction of the amount in chicken liver—and still has a decent amount of iron.

Pick the darkest parts of poultry. If your meat intake consists mostly of skinless chicken breast, try to develop a taste for the darker parts of the bird, such as the leg or thigh. Ounce for ounce, they contain more total iron than the breast, and more of that iron is the heme type. Forty percent of the iron in a chicken drumstick and 32 percent of the iron in the thigh is heme, compared with 29 percent in the breast.

True, dark meat is higher in fat than white meat. But if you consume it in sensible 3-ounce portions and watch your overall fat and calorie intake, there's no cause for concern.

Get in the game. Take a walk on the wild side and try game meats such as venison, rabbit, bison, or buffalo. Game is often significantly lower in fat than even the leanest beef, pork, lamb, or veal—and it contains as much or more iron. Two examples: a 3-ounce portion of venison contains 134 calories, 2.7 grams of fat, and a whopping 3.8 milligrams of iron. The same portion of bison contains 122 calories, 2 grams of fat, and 3 milligrams of iron. Game meats are available at some supermarkets, at specialty stores, or by mail order from catalogs or the Internet.

Go to C. If you dislike dark-meat poultry, then eat your skinless breast with foods that are rich in vitamin C, such as tomatoes, broccoli, spinach, red bell peppers, brussels sprouts, and snow peas. Vitamin C "captures" iron and keeps it in the form that your body can most easily use.

Pick the leanest pork. Go for the tenderloin, says Dr. Epley. A 3-ounce serving contains 139 calories and 4.1 grams of fat. Other lean cuts (based on a 3-ounce serving) include extra-lean boneless ham (123 calories, 4.7 grams of fat), boneless sirloin chops (164 calories, 5.7 grams of fat), and boneless loin chops (173 calories, 6.6 grams of fat).

Shop for chops. According to the Utah State University study, 80 percent of the 1.7 milligrams of iron in lamb chops is heme. The beautiful part is that a well-trimmed 3-ounce broiled chop contains just 184 calories and 8.2 grams of fat.

Soak your meat. To add flavor, marinate lean meats such as eye of round, top round, and pork tenderloin before cooking. Try this marinade for beef, pork, or lamb: ⅓ cup of dry white wine; ¼ cup of reduced-sodium soy sauce; 1 tablespoon each of honey, minced fresh ginger, and chopped scallions; 1 small clove of garlic, minced; 2 teaspoons of Worcestershire sauce; and a big pinch of black pepper. Pour over the meat, cover, and refrigerate overnight for the next day's meal.

Milk: More Than Just a Bone Builder

Power Maker #9: For sturdier bones, stronger muscles, and healthier nerves, include a generous source of calcium—like milk, cheese, or greens—in every meal.

You've told your kids a million times: "No more soda—you need to drink more milk."

But what about you?

If you're like most women, you drink barely more than a cup of milk a day, depriving your body of the nutrients—particularly calcium—it supplies.

"We have a huge calcium crisis in this country," says Rachel K. Johnson, R.D., Ph.D., associate dean for research and associate professor of nutrition and food sciences at the College of Agriculture and Life Sciences at the University of Vermont in Burlington. Only 16 percent of us get at least two servings of dairy foods a day (the USDA recommends two to three), with more than half of us getting less than one serving. Overall, 43 percent of women get less than 60 percent of the Daily Value for calcium.

Our kids should be chastising *us*!

You know calcium helps protect against osteoporosis and other bone disorders, but did you know that it can also lower your blood pressure, stave off gum disease and subsequent tooth loss, protect against certain kinds of cancer, and help you lose weight? Read on.

Don't Worry, It's Not Fattening

One of the main reasons that women shy away from milk and other dairy products is the fear of gaining weight. But, in fact, drinking your milk can actually help you lose weight.

When researchers at Purdue University in West Lafayette, Indiana, followed 54 young women for 2 years, they found that those who consumed fewer than 1,900 calories and an average of 1,000 milligrams of calcium a day (mainly from dairy products such as fat-free milk, low-fat yogurt, and regular cheese) lost 6 to 7 pounds of body fat over the 2 years, without exercising more. Those who consumed only 500 milligrams of calcium a day actually gained about 2 to 3 pounds of body fat, although they too kept their total calories below 1,900.

"We thought it was a fluke," said Dorothy Teegarden, Ph.D., assistant nutrition professor and lead researcher. Then she heard about the work of Michael B. Zemel, Ph.D., director of the Nutrition Institute at the University of Tennessee in Knoxville. He found that increasing the level of calcium in fat cells acts like a key, turning on the genes that make the enzymes that produce fat. At the same time, it suppresses the system that breaks down fat.

When you have low levels of calcium in your diet, a special hormone kicks in to pull the mineral from your bones and push it into your fat cells. The hormone—along with a form of hormonal vitamin D—stimulates those fat cell genes. If you keep your dietary levels of calcium high, the hormone doesn't turn on, so fat is burned normally.

The reason our bodies work this way probably dates back to our cave-dwelling ancestors, says Robert P. Heaney, M.D., professor of medicine at the Osteoporosis Research Center at Creighton University in Omaha, Nebraska. Even though they didn't have dairy cows, our forebears got tons of calcium in nearly everything they ate—which consisted mainly of leafy plants and tubers. A decline in calcium signaled a decline in food, prompting the body to hang on to every bit of fat that it could.

Dr. Zemel tested his theory on mice bred with the so-called obesity gene. Half got extra calcium in the form of nonfat dry milk or supple-

POWER

MILKSHAKE

TROPICAL SMOOTHIE

If drinking milk just isn't your thing, get the same benefits from a creamy, low-fat shake like this one. You get over 40 percent of your calcium requirement in a 1½-cup serving, thanks to both nonfat dry milk and yogurt. Extra bonuses: The mango is an excellent source of vitamin A (from beta-carotene) and vitamin C, and the pineapple is also high in vitamin C.

1	cup low-fat plain yogurt
1	cup mango cubes
1	small banana, sliced
½	cup pineapple chunks
¼	cup nonfat dry milk
1	tablespoon lime juice

In a blender, combine the yogurt, mango, banana, pineapple, milk, and lime juice. Blend until smooth.

Makes 3 cups

Per 1½ cups: 230 calories, 10 g protein, 45 g carbohydrates, 2.5 g fat, 9 mg cholesterol, 3 g dietary fiber, 129 mg sodium

Note: For a thicker, icy-cold drink, freeze the fruit first (keep a supply of fruit chunks in the freezer for instant smoothies).

ments, while the rest were on low-calcium diets. Over 6 weeks, those getting the dry milk gained 30 to 50 percent less fat than those on the low-calcium diets. Even more interesting, those getting their calcium from milk gained less weight than those getting it from supplements.

Then Dr. Zemel looked at national data on dietary habits and weight and found that women who got about 1,400 milligrams of calcium a day from 3.4 servings of dairy foods were 80 percent less likely to be fat than those who only got 484 milligrams a day from 1.3 servings of dairy foods.

"Calcium accounts for only two-thirds of the benefits of low-fat dairy products," says Dr. Zemel says. "Something else is at work."

"Young women who fear dairy products because they're worried that they will get fat ought to think again," adds Dr. Zemel. "Not only will eating dairy foods not make them fat, but it may make them lean." Lean and healthy, that is.

What Dairy Products Offer That Supplements Don't

Supplements can help meet your daily requirements for calcium—about 1,000 milligrams for women up to age 50 and 1,500 milligrams after that. But they don't provide the overall benefits of dairy products.

DO DAIRY PRODUCTS AGGRAVATE ASTHMA?

Among the advice women hear or read from time to time is the suggestion to eliminate dairy products from their diets to reduce the wheezing, coughing, and chest tightness associated with asthma. Some women try this, and it seems to work. But it may be a placebo effect. Little research exists to link dairy food consumption to respiratory symptoms.

"Our research has shown that a significant number of people with asthma are unnecessarily restricting their diets and are at possible risk of developing nutritional deficiencies," says Rosalie Woods, Ph.D., a dietitian and research fellow in the epidemiology and preventive medicine department at Monash Medical School in Victoria, Australia.

She tested 20 subjects with asthma, including 13 women, 10 of whom thought their asthma got worse with dairy products. There was no significant difference between how well the women could breathe when they drank about 1⅓ cups of milk compared to when they drank a placebo.

A previous study for diagnosis of cow's milk allergy found that most people who thought that they were hypersensitive to milk could actually tolerate dairy. While a few people have a genuine problem with milk, many do not, says Dr. Woods. A blind food challenge test is the only way to identify a true milk allergy.

Dairy foods currently provide us with 20 percent of our protein, 31 percent of our riboflavin, 18.5 percent of our potassium, 19 percent of our zinc, 16 percent of our magnesium, 17 percent of our vitamin A, and 10 percent of our vitamin B_6. In fact, an Australian study found that women who increased their calcium intake with dairy products also increased consumption of 11 other nutrients.

Dairy products also contain little-known substances like sphingolipids, which researchers say have profound effects on regulating cell growth and death, critical elements in the progression of cancer. Dairy foods also supply conjugated linoleic acid, or CLA, a fat found only in dairy products and certain types of meat.

Preliminary data from a study on guinea pigs suggests that CLA may reduce asthmatic and allergic responses to certain foods. It has also reduced breast, stomach, colon, and skin cancers in several different animals and in test tubes. When CLA was fed to mice, the results led researchers to speculate that it may play a role in protecting against postmenopausal bone loss.

Even the scientists aren't sure why they often see better results when their subjects, be they mice or moms, get their calcium from food. "Sometimes it's the way nutrients are packaged that gives us the interactions," says Dr. Zemel.

Calcium and Old Lace

If you put a chicken bone in a jar of vinegar and let it sit for a few days, the bone turns rubbery. You can bend it nearly double without breaking it. The acid in the vinegar leaches all the calcium out of the bone.

Ninety-nine percent of the calcium our bodies absorb heads straight to our bones. Without it, we'd be as rubbery as that chicken bone. While low calcium intake isn't the only risk factor for osteoporosis, it's one of the few we can control.

In our twenties and thirties, we don't worry much about future fractures. Yet half of all women will experience an osteoporosis-related fracture in their lifetimes.

Think of our bones as a savings account for calcium. The bank account opens as soon as we're born. If we don't get enough calcium as a child, we'll still grow, but our bones will begin undermining themselves almost immediately, snatching bone from the inside to support bone

TOO MUCH PROTEIN
AND SALT LEACH CALCIUM

When your calcium intake is substandard, salty high-protein foods like fried chicken can cause you to lose more calcium in your urine. "If you have an order of fast-food chicken for lunch, you get as much as 2,200 milligrams of sodium in one serving, which washes out 40 milligrams of calcium," says Robert P. Heaney, M.D., professor of medicine at the Osteoporosis Research Center at Creighton University in Omaha, Nebraska. "You need a high-calcium diet to compensate for that." The bottom line is that if you eat a high-protein, high-salt meal, you should wash it down with milk or another good source of calcium.

lengthening, leaving weak, brittle bones as we age. (If you look at an electron photograph of osteoporotic bone, it looks as fragile as old lace.)

If our bones are well-capitalized with calcium, then estrogen is like a safe, protecting the calcium stores in our bones and enhancing calcium absorption from our intestines, among other effects.

Around age 50, menopause creates a run on the bank. We begin losing bone at the rate of 1 to 3 percent a year for the first 5 to 6 years after our last menstrual periods. That's why hormone-replacement therapy is so effective at preventing and treating osteoporosis.

But calcium has a strong effect on bone even after menopause. Although we can't restore bone already lost, we can maintain what's left. In a study of 84 elderly women, researchers in Western Australia found that those who took about 1,900 milligrams of calcium supplements a day for 4 years didn't lose any bone in their hips or ankles. Those who didn't take calcium supplements at all lost a significant amount of bone.

And it's not just the bones in your hips, legs, and arms that are affected. Researchers at the University of New York at Buffalo found that men and women who had calcium intakes of less than 500 milligrams a day were more likely to lose their teeth than those who consumed more. A similar study showed that postmenopausal women who lost teeth also lost bone density in their hips and the rest of their bodies at a faster rate than those who didn't lose teeth.

Cardio-Protection from the White Stuff

While most women are aware that calcium or the lack of it plays a role in osteoporosis, very few know that it can help control blood pressure. But more and more doctors are now convinced that calcium has an anti-hypertensive effect in some people, especially if they are salt-sensitive, says Dr. Zemel.

The effects on blood pressure regulation are stronger with food sources of calcium. "You get twice as big a reduction in blood pressure with dietary calcium as has ever been reported for calcium supplements," says Dr. Heaney.

When 153 men and women were put on a special diet rich in fruits, vegetables, and low-fat dairy products, blood pressure fell within days—more than in subjects who were on a similar low-fat, high-fiber diet without dairy foods. If everyone in the country ate similar diets, including two to three dairy products a day, says Dr. Heaney, 27 percent fewer people would have strokes, a frequent end result of high blood pressure.

Here are some other cardiovascular effects from calcium and dairy products.

Lower levels of cholesterol. When researchers at the University of Kentucky fed volunteers just over 1 cup of yogurt a day for 4 weeks, they found that their overall cholesterol levels dropped as much as 3.2 percent compared to those of a control group. Since every 1 percent reduction in

VITAMIN D, THE EXECUTIVE ASSISTANT

Without vitamin D, you can't absorb calcium, and the only sources are dairy products, sunlight, and cod-liver oil. If you live in a northern climate, you'll have a hard time getting enough vitamin D even if you stay in the sun all day in the winter, says Connie Weaver, Ph.D., professor and director of the department of foods and nutrition at Purdue University in West Lafayette, Indiana. "In winter in Boston, for instance, the sun doesn't come down straight enough to activate the synthesis in your skin." That's why researchers found Bostonian women lose calcium from their bones during the winter. Consuming dairy products fortified with vitamin D can help.

serum cholesterol concentration is associated with an estimated 2 to 3 percent reduction in risk for heart disease, a regular intake of yogurt containing a strain of *Lactobacillus acidophilus* could reduce the risk for coronary heart diseases by 6 to 10 percent, say the study's authors. A comparable study by Brazilian researchers found similar results.

Reduced overall risk of heart disease. When researchers analyzed data from 34,486 postmenopausal Iowa women who had no history of heart disease, they found that those who consumed relatively high levels of calcium—at least 1,400 milligrams a day in either low-fat dairy foods, supplements, or both—had one-third the chance of dying from heart disease that women who had low amounts of calcium had.

Cancer Guards in the Dairy Case

Dairy foods seem to protect women at the cellular level.

Reduced odds of breast cancer. When Finnish researchers followed for 25 years the relationship between dairy consumption and breast cancer in 4,700 women, they found that drinking about 3 cups of milk a day could cut a woman's risk of breast cancer by more than half compared to women who drank less than 1½ cups a day. The possible reasons that researchers suggest are the lactose or calcium in dairy products, which some studies suggest may reduce breast cancer risk, or the CLA (conjugated linoleic acid) found in milk. This is a fatty acid shown to suppress breast cancer tumors in animals.

Lower risk of colon cancer. Colon cancer is the second leading cause of death from cancer in this country, almost surely due in part to the fact that with low calcium intake, we can't get rid of some of the noxious substances responsible, according to Dr. Heaney. "Natural residues from digestion can stimulate the growth of cancer, but calcium neutralizes those residues so that they don't have that effect."

A number of studies bear this out. For instance, in one study volunteers with a history of colon polyps (benign tumors that often turn cancerous) received either a placebo or 1,200 milligrams of calcium supplements. The supplement group fared better: After 4 years, 7 percent fewer people taking supplements developed another polyp, and as a group they developed fewer polyps than those taking a placebo. In effect, they reduced their risk of polyps by 19 percent.

In another study of 70 men and women at risk for colon cancer, those

A CHEESE FANATIC'S GUIDE TO THE GALAXY

When *Prevention* magazine surveyed women about their favorite foods, "real cheese" ranked high among foods women would love to eat more of, if fat and calories were of no concern.

No need to eschew cheese forever. Just use this handy guide to know what you're getting when you help yourself to the real thing.

TYPE	SERVING SIZE	CALORIES	FAT (g)	CALCIUM (mg)
Brie	1 oz	93	8	51
Cheddar	1 oz	113	9	202
Cottage cheese (1%)	½ cup	82	1	69
Cream cheese	1 Tbsp	51	5	12
Feta	1 oz	74	6	138
Parmesan, grated	1 Tbsp	27	2	82
Swiss	1 oz	105	8	269

receiving 1,200 milligrams of calcium from low-fat dairy foods saw some precancerous cells lining their colons return to normal, while overall growth of precancerous cells slowed.

A buffer against rectal cancer. Researchers at the University of Minnesota in Minneapolis analyzed food surveys from 34,702 postmenopausal Iowa women. After adjusting for numerous factors, including age, total calories, and smoking, they found that women who got at least 1,287 milligrams of calcium a day (the amount in about 4 cups of milk) were 41 percent less likely to develop rectal cancer during a period of 9 years.

Even Your Kidneys Benefit

If you've been diagnosed with kidney stones, you've likely been advised to avoid calcium supplements. Calcium-rich food, however, may actually be protective. If you've ever had a baby, you have an idea of the kind of pain involved in passing kidney stones. Calcium, however, acts to prevent them. "With a high-calcium diet, the calcium in our food works

A REFRIGERATOR-DOOR GUIDE TO MILK

Whole milk, fat-free milk, goat's milk, soy milk. What's the difference? Here's a quick guide to help you sort out your options for nutrition and taste.

TYPE	CALCIUM (mg per cup)	TASTE	FAT (g per cup)
Whole cow's milk	290	What you grew up with	8
Fat-free cow's milk	302	Slightly watery	Less than 1
Lactose-free milk	500	Slightly sweeter and richer taste than fat-free cow's milk	0
Low-fat buttermilk	285	Slightly sour	2
Goat's milk	327	Slightly sweeter than cow's milk; tastes like hazelnuts	10
Regular soy milk	10 (if fortified, as much as 400)	Unique creamy, nutty, or faintly sweet taste; also comes in flavors	5
Fat-free soy milk	10 (if fortified, as much as 400)	Unique creamy, nutty, or faintly sweet taste; also comes in flavors	0
Low-fat rice milk (Pacific Foods)	150	Light and sweet; also comes in cocoa and vanilla	2
Fat-free rice milk (Pacific Foods)	150	Light and sweet; also comes in cocoa and vanilla	0
Oat milk (Pacific Foods)	20	Slightly sweet; also comes in vanilla	1.5

with the acid in our intestines to prevent absorption of oxalic acid," says Dr. Heaney. (Oxalic acid is one of the primary risk factors for stones.)

"That's not surprising," he says. "Nutritionists have long known that you treat a syndrome known as intestinal hyperoxalosis—which results in huge quantities of oxalic acid being produced—with a very high calcium intake, as high as 8 grams of calcium carbonate per day."

BENEFITS	DRAWBACKS
All the benefits of the various vitamins and minerals contained in milk	The fat
No fat; all the benefits of whole milk	Some don't like the thin, watery taste, but new manufacturing methods are rendering creamier, thicker fat-free milks
No gas, bloating, or diarrhea from lactose intolerance	None
Lower in fat than whole cow's milk	None
Higher levels of several vitamins and minerals, including vitamin A, niacin, and potassium	The fat; you can't pick it up at the mini-mart
The benefits of soy, including reduction in the rates of certain cancers and cardiovascular disease, osteoporosis, and autoimmune disease; lactose-free	The taste, and unless it's fortified, you're missing out on the calcium
The benefits of soy, including reduction in the rates of certain cancers and cardiovascular disease, osteoporosis, and autoimmune diseases; lactose-free	The taste, and unless it's fortified, you're missing out on the calcium
Good for those who are lactose intolerant; some brands are gluten-free; less sodium than soy milk	More carbohydrates and less protein than soy; sweetness not ideal for cooking
Good for those who are lactose intolerant; some brands are gluten-free; less sodium than soy milk	More carbohydrates and less protein than soy; sweetness not ideal for cooking
Good for those who are lactose intolerant; adds more fiber to your diet	Much lower in calcium than other types of milk

In the Iowa study, researchers found that the women who developed kidney stones ate 250 milligrams a day less calcium than women who didn't get stones. The data suggest that the results are due to the intake of dietary calcium (milk, cheese, and yogurt), not supplements. Harvard researchers found that women who took calcium supplements *increased* their chance of developing kidney stones. In that study, those who took in about 1,100 milligrams of dietary calcium were 35 percent less likely to develop stones than those eating just 430 milligrams of calcium. The Harvard researchers speculate that there may be something in the dairy products other than calcium that is responsible for the lower risk, perhaps phosphorus.

Female-Friendly Food

Then there are the women-only effects of calcium, like preventing PMS and improving fertility.

In a multicenter study, 466 women with severe premenstrual syndrome were split into two groups. One group received 1,200 milligrams of calcium supplements a day in the form of four Tums E-X tablets, while the other group took a look-alike placebo over the course of three menstrual cycles. In nearly every type of premenstrual symptom, from mood swings, depression, and irritability to cramping, lower-back pain, and bloating, the women receiving calcium supplements improved. Overall, the women who took the calcium reduced their symptoms 48 percent compared to 30 percent in the placebo group, results comparable to those found using prescription antidepressant and antianxiety medications.

DON'T GIVE UP ON LOW-FAT CHEESE

One noticeable difference between regular cheese and many low-fat varieties is that the reduced-fat stuff doesn't melt. Grilled cheese sandwiches just aren't the same. The reason is simple: There's no oil on the surface of the cheese, says David M. Barbano, Ph.D., professor of food science and director of the Northeast Dairy Foods Research Center at Cornell University in Ithaca, New York. Nearly 50 percent of the fat in regular mozzarella oozes out as oil during cooking (that's why you need to blot that pizza with a paper napkin). By simply spraying fat-free cheese with vegetable oil spray—adding back just a teensy bit of fat—researchers were able to get low-fat and fat-free mozzarella cheese to melt and otherwise behave like its full-fat cousins. This will probably work with any kind of low-fat cheese.

The interaction of calcium and the calcium-regulating hormones on your neurotransmitters may affect premenstrual symptoms, says Susan Thys-Jacobs, M.D., an endocrinologist and assistant professor of medicine at St. Luke's–Roosevelt Hospital Center in New York City.

Premenstrual pain may be moderated by calcium's effects on smooth muscle, suggests James Penland, Ph.D., research psychologist at the USDA Human Nutrition Research Center at Grand Forks, North Dakota, who also researched calcium and menstrual symptoms. The mineral makes smooth muscles—like those found in the uterus—work better.

Most exciting, says Dr. Thys-Jacobs, are the results of a small study she conducted on 13 women with polycystic ovarian syndrome, a disorder characterized by absent or irregular menstruation, excess body hair, extreme overweight, and infertility.

> ## MASKED DISASTER
> ### Cream Cheese
> Don't kid yourself into thinking cream cheese counts as a calcium-rich dairy choice. A tablespoon of regular cream cheese has a measly 12 milligrams of calcium but 5 grams of fat. A better bet for your bagel is 2 tablespoons of 1% cottage cheese, which has 17 milligrams of calcium and less than 0.5 gram of fat.

By adding vitamin D and calcium to their diets, their menstrual cycles normalized in 2 months for seven of the women, with two becoming pregnant.

"Calcium seems to play a major role in development of the egg cell in the ovary," says Dr. Thys-Jacobs. "Perhaps if you don't have enough calcium and vitamin D, these cells go into a stage of arrest: They stop maturing and stop differentiating."

Although the results are very preliminary, Dr. Thys-Jacobs says that they have potentially important results for women who have trouble getting pregnant.

Are You Really Lactose Intolerant?

Yeah, yeah, yeah, you're saying. I know milk is good for me. But I can't drink it. I'm lactose intolerant. Well, maybe you are, and maybe you aren't.

"One out of three women who think that they're lactose intolerant are not," says Fabrizis Suarez, M.D., Ph.D., assistant professor in the department of food science and nutrition and a faculty member in the department of medicine of the University of Minneapolis in Minnesota.

Lactose intolerance occurs when you lack the enzyme that digests lactose, a sugar found in dairy products. People who are lactose intolerant often have bloating, gas, and diarrhea when they drink milk and other dairy products.

But Dr. Suarez's studies show that most adults can handle 2 cups of milk a day with no problem if they drink the milk in two widely divided doses and with other foods. In fact, his research shows that drinking milk and eating other lactose-containing dairy foods may actually improve your ability to digest the sugar.

Even women who are somewhat lactose intolerant, he says, should be able to consume 1,500 milligrams of calcium from dairy sources without major symptoms.

Here's how to avoid some of the symptoms.

Start small. Try ½ cup of milk with a meal and gradually build up.

Say cheese. Hard cheeses like Cheddar, Colby, Swiss, and Parmesan have very low levels of lactose.

Spoon it up. The live and active cultures in yogurt help digest lactose, and ice cream has less lactose than milk.

Go chocolate. Chocolate milk may be easier on your stomach.

Hit the drugstore. Use an over-the-counter lactase digestive aid.

Get on the Dairy Train

Ready to take on the white stuff? Then follow some of these suggestions.

CALCIUM ALTERNATIVES

While dairy products are still the best sources of calcium per calorie (1 cup of fat-free milk has 302 milligrams), you can get calcium from other foods—but only if you eat enough of them. Don't depend on spinach as a calcium source, though: You absorb very little because of the binders it contains.

FOOD	SERVING SIZE	CALCIUM (mg)	SERVINGS NEEDED TO EQUAL 1 CUP OF FAT-FREE MILK
Green beans, snap, cooked	½ cup	33	More than 10
Broccoli, cooked, chopped	½ cup	36	More than 8
Figs, dried	3	82	Almost 4
Kale	1 cup	91	More than 3
Blackstrap molasses	1 Tbsp	172	About 2
Sardines with bones (canned in oil)	3 oz	325	Less than 1
Tofu	½ cup	434	Less than 1

Go low-fat. That means 1% or fat-free milk—not 2%, which the FDA has forbidden milk manufacturers from calling low-fat. Low-fat dairy products have exactly the same amount of calcium and other minerals as the regular stuff.

Go with what you love. That's ice cream, right? Or frozen yogurt. Or ice milk. For the 265 calories in a cup of vanilla ice cream, you'll reap 169 milligrams of calcium. How about a milkshake instead of a cola with that hamburger? One cup gives you 203 milligrams of calcium. Make it with fat-free milk, and lower the calories. Can't stand low-fat ice cream? Try chocolate-flavored. When researchers conducted taste tests, more than 100 students at the University of Missouri found "no significant difference" in the flavor of low-fat versus regular chocolate ice cream.

Tote it. Slip a few calcium-rich, low-fat cheese sticks into your purse when you run errands, take the yogurts with spoons right in the lids to soccer games, or try boxed milk that doesn't need refrigeration.

Hide it. Add nonfat dry milk powder or solids to casseroles, meat loaf, soups, and other dishes. Each teaspoon provides about 94 milligrams of calcium, and you can add up to 5 tablespoons—containing 1,410 milligrams, or an entire day's worth of calcium. Use fat-free milk instead of water when making soups and oatmeal.

Some coffee with that milk? Fill your cup almost to the top with milk and *then* add coffee. Not only will you get nearly one-third of your daily calcium requirement, but you'll neutralize the ability of the caffeine to interfere with calcium absorption.

Add syrup. One reason women don't drink milk is because they just don't like the way it tastes, says Alma J. Blake, R.D., Ph.D., assistant professor of nutrition and food science at the University of Maryland in Baltimore, who surveyed 100 women about their milk-drinking habits. But many women love chocolate, so it came as no surprise that in a taste test, women preferred chocolate milk to strawberry milk. Dr. Blake speculates that because many parents commonly add flavoring to milk in order to get children to drink it, this may influence their taste preferences as adults. So go ahead, add chocolate syrup, vanilla extract, or one of the flavorings made for coffee. Even use a teaspoon of sugar if that's what it takes.

Dunk it. Cut up fruit and vegetables and dunk them in low-fat, flavored yogurt for a healthy, calcium-packed snack. "One cup of yogurt probably has the most significant amount of calcium you can get in one item," says Lorna Pascal, R.D., a nutrition consultant at the Dave Winfield Nutrition Center at Hackensack University Medical Center in New Jersey.

Make super milk. Add a couple of tablespoons of nonfat dry milk to your glass of milk to up the calcium and other nutrients.

Finish your milk. In the bottom of your bowl of cereal, that is. "If you leave the milk, you're not getting the benefits," says Pascal.

Have dessert. Make or buy fat-free puddings for dessert. Each ½-cup serving contains ½ cup of milk.

Protein and Carbohydrates: Find the Safe Balance for You

Power Maker #10: When it comes to calculating your protein and carbohydrate needs, we have one word for you: Don't. Instead, follow the "plate rule": Vegetables should fill 75 percent of your plate; meat, 25 percent.

Steak houses are sizzling. Low-carb, high-protein-diet books are bestsellers. And the shelves of drugstores and health food stores groan under the weight of over 100 new protein-fortified products—everything from the standard power bars to protein-fortified cookies.

In recent years, protein has made a comeback and carbohydrates have lost favor—at least among the pro-protein champs, who blame carbohydrates for the fattening of America.

Their theory is that a high-carb diet encourages the body to store fat. A few high-protein zealots are so down on whole grains—and even some fruits and vegetables—that you half expect them to blame carbohydrates for tax hikes, high crime, and bad hair days.

With all this renewed fanfare espousing the power of protein, many women jumped on the pro-protein bandwagon. Our advice: Don't!

123

"While protein is essential to good health, we need a surprisingly small amount of it. Many women already eat far too much," says Ellen Glovsky, R.D., Ph.D., a nutritionist at the Boston University Nutrition Group, which is affiliated with Boston Medical Center.

A high-protein diet also tends to be high in cholesterol and fat, particularly saturated fat. Further, "a calorie is a calorie, and extra calories from protein go to your thighs as surely as any other extra calories," says Dr. Glovsky.

In short, she says, "Carbohydrates aren't the enemy. And protein isn't a miracle. Both are vital to a woman's physical health." What you need to do is consume the right balance between the two and be discriminating in your selection of each.

Here, then, is a woman's guide to protein and carbs—what they do, how much you need, and how to get the most from both.

Protein: The All-Purpose Nutrient

Protein is the little black dress of nutrients. It comes in a dazzling array of styles. It's versatile. And you really can't live without it.

Your cells contain protein, which is used for carrying out an astonishing number of functions. It helps to grow and repair body tissues, make disease-fighting antibodies, and facilitate chemical reactions. One type of protein delivers oxygen to your cells; others carry vitamins and minerals. Like those "it slices, it dices" gizmos on the infomercials, protein does it all.

Proteins are made of amino acids, and amino acids might be likened to the letters of the alphabet. Like letters, amino acids can be arranged in an infinite number of combinations, all of which determine protein's unique functions. While our bodies can make most of these amino acids, nine are found only in food.

Meat, eggs, and other animal foods, which contain these nine essential amino acids, are complete proteins. The protein in plant foods is incomplete—it lacks one or more of the essential amino acids. But this doesn't mean you need meat at every meal. A small amount of complete protein during the day is sufficient. Also, if you eat a wide variety of plant foods, the amino acids missing in one food will be provided by another.

A Sorority of Meatheads

"I would say that the average woman gets more than twice the protein she needs," says Lisa Young, R.D., Ph.D., adjunct professor in the department of nutrition and food studies at New York University in New York City. The Daily Value of protein is 50 grams, and you can get close to that amount in just one 6-ounce can of water-packed tuna and two pieces of whole grain bread.

WHAT ABOUT PROTEIN DRINKS?

You've seen those high-protein weight-loss drinks and powders that claim to burn fat. Do they?

No, says David Pearson, Ph.D., an exercise physiologist at Ball State University in Muncie, Indiana. "There are no 'fat-burning foods,' and high-protein weight-loss drinks don't burn fat either," he says. The fat-burning claim may stem from a small grain of truth—that muscle burns more calories than fat. Well, it does. But glugging down a glass of collagen, amino acids, or generic "protein" won't help you build muscle. "This is theoretical physiology stretched as far as it will go," he says.

Consider, for example, the "hydrolyzed collagen" added to some high-protein powders. "In layman's language, hydrolyzed collagen—or collagen hydrolysate—is plain old gelatin, the cheapest form of protein there is," he says.

The bottom line on protein supplements is to skip them. "As always, weight loss comes down to the basics—eating less and exercising more," says Dr. Pearson.

WHY HIGH-PROTEIN DIETS ARE DANGEROUS

Chances are you've tried a high-protein diet. And why not? On one plan, you're allowed—heck, encouraged—to feast on hard salami, grilled chicken sandwiches with cheese and bacon, and pork rinds.

We hate to break it to you, but while you probably will lose weight initially on this fare, you'll almost certainly find it again. In one survey of 1,000 people, 40 percent said they tried a high-protein diet to lose weight—and 40 percent of those dieters said the weight came back.

High-protein diets work because they are very low in calories. "Some are as low as 800 calories a day," says Constance Geiger, R.D., Ph.D., research assistant professor in the division of foods and nutrition at the University of Utah in Salt Lake City.

Further, the "weight" you lose during the first couple of weeks on a high-protein diet is mostly water, not fat. When they're stored in our bodies, carbohydrates—the body's primary source of energy—hold water, says Susan Nitzke, R.D., Ph.D., professor of nutritional sciences at the University of Wisconsin in Madison. So as you use up the last of your stored carbohydrate fuel, you'll have a false sense of success—you'll feel lighter but won't necessarily be leaner.

But here's the scary part: High-protein diets can also jeopardize your health. They can cause headaches, dizziness, fatigue, and nausea, says Dr. Nitzke. One cause is ketosis. It occurs when the body, desperate for carbohydrate fuel, turns to fat and breaks it down too quickly.

What's more, these diets are astronomically high in fat—especially saturated fat, says Dr. Geiger. Research shows that the more saturated fat you consume, the higher your risk for heart disease.

High-protein diets are especially hard on the liver and kidneys, which must work harder to break down and eliminate all that protein and fat, says Dr. Nitzke. Pregnant women and women with kidney problems or diabetes—who are vulnerable to kidney disease—should not embark on a high-protein diet without medical supervision, she says.

Most of the excess protein that most of us eat comes from meat. Just 3 ounces of lean ground beef packs 21 grams of protein—and restaurants routinely serve burgers made with double or triple that amount. So it's easy to see how meat can put you into protein overload.

Worried that you won't get enough protein if you cut back on meat? Don't be. Even the conservative American Dietetic Association says that we can get enough protein from plant foods alone, providing that we eat a variety of them and consume enough calories.

"Legumes, particularly lentils, lima beans, and chickpeas, are excellent sources of protein," says Carmen Conrey, R.D., senior clinical dietitian at the Johns Hopkins Weight Management Center in Baltimore. "Whole grains such as brown rice and barley also contain protein." And unlike animal protein, beans and grains are packed with fiber—and they won't cause a plaque pileup in your arteries.

Carbohydrate: Energy to Burn

Jelly beans. Whole wheat bread. Cupcakes. Broccoli. As different as they may seem, all are carbohydrates, the substances from which you extract the "juice" that makes you run.

That juice is glucose, or one of the sugars most important in nutrition. Glucose is the main source of fuel for your brain, which uses up to 600 calories' worth of glucose a day. Glucose is stored in your liver and muscles as glycogen, which your body converts back to glucose when you need it—during exercise or when you're under serious stress. (Along with a pounding heart and sweaty palms, you get a burst of glucose during the fight-or-flight reaction, the body's automatic response to stress.)

There are two types of carbohydrates: simple and complex. Simple carbohydrates are found in foods like fruit, sugar, and milk. Complex carbohydrates are found in the fibers and starches in plant foods. Whole grains, potatoes, and pasta contain complex carbs, as do vegetables and legumes.

Both simple and complex carbohydrates end up as glucose. So does it matter whether you tank up with jelly beans and low-fat pastry or beans and brussels sprouts? You bet it does, says Conrey. You can't prevent heart disease or cancer on a diet of white flour and sugar. It's the slew of protective substances in fruits, vegetables, legumes, and whole grains that keep you healthy and prevent disease. Plus, complex carbs are usually lower in fat than the refined simple carbs.

Carbo-Loading for Health

Slightly more than half of your total daily calories—55 to 60 percent—should come from carbohydrates, primarily the unrefined kind, says Conrey. So eat more fruits and vegetables, beans, and whole grains.

It's particularly important to heed the whole grain message, says Constance Geiger, R.D., Ph.D., research assistant professor in the division of foods and nutrition at the University of Utah in Salt Lake City. (For details, see Grains: Powerhouses of Nutrition on page 62.)

Here is your step-by-step strategy for carbo-loading the healthy way. In each category of food, opt for the lower number of servings if you are not very active, and opt for the upper number if you are active.

Fruit: Get two to four servings a day.

One serving equals: One whole, medium fruit; half of a grapefruit or ½ cup of berries; ½ cup of chopped, cooked, or canned fruit; ¾ cup of fruit juice; ¼ cup of dried fruit.

Smart picks and tips: Select pink grapefruit if available—it's higher in the anti-cancer phytonutrient lycopene than the white variety. Eat lots of berries, particularly strawberries. They are loaded with ellagic acid, a compound that's been found to decrease the risk of cancer. Instead of drinking fruit juice, eat whole fruit, recommends Conrey. You'll get a dose of fiber along with other nutrients.

Vegetables: Get three to five servings a day.

One serving equals: 1 cup of raw leafy vegetables; ½ cup of cooked or canned vegetables; one medium sweet or white potato; ¾ cup of vegetable juice.

Waistline

The ideal proportion of carbohydrates, fat, and protein: 55 to 60 percent carbohydrates (mostly complex carbohydrates), 25 to 30 percent fat, 12 to 15 percent protein.

What the average woman actually eats: 50 percent carbohydrates, 35 percent fat, 15 percent protein.

UPGRAIN YOUR DIET

I t's simple to switch to 100 percent whole grain bread and cereal. But are there tasty alternatives to other refined products? Yes, there are. Here are a few to get you going with the (whole) grain.

INSTEAD OF . . .	TRY THIS . . .
A doughnut	Half of a large toasted cinnamon-raisin bagel
Ritz crackers	Whole wheat crackers
A multigrain cereal bar	A microwaved apple, pear, or banana topped with cinnamon and raisins
Regular spaghetti	Whole wheat spaghetti
Nacho chips	Hard, whole wheat pretzels

Smart picks and tips: When it comes to vegetables, fresh is best—if you use them right away. But buy frozen veggies if fresh ones tend to languish in your crisper. (The frozen may contain more nutrients than days-old "fresh" vegetables.) Make salads with dark greens, such as romaine lettuce and spinach, rather than pale iceberg lettuce—they pack more nutrients. Try to eat at least one dark leafy green a day. Kale, spinach, mustard greens, turnip greens, and Swiss chard contain phytonutrients found to help prevent heart disease and cancer and to protect against macular degeneration, a debilitating eye disease. Use sweet potatoes more than white potatoes; they're an excellent source of beta-carotene.

Breads, grains, and cereals: Get 6 to 11 servings a day.

One serving equals: One slice of bread; ½ to 1 cup of cold cereal (check labels for the amount that will provide approximately 70 to 90 calories); ½ cup of cooked cereal such as oatmeal; ½ cup of cooked pasta; ½ cup of cooked rice; half of an English muffin or bagel.

Smart picks and tips: Choose whole grain everything—bread, cereal, pasta, snack crackers—says Dr. Young. Check the product's list of ingredients; the first word should be "whole," as in whole wheat. If it isn't, that brand is using all or mostly white flour. Be wary of "wheat," "seven-grain," and "stone-ground" loaves; most are made with white flour. Bread should contain at least 2 grams of fiber per slice; cereals, at least 3 grams of fiber per serving.

Fats: Are You Getting Enough of the Right Kind?

Power Maker #11: Use regular, not fat-free, salad dressing, preferably made with olive or canola oil, which protects women against heart disease and helps the body absorb nutrients found in vegetables.

Admit it: You're more likely to count grams of fat than calories or cholesterol these days. Your refrigerator and pantry are crammed with more low-fat and fat-free prepared foods than a test kitchen. And when you do bring home the regular version of a food, like real ice cream, your kids go into shock.

Nutrition professor Alice H. Lichtenstein, D.Sc., professor of nutrition at the Jean Mayer USDA Human Nutrition Research Center on Aging at Tufts University in Boston, calls it our national obsession with fat intake.

And the worries start young: A poll of schoolchildren found that 81 percent thought that the healthiest diet of all was one that eliminated all dietary fat.

The truth is, banishing fat is one of the *least* healthy things they could do.

Low-Fat Myths

Fat has been indicted for causing heart disease, breast cancer, and obesity. But the connections are just not that clear.

Heart disease. It's true that a high-fat diet has been implicated in heart disease. But it's the *kind* of fat we're eating in high-fat diets that's most closely related to heart disease. In one study, Harvard School of Public Health researchers including Frank B. Hu, M.D., Ph.D., professor of nutrition at Harvard University, investigated replacing "bad" fats—saturated fats (like those found in red meat) and trans fatty acids (the manmade version found in margarine)—with "good" fats like olive, canola, and fish oils. Changing the type of fat did a better job of preventing coronary heart disease in women than did reducing overall fat intake.

Breast cancer. Some time back, researchers noticed that women from Asian countries and other areas with traditionally low-fat diets had low rates of breast cancer but developed breast cancer at rates equal to Americans when they moved here and began eating our diet. They assumed that the fat in our diet was to blame. Wrong. "Fat intake doesn't make any difference in the incidence of breast cancer," says Michelle D. Holmes, M.D., Ph.D., an instructor in medicine at Harvard Medical School who has researched this area. In fact, some studies suggest that intake of good fats like olive oil may *reduce* the risk of breast cancer.

Overweight. Contrary to what you (and many others) have come to believe, fat molecules in food are not transformed directly into body fat, nor do they go directly from our mouths to our butts, stomachs, and thighs. In other words, the ice cream you ate last night has not necessarily taken up permanent residence on your hips.

It's true that any excess calories are stored as fat. But those calories can come from carbohydrates, protein, or fat.

Dietary fat does contribute to overweight in another way, however: It has more calories per gram than protein or carbohydrates. Compared to 4 calories in each gram of carbohydrate or protein, there are 9 in fat (and 7 in alcohol). So if too much of your food is high in fat and you don't reduce the amount of food you eat, you're going to get too many calories and—voilà!—get fat.

Hence our low-fat paranoia.

Good Intentions Gone Too Far

Even women who aren't particularly health conscious can probably re-cite the recommendations for fat intake: between 25 and 30 percent of our overall diet. But for many, "less fat" automatically translates into "no fat."

It's a message that's been taken to the extreme in such diets as Dr. Dean Ornish's very low fat diet, with less than 10 percent of calories coming from fat, or the Pritikin Diet.

While no one is suggesting that we begin loading up on butter, whole milk, and french fries every day, neither should we focus solely on re-ducing overall fat intake, says James O. Hill, Ph.D., associate director of the Center for Human Nutrition at the University of Colorado Health Sciences Center in Denver. "It surprises me that people don't give a bal-anced view of this," he says. "They attribute so many positive and nega-tive things to fats, and the truth is really somewhere in the middle."

Your Body Needs Fat

We need fat—to help us feel full, so food tastes better, to get essen-tial vitamins into our bodies, and to protect our hearts, immune sys-tems, and even psyches. Fat is the reason bacon and hamburgers smell so good on the grill, why the aromas of sautéed onions and stir-fried vegetables can make our stomachs growl.

Without fat, vitamins A, D, E, and K can't get into our cells. Horse-back riding would hurt, and we'd be cold all the time. Although some fat has been shown to increase our risk of heart disease, other types can protect us.

And get this: Too little fat in our diets may be harmful, not helpful, to heart health. Some studies show that very low fat diets may raise levels of a dangerous form of cholesterol, called LDL, while significantly lowering high-density lipoprotein (HDL), our "good" cholesterol, says Mary Flynn, R.D., Ph.D., assistant professor of medicine at Brown Uni-versity in Providence, Rhode Island, and coauthor of *Low-Fat Lies, High-Fat Fraud.*

When all is said and done, what really counts is how much of various kinds of fat you eat. Most foods that contain fat, even vegetable oils, con-tain various proportions of saturated, monounsaturated, and polyunsat-urated fat. Each act differently in your body.

POWER

SALAD DRESSING

TOMATO "VINAIGRETTE"

If fat-free salad dressings leave you cold, listen up. The olive oil in a typical vinaigrette is packed with disease-fighting monounsaturates—something fat-free dressings lack. To keep calories low in homemade dressing, replace part of the oil with water and then kick up the flavor with herbs. The generous dollop of tomato paste used here also heightens flavor—and adds lycopene that helps prevent heart disease and cancer.

This dressing is infinitely variable. You easily can replace the basil with marjoram, oregano, tarragon, dill, or other herbs (and by all means use fresh herbs if you have them). For a Tex-Mex flair, use lime juice and chopped cilantro—perfect for jazzing up a bean salad or sliced avocados (more monounsaturates).

$\frac{1}{2}$ cup water

2   tablespoons tomato paste

2   tablespoons lemon juice

1   tablespoon grated onion

1   clove garlic, crushed

$\frac{1}{2}$ teaspoon dried basil

$\frac{1}{4}$ teaspoon salt

$\frac{1}{8}$ teaspoon ground black pepper

$\frac{1}{3}$ cup olive oil

In a blender, combine the water, tomato paste, lemon juice, onion, garlic, basil, salt, and pepper. Blend until smooth. With the blender running, slowly add the oil.

Makes 1 cup

Per tablespoon: 43 calories, 0 g protein, 1 g carbohydrates, 4.5 g fat, 0 mg cholesterol, 0 g dietary fiber, 50 mg sodium

Note: Store leftover dressing in a covered container in the refrigerator for up to 3 days. Shake the container or whisk the dressing before using.

Saturated Fat: More Than a Smidgen Is Superfluous

Animal products like hamburger and dairy products, as well as palm and coconut oils, have the highest concentrations of saturated fat. This type of fat has more hydrogen atoms than other types of fat. It's heavier and stickier in a sense, and it's solid at room temperature.

MASKED DISASTER

Reduced-Fat Milk and Burgers

According to the label, reduced-fat milk is just 2 percent fat. And ground beef is just 20 percent fat. So they should qualify as ways to keep your fat intake at 25 percent, right?

Those percentages are by weight, not by percentage of calories. In actuality, 2% milk has 35 to 37 percent of calories from fat, and 20% ground beef has 60 percent of calories from fat.

Your best bets are to opt for 1% or fat-free milk, with only 20 percent or fewer calories from fat, or ground sirloin or round, at 92 percent lean, for 40 percent of calories from fat.

Eating foods high in saturated fat seems to increase our risk of heart disease and stroke. That's because saturated fats raise levels of LDL, the "bad" cholesterol that attaches itself to the walls of our arteries, where it can build up hard deposits, blocking blood-flow and leading to heart disease.

The saturated fat in foods has a far greater effect on blood levels of cholesterol in our bodies than does the cholesterol in foods, which, contrary to popular belief, is not a type of fat. Even just one meal high in saturated fats can spark a dramatic rise in a blood component that can, over time, increase the risk of death from heart disease and stroke.

"Our bodies need some saturated fat, and it's almost impossible to avoid in a normal diet," says Glenn A. Gaesser, Ph.D., professor of health and physical education at the University of Virginia in Charlottesville. "But you don't need to consume any extra saturated fat."

Foods like lard are virtually all saturated fat, while some oils—like canola oil—contain very little, about 7 percent. So it's difficult to avoid saturated fat completely. Nevertheless, no more than 7 percent of your calories should come from saturated fat, and preferably less, Dr. Gaesser says. We currently get about 11 percent of our daily calories from saturated fat. The difference is equal to about three pats of butter.

Monounsaturated Fat: The Elixir of Life

The predominant fat in canola and olive oils is monounsaturated fat. In various studies, olive oil has been shown to reduce the risk of developing high blood pressure, arthritis, cataracts, and osteoporosis. Monounsaturated fats are considered one of the critical elements in the so-called Mediterranean diet, which, while deriving a relatively high proportion of calories—up to 40 percent—from fat, seems to result in extremely low levels of heart disease.

One of the reasons, Dr. Flynn says, is that the primary fat used is olive oil.

Monos also improve overall cholesterol levels—one of the greatest indicators of your risk for heart disease. In addition to lowering levels of bad LDL, they appear to raise levels of good HDL. HDL is important because it acts like the street cleaner of the bloodstream, sweeping away bad LDL particles and returning them to the liver for processing, says Dimitrios Trichopoulos, M.D., professor of cancer prevention at Harvard University. Some studies also report that olive oil may reduce the risk of several kinds of cancer, including breast and colorectal cancers.

As for how much monounsaturated fat is healthy, Dr. Hu says, "There really is no upper limit, as long as your total intake of fat is balanced with your physical activity."

Polyunsaturated Fats: A Mixed Bag

Typically found in vegetable oils, nuts, fish, and some leafy green vegetables, polyunsaturated fats are the good fats—sometimes.

Years ago, nutritionists touted polyunsaturated oils as the best, sparking a boom in purchases of margarine over butter and vegetable oil over lard. While they're better than saturated fats, they're not as good as monounsaturated fats. Polys tend to lower overall cholesterol by lowering levels of bad LDL. But they also lower levels of good HDL.

Some researchers think that's because with less LDL, the body needs less HDL. Others disagree, particularly when it comes to postmenopausal women who are at greatest risk of heart disease. HDL levels of 50 or lower are truly dangerous, almost regardless of LDL levels.

Omega-3's: The Good Polys

You can avoid the HDL-lowering effects of polyunsaturated fats if you increase the amount of one kind of poly: omega-3 fatty acids.

These are one of two types of critical fatty acids found in food, which our bodies can't make: omega-3 and omega-6. Together, they are vital for brain development, the health of our eyes, immune function, and bone repair, says Robert Wildman, R.D., Ph.D., assistant professor of nutrition at University of Louisiana at Lafayette.

The problem is that omega-6 fatty acids tend to oxidize in our bodies, throwing off cell-damaging forces known as free radicals that cruise

TAKE IT EASY WITH FAKE FATS

It sounds too good to be true—foods that taste the same as their high-fat cousins, but whose fat passes harmlessly out of your body instead of heading to your backside.

Food manufacturers have come up with several kinds of fat that pass through your body unabsorbed. But are they safe? Here's the scoop.

OLESTRA. A combination of sugars and vegetable oil, this can be heated and is used in snack foods like potato chips.

Because Olestra is not absorbed by the body, it interferes with absorption of vitamins like A, D, E, and K, which depend on fat for absorption. The same goes for phytonutrients like carotenoids, found in fruits and vegetables, if they are consumed along with Olestra.

Some people report increased flatulence, diarrhea, and stomach cramps from Olestra. But several studies with thousands of volunteers found that Olestra had no more negative effects on the digestive system than any other kind of fatty snack food.

NUTRIM. A cross between barley and oat bran, this is used in baked goods, ice cream, salad dressings, and sauces. You need less to achieve the same results as with other fat substitutes, and it's less expensive. Nutritionally, it offers no particular disadvantages.

around our bodies trying to steal electrons from other cells, damaging healthy cells in the process.

Free radicals have been implicated in aging, cancer, and heart disease. They cause LDL to stick to artery walls, leading to heart disease. Some evidence indicates that polys may increase the risk for breast cancer.

Omega-3 fatty acids, however, found primarily in fatty fish like sardines, halibut, and salmon, make platelets in the blood smoother, more slippery, and less likely to stick to arteries.

It's important, however, that you not only get more omega-3 fatty acids but also balance the omega-6 fatty acids. To do that, simply reduce the amount of omega-6 fatty acids—found in many vegetable oils like

OATRIM. One of several fiber-based, carbohydrate fat substitutes, this is used in baked goods. It has no reported digestive side effects, and it imparts some of the same health benefits as fiber. It may not impart the same rich taste as real fat, however.

SIMPLESSE AND TRAILBLAZER. Protein-based fat substitutes, often used in dairy products and mayonnaise, these provide just a bit of extra protein—without loss of nutrients.

SALATRIM. This is a partially digestible fat similar to Olestra, with similarly reported side effects, although it doesn't interfere with the absorption of fat-soluble vitamins and nutrients. This pseudo-fat has about half the calories of true fat and is used in salad dressings.

Ironically, eating fat-free products may end up making you fat, expressly because of their lack of fat. "Fat does act as an appetite signal, telling your brain that you're full," explains Stanley Segall, Ph.D., professor of nutrition and food science at Drexel University in Philadelphia. No fat, no signal to brake. "People tend to eat more when they're eating fat-free substitutes, partly because they don't feel full, and also because they don't feel guilty."

Your best bet is to check out the fat-free aisle at the grocery store, otherwise known as the produce section.

sunflower, safflower, corn, and soybean oils—and increase the amount of omega-3 fatty acids in your diet.

Optimal omega-3 intake is at least 500 milligrams a day of the omega-3's found in fish—under 1 percent of your overall daily fat intake. No more than 10 percent of your total calories should come from polyunsaturated fats, according to the American Heart Association.

Sound complicated? It's not. Simply make two changes: Increase the amount of cold-water fish in your diet, especially salmon, mackerel, or tuna. And substitute olive or canola oil for other cooking fats. Your Day-to-Day Power-Eating Plan on page 541 shows you how to do this.

Trans Fats: Saturated Fats in Disguise

Take an otherwise innocuous polyunsaturated fat, whip it up with some hydrogen to make it solid at room temperature, and presto! You've created trans fatty acids, found in many prepared foods like cakes and cookies, and in meat, dairy products, and margarine.

If you're like many women, you may have switched from butter to margarine years ago, thinking you were doing your heart a favor. The problem is that trans fats have been implicated in heart disease and possibly in breast cancer. A large Brandeis University study on trans fats showed that they may even be worse than saturated fats: Not only do they raise damaging LDL levels as do saturated fats, they also appear to lower HDL levels.

Basically, the more liquid a fat is, the less it is composed of trans fatty acids. Soft margarine, or tub margarine, has fewer trans fatty acids than stick margarine, for example.

Even though there is no official limit on the amount of trans fatty acids we should get, Dr. Hu says we should eliminate them altogether.

Waistline

Ninety percent of women consume low-fat, reduced-fat, or fat-free beverages.

THE LOWDOWN ON LOW-FAT FOODS

Think you'll get the fat out—and lose the weight—by switching to prepared low-fat or fat-free foods? Think again. Despite the proliferation of such items on grocery shelves, Americans have only gotten fatter.

"With the emphasis on low-fat and fat-free, people thought calories didn't count," says Glenn A. Gaesser, Ph.D., professor of health and physical education at the University of Virginia in Charlottesville and author of *Big Fat Lies*.

But calories still count. In the Nurses' Health Study at Harvard University, the more sugar-free diet products the women ate, the more likely they were to gain weight. They thought sugar-free meant calorie-free, so they ate even more.

As for fat-free goodies, in order to enhance the taste, manufacturers loaded them up with sugar, to the point where some have even more calories than their fattier counterparts.

"It's not unusual to discover people on fat-free diets consuming more calories than those on the fattier diets," says Stanley Segall, Ph.D., professor of nutrition and food science at Drexel University in Philadelphia.

The real goal behind reducing our fat was to consume more of our calories in the form of fruits, vegetables, and whole grains, not to make up the difference with fake-fat, high-sugar, calorie-dense cakes and cookies, says Alice H. Lichtenstein, D.Sc., professor of nutrition at the Jean Mayer USDA Human Nutrition Research Center on Aging at Tufts University in Boston.

In other words, just because something is low-fat or fat-free doesn't mean it's low-calorie or your best choice.

But as with saturated fat, that's not entirely practical: Some otherwise healthy foods—like whole grain crackers—contain some hydrogenated oil, and therefore, trans fats. So nutrition experts recommend counting trans fats as part of your saturated-fat budget.

At this time, nutrition labels on food don't list trans fats. But it's easy to figure out how much a given food has. Just add the total amount of saturated, polyunsaturated, and monounsaturated fats and subtract it from the total amount of fat. That's the amount of trans-fat grams.

Finally, don't switch back to butter just to avoid trans fats in margarine. Butter has 8 grams of saturated fat per tablespoon, more than the combined total of trans and saturated fats in a tablespoon of stick margarine. And now there are two new margarines that have been formulated to be trans-free, Benecol and Take Control, which tout their cholesterol-lowering benefits.

Out with the Bad, In with the Good

For all our focus on low-fat diets, the amount of fat in our diets has actually been increasing, with the average woman consuming 65 grams of fat a day. On an 1,800-calorie diet with no more than 25 percent of our calories coming from fat, we should get 50 grams or less.

And that should be 50 grams of *good* fat.

If you're like many women, you've probably already switched to fat-free milk and dairy products. And you know that you should trim visible fat from pork and beef and remove the skin from poultry. Here's what else you can do.

- Switch from butter to non–trans fat margarines or, better yet, dip your bread in olive oil.

- Use wine; lemon, orange, or tomato juice; herbs; spices; fruits; or broth instead of butter or vegetable oils when cooking.

- Switch from vegetable oil to canola or olive oil and use liquid fats whenever possible.

- Increase the amount of fruits and vegetables in your diet instead of substituting fat-free foods for their high-fat counterparts.

- Check ingredient lists for partially hydrogenated oil of any kind. These foods contain trans fats. Keep them to a minimum.

- Avoid fried foods—particularly fast-food french fries. Most are fried in partially hydrogenated vegetable oil, that is, trans fats.

Liquids of Life:
Good, Better, Best

I ts bouquet could best be described as insipid, with perhaps just a whisper of iron. Upon the tongue, the initial taste is one of a crystal clear stream, with overtones of moss, or perhaps an oak leaf. It swallows cleanly with no overt aftertaste, leaving just the slightest hint of swimming pool in the back of the throat.

So it's not a fine Bordeaux. But water, just plain water—even from the tap—is worth more to your body than the rarest Burgundy is to a wine collector. It's one of nature's most important nutrients, and one of which most women don't get nearly enough.

On average, we drink 4.7 cups of water-based liquids—juice, soda, coffee, and so on—a day. Less than half is plain water. Yet you need at least 9 cups of fluid a day, more if you're doing anything more strenuous than working at a keyboard. And new research shows that at least 5 cups of that should be plain water.

"The biggest problems that I see among women whom I advise is that they won't exercise and they won't drink their water," says Anne Dubner, R.D., a Houston-based nutritionist and a spokesperson for American Dietetic Association. "They say that they don't like water or they forget or they aren't thirsty."

What they don't understand, say Dubner and other nutritionists, is that water does much more than quench thirst. On a day-by-day basis, it keeps you alert, cools you off, and makes your skin glow. It helps prevent diseases ranging from cancer to kidney stones. It can even help you lose weight. It all starts with the first sip.

Invisible but Essential

We're made up of so much water that it's a wonder we don't squish when we walk. The average woman's body is made up of 50 to 55 percent water, a bit less than a man's because we have more fat, and fat contains less water.

Water is an essential nutrient. And unlike other essential nutrients such as vitamins and minerals, where a deficiency may take weeks or months to develop, you can only go a few days without water.

Even without serious sweating, you can lose nearly 4 percent of your body weight every day in water. So your "daily value" for water is figured not on how much you weigh, but on how many calories you burn. For the typical woman who burns 1,800 to 2,200 calories a day, that equates to 9 cups. In hot weather, you need half again as much. And add another cup for every 240 additional calories you burn.

POWER-EATING TIP

To stay hydrated on airline flights, drink at least one 8-ounce glass of water for every hour that you are in the air. Airplane air is some of the driest around.

Are You Really Tired—Or Just Dehydrated?

If you are experiencing headache, fatigue, dizziness, and maybe a burning sensation in your stomach, don't blame it on stress. It could be that you are slightly dehydrated.

When you don't drink enough, your cells start drying out. To quench their thirst, they suck fluid from the bloodstream, which leaves your blood thick and sludgy, like refrigerated olive oil. Thus your heart has to pump harder to push the blood through, which can tire you out more than a toddler on caffeine.

Frequent colds may be another side effect of dehydration. The mucus that coats your throat contains antibodies and can trap cold viruses. But if you're even minimally dehydrated, the viruses have a better shot at survival because your dried-out tissues aren't producing enough mucus.

And forget about waiting until you're thirsty to drink. By then, you have already dehydrated 0.8 to 2 percent of your total body weight. At a dehydration level of just a little more than 3 percent, you are dangerously low on fluid and need medical attention.

Bathroom Breaks

If you drink all this water, you are bound to find yourself making hourly trips to the bathroom. "That's a good thing," says Susan Kleiner, R.D., Ph.D., assistant professor of nutrition at the University of Washington in Seattle and author of *Power Eating*. "It gets your blood moving. Your mind works better when you get up."

POWER-EATING TIP

If you are going to the bathroom every 2 to 4 hours, you are probably drinking enough. While you're there, check your urine. It will be pale yellow or clear if you're getting enough water.

Not Just Any Beverage Will Do

Like many nutritionists, Dr. Kleiner used to tell women that any fluid that didn't contain alcohol or caffeine counted as water. No more. A growing body of evidence says that water alone—plain H_2O—helps to reduce a woman's risk of developing certain cancers and other diseases.

Urinary tract cancer. When researchers in Hawaii compared 66 women with bladder, renal pelvic, and urethral cancers to cancer-free women, they found that the more a woman drank—particularly if her drink of choice was water—the lower her risk of cancer (about 30 percent lower).

Similarly, researchers analyzing data on 47,900 men found that those drinking 6 cups of water a day cut their risk of bladder cancer in half compared with men drinking only 1 cup a day. It makes sense: The less you drink, the more carcinogens concentrate in your urine and the more time the toxins spend in contact with your bladder.

Colon cancer. Seattle researchers found that women who drank more than five glasses of water a day had a 45 percent decreased risk of colon cancer compared with those who drank two or fewer glasses.

"Not just any beverage—*water*," emphasizes Emily White, Ph.D., of the Fred Hutchinson Cancer Research Center at the University of Washington, who worked on the study. In this case, it could be that with lower water intake, you are more likely to be constipated. Just as traffic backed up in a tunnel poisons the air, this kind of obstruction in your colon increases the chance that tumors will develop.

Researchers aren't sure why the effects seem so much stronger for water than for other fluids.

Breast cancer. When researchers in England compared 100 women with newly diagnosed breast cancer with 100 women without breast cancer, they found that the women who didn't drink water regularly had a fourfold increase in risk for breast cancer.

One reason is that cell reactions require certain ingredients in certain proportions, suggests study leader Jodi Stookey, a Ph.D. candidate and adjunct faculty member at the University of North Carolina in Chapel Hill. If the cells are parched and shrunken, some of those reactions can be slowed or stopped, while others might be stimulated. So thirsty cells might not be reading their DNA codes correctly and, as a result, might be making mistakes in building the proteins required for normal cell life.

Successive damage like this could lead to cancer, she says. She speculates that dehydration may be one reason that airline attendants have higher rates of breast cancer than the general population.

Waistline

The average woman drinks about 26.5 gallons of diet soda a year but only about 14 gallons of plain water a year.

Heart disease. For decades, researchers have noticed major differences in the rates of heart disease around the country. One hypothesis is that the hardness of the water—measured by the amount of trace minerals in it—protects against heart disease. Some studies have shown that hard water may reduce the risk of heart attack and strokes by as much as 10 percent.

One way in which drinking water might protect against cardiovascular diseases is by replenishing the body's stores of magnesium and calcium, says Joshua I. Barzilay, M.D., faculty member of the endocrinology department at Emory University in Atlanta and author of *The Water We Drink: Water Quality and Its Effects on Health*. Magnesium is an essential element that helps maintain cells' ability to conduct electrical signals, particularly important in the heart, which might be considered the body's electrical power plant. Low intakes of calcium are associated with high blood pressure, the major cause of heart disease in this country, says Dr. Barzilay. It's thought that calcium contributes to heart health by affecting the way muscle cells contract.

When researchers in Sweden studied water consumption among 1,746 women who had various chronic diseases, their data suggested that the women who drank water with higher levels of magnesium and calcium lowered their risk of dying from heart disease by 40 percent.

POWER-EATING TIP

For heart-healthy calcium and magnesium, drink at least one bottle of mineral water a day.

Osteoporosis. Although milk and other dairy products are the most plentiful sources of dietary calcium, calcium in water is also an important protectant against osteoporosis and other bone disorders. In a French study of 4,434 elderly women, an increase of 100 milligrams per day of calcium in their drinking water made their thighbones denser than a similar increase in calcium from other dietary sources, like dairy products. Calcium-rich mineral water, researchers concluded, may be a good alternative for older women who eat few dairy products.

"Water will never be your main source of calcium," says Dr. Barzilay, but since most women don't get enough calcium anyway, "you may actually be making a significant increase in your percentage of calcium intake—up to 15 percent more—by choosing mineral water." Gerolsteiner Sprudel sparkling mineral water, for example, supplies 80 milligrams of calcium per 8 ounces. San Pellegrino sparkling mineral water contains 50 milligrams of calcium per 8 ounces.

Urinary tract infections (UTIs). Cranberry juice is a known guardian against UTIs. But did you know that plain water is equally powerful? Like power-washing your house strips mold and mildew before they can damage your siding, drinking nine 8-ounce glasses of water a day whisks away bacteria before it can cause infection.

Kidney stones. Even Hippocrates used to recommend gulping goblets of water to reduce kidney stone recurrences. Now science backs up his hunch. In a 5-year Italian study of 300 people who'd had kidney stones, researchers asked half of them to drink extra water every day, while the rest didn't change their water consumption. Eighty-eight percent of those who drank more water were stone-free after 5 years, compared to 73 percent of the untreated group. And it took longer for the people who drank extra water to have a recurrence than it did those who didn't up their water intake.

POWER-EATING TIP

If you're prone to kidney stones, make sure your liquid consumption includes, at the very least, five 8-ounce glasses of water a day.

Weight Control from Your Tap

If you let yourself get dehydrated—either accidentally through exercise or on purpose by crash-dieting or using diuretics—you'll lose water weight. That's not good.

First of all, you'll regain the weight when you start to drink water again. But dehydration backfires in another way: It affects the way we metabolize our food, says Wayne Askew, Ph.D., professor of nutrition and director of the division of foods and nutrition at the University of Utah in Salt Lake City. In one study, he found that volunteers who were already dehydrated due to the use of diuretics burned fewer calories after a period of stationary cycling than they were burning before the exercise started.

POWER-EATING TIP

Freeze a partly filled bottle of water, then add more water just before you leave the house. The body absorbs cold water faster than warm, and funny tastes aren't as apparent in cold water. Even better, you burn about 123 calories a day to warm 8 pints of ice water to body temperature. Over the course of a month, that's a pound lost.

Drink two glasses of water before every meal. Not only will it keep you hydrated, but a Dutch study showed that drinking two glasses of water can make you feel less hungry, possibly reducing your food intake and aiding weight loss.

MASKED DISASTER

Cappuccino Grande

Not only is coffee a diuretic, but some specialty coffees are like liquid dessert. A typical 16-ounce cappuccino—a *grande*—has 180 calories and 9 grams of fat. In comparison, 16 ounces of regular coffee with 1 tablespoon of fat-free milk has 15 calories and no fat.

Switch to a frosty mug of fat-free milk with a splash of coffee, and you'll get about half the calories and a fraction of the fat. As a bonus, you'll get 302 milligrams of calcium.

Is Your Water Safe to Drink?

Bottled water has become such a cliché in this country that some restaurants put silver holders on their tables for the plastic containers. It's particularly popular with women, who are 23 percent more likely to drink bottled water than men.

"It's the ultimate health beverage," says Gary Hemphill, vice president of the Beverage Marketing Association in New York City, which tracks the bottled water industry. "There are no calories, no additives, and the bottle is portable, so it can be taken just about anywhere."

At least 25 percent of bottled waters sold in this country are nothing more than purified tap water, says Mike Miller, general manager of the bottled water division of NSF International, an independent, not-for-profit company based in Ann Arbor, Michigan, that evaluates bottled water and water filtration systems. The FDA has three separate regulations covering its production, and there has never been a single disease outbreak caused by bottled water in the United States.

The same can't always be said of public water. Although many experts, including Miller, say that the United States has one of the safest public water supplies in the world, problems can, and do, happen. Over the years, isolated incidents have occurred involving contamination by parasites, gasoline additives, *Escherichia coli* bacteria, pesticides, and lead that occasionally turn up in some water systems.

Most water is disinfected with chlorine, the same stuff that keeps your swimming pool crystalline. But some studies have found a slight association between chlorine by-products in drinking water and some cancers. A study of 28,237 Iowa women found a slight increase in colon cancer among women who drank chlorinated water, but, says Timothy Doyle, an epidemiologist with the Centers for Disease Control and Prevention, the results were very weak.

POWER-EATING TIP

If you're worried about the health effects of chlorine, try a home filtering product on your tap or to filter the water into a pitcher, like the Brita or Pūr water filters. NSF International evaluates such filters for their effectiveness and posts results on their Web site at www.nsf.org.

To learn how safe your local water is, read the Consumer Confidence Report for your local water supplier, available in local libraries and schools. You should also receive a copy of the report each year with your water bill. Or check out the Environmental Protection Agency's Web site: www.epa.gov.

When Bottled Is Best

Choose bottled water over tap water in the following cases.

You prefer the taste. Even if it's just municipal water in that bottle, manufacturers usually use extra filtering, reverse osmosis, and

WHAT ABOUT FLUORIDE?

Kids aren't the only ones who need fluoride. "It's important for adults, too," says Susan Kleiner, R.D., Ph.D., assistant professor of nutrition at the University of Washington in Seattle. "Our teeth actually remodel themselves throughout our lifetime, just like our bones, so you must have fluoride available."

If you use a water filter (like a Brita or Pūr filter), rest assured: It doesn't filter out the fluoride. And some bottled water manufacturers are adding fluoride to their products.

other processes to purify water and rid it of the chlorine taste, Miller says.

You have a compromised immune system. Bacteria that would simply send most of us to the bathroom a few extra times could send you to the hospital.

Other Sources to Consider

In reality, the chances of your drinking nothing but water all day are about as slim as a supermodel. So here's what you need to know about other sources of fluid.

Coffee, tea, and other caffeinated drinks. They are diuretics—that is, they step up urination. If you drink 3 cups of coffee a day, in that same time period, you could lose up to 2.4 pounds of water, nearly 2 percent of your body weight.

The more you habitually drink caffeinated and alcoholic drinks, the less likely you are to realize that you are thirsty. If you must drink tea or coffee, switch to the decaffeinated kind. Keep in mind, though, that they still contain some caffeine. To reach your 9 cups a day, caffeine-free herb teas are a better choice.

Beer, wine, or liquor. Alcohol depresses production of the antidiuretic hormone (ADH), which usually tells the kidneys to reabsorb water. Without ADH sending its messages, the kidney snoozes and water loss increases. If you drink a 5-ounce glass of wine, you will pass almost that same amount as urine.

POWER-EATING TIP

Alcoholic beverages don't count as part of your daily liquid intake. In fact, you need to drink even more water to counteract the diuretic effect of each alcoholic drink you down. Drink 1 cup of water for every cup of caffeinated or alcoholic liquid you sip.

Milk. Fat-free milk is 90 to 99 percent water and has just 86 calories a cup, not to mention that it is a significantly better source of calcium than mineral water.

Juice. It's fine if part of your daily liquid quota comes from juice, provided you watch the sugar.

Stick to juices that are nearly all fruit juice and dilute them with water to reduce calories and improve your fluid intake. Avoid soda: A regular cola has about 150 calories and the equivalent of 9 teaspoons of sugar—about as much as a candy bar. Plus, the dark-colored sodas—both diet and regular—are high in phosphorus, which some studies show can leach calcium from the bones.

Sports drinks. These usually have about half the calories of juice and soda. But be careful: The sodium in sports drinks actually enhances thirst, so you'll want to drink even more. "Unless you are sweating a whole lot—as when you exercise for an hour or more—you don't really need these concentrated beverages," explains Dubner.

To make your own sports drink, combine 8 ounces of water (avoid carbonated water, which can make you uncomfortable during or after exercise), 1 teaspoon of lemon juice, ¼ teaspoon of salt, and 4 teaspoons of sugar. Mix well.

MASKED DISASTER

Bottled Iced Tea

A typical 16-ounce bottle of lemon-flavored iced tea packs a walloping 200 calories, nearly 11 teaspoons of sugar, and 48 milligrams of caffeine.

A cold glass of sparkling mineral water with lemon contains no calories, no sugar—and no caffeine.

POWER

FRUIT SLUSH

STRAWBERRY-WATERMELON SLUSH

It's liquid ambrosia (and a fun change from plain water). Keep a supply of strawberries and watermelon cubes in the freezer for quick drinks, and you'll have no trouble getting your recommended 9 cups of fluid a day. Plus, the fruit has lots of vitamin C (160 percent of the Daily Value in 1½ cups), fiber, and other nutrients. Calcium-fortified orange juice gives an extra boost of the bone-strengthening mineral.

- 4 ice cubes
- 6 frozen strawberries
- 2 cups frozen seedless watermelon cubes
- ¾ cup calcium-fortified orange juice
- 1 tablespoon lime juice

In a blender, combine the ice cubes, strawberries, watermelon, orange juice, and lime juice. Blend until smooth.

Makes 3 cups

Per 1½ cups: 112 calories, 2 g protein, 26 g carbohydrates, 0 g fat, 0 mg cholesterol, 3 g dietary fiber, 6 mg sodium

Note: To freeze melon chunks, lay the chunks on a baking sheet and cover with plastic. Place in the freezer for about 1 hour. For best quality, store the fruit in plastic freezer containers and use it within 2 to 3 months.

Food. Some foods are basically just rearranged water molecules. Lettuce, watermelon, broccoli, and grapefruit are all more than 90 percent water. Carrots and cottage cheese weigh in close behind with 88 percent and 79 percent, respectively.

Water-based food is good for about 35 percent of your daily water requirement.

Your Daily Water Plan

Remember, if you wait until you are thirsty to drink, it's already too late.

"You need to have a water plan, just like you have a food plan," says Dr. Kleiner.

• Keep a glass of water on your bedside table and drink it all down before you even get out of bed.

• Put it in a pitcher. Dr. Kleiner keeps water pitchers with filters on her desk, in her kitchen, and in the refrigerator. Each pitcher holds about 8 cups of water and is a constant reminder to drink.

• Never walk by a water fountain without stopping, says Dubner. Figure that 10 big gulps equals 1 cup of water.

• Squeeze lemon or lime wedges into tap or bottled water to give it extra zing—and yourself an extra dose of vitamin C and antioxidants.

• Make sure that you include water any time you have a snack, says Dubner. Maybe even choose salty snacks like pretzels that will make you thirsty.

• Start meals with soup. They're mostly water.

• Fill up your water glass or bottle every time you get up to go to the bathroom. Remember: water out, water in.

• Flavor water by freezing fruit juice in ice-cube trays and adding a couple to a glass of water.

• Drink on schedule. Write it on your calendar, or program the alarm on your watch to beep every hour. Each time you are reminded, drink a cup of water.

Sugar: How Bad
Is It, Really?

Power Maker #13: To limit sugar intake, don't add sugar to cereal, coffee, tea, or sliced fruit; sweeten foods by adding vanilla, cinnamon, or nutmeg instead of sugar; drink water, not soda; and read labels carefully.

To a baby, breast milk is as sweet and luscious as ice cream. No wonder some babies latch on to the breast like Super Glue. It's nature's way of making sure that we get what we need from day one.

We are genetically programmed to like sweets. The hardwiring starts even before we're born: When liquid sugar is introduced into the placenta, the fetus immediately starts sucking.

Back in the pre-cheesecake, live-in-a-cave days, preferring sweet to sour had its benefits: The sweeter the food, the more we would eat. The more we ate, the more we weighed—important back when food was hard to come by and hunting for it took stamina. Also, sweet plants were less likely to be poisonous than bitter ones.

But today, most of us need the extra calories about as much as a pregnant woman needs a diaphragm, and we're pretty savvy about not eating those mushrooms growing in the backyard.

Yet when it comes to our favorite foods, we still favor sweets. When sugar-and-fat guru Adam Drewnowski, Ph.D., director of the nutritional sciences program at the University of Washington in Seattle, asked nearly 400 obese women to write down their 10 favorite foods, ice cream, doughnuts, cakes, and cookies topped the list. Compare that to men, who choose foods like steak, hot dogs, and eggs.

Heightened senses of taste and smell may make women better at picking out sweet tastes than men, says Paula J. Geiselman, Ph.D., of Pennington Biomedical Research Center at Louisiana State University in Baton Rouge. When she fed women chocolate puddings ranging from bland to make-your-teeth-cringe sweet, the women invariably chose the sweetest pudding.

We get about 20 teaspoons of added sugar a day, not counting the natural sugars in milk and fruit. That's the equivalent of nearly two 12-ounce sodas a day—about twice the limit that the USDA recommends. It's also a whopping 320 calories.

Plus, sugar won't do the things other foods like fruits and vegetables and whole grains will do, such as protect against heart disease and some cancers. If one-quarter of your calories come from the sweet stuff, then something else is getting short shrift. So generally, nutritionists recommend that we get no more than 10 percent of our daily calories from added sugar.

Sugar Is Sugar

Brown or white, cubed or superfine, liquid or solid, fructose or sucrose, all sugars have the same nutritional benefit—zilch.

That's why nutritionists condemn sugar as a source of "empty calories."

True, sugar is a carbohydrate, a combination of carbon, hydrogen, and

Waistline

The average woman consumes just over 2 cups of added sugar each week, including sugar in processed foods. You could spread those 1,703 calories over the entire week or save up for one big splurge on Saturday night and scarf down seven pieces of cheesecake.

CRAVE SUGAR? GET SOME SUN

Next time you need a sugar fix, go for a walk in the sun. Some people may crave sweets when their serotonin levels are low. Dark days cause serotonin levels to go down, which makes appetites go up. Bright light increases serotonin levels, which should calm cravings.

oxygen that supplies energy—a.k.a. calories. And conventional wisdom urges us to eat more carbs and fewer fats. The problem is that sugars—fructose, sucrose, galactose, glucose, lactose, and maltose—are simple carbohydrates. They're made of short chains of single or double molecules. But what you need to be packing in are complex carbohydrates—starches and fibers consisting of large chains of molecules—like whole grains and vegetables. Complex carbohydrates supply not just energy, but vitamins, minerals, and other helpful substances as well.

And in fact, when British researchers looked at the diets of 1,600 men and women over a 1½-year period, they found that the more sugar was in the diet, the less fruits and vegetables were.

It's not surprising, says Christina Stark, R.D., a nutritionist at Cornell University in Ithaca, New York. "If you look at the Food Guide Pyramid, there are a lot of recommended foods that you should eat. If you eat a lot of sugar, you won't be able to eat all of those and still keep your calories reasonable."

It doesn't matter what kind of sugar you choose. One is just as much a nutritional wasteland as another.

"It's so funny, this propensity for people to buy naturally milled versus refined sugar," says Richard S. Surwit, Ph.D., chief of the division of medical psychology at Duke University in Durham, North Carolina. "All sugars are naturally refined. Do you know what they do to make that 'sugar in the raw'? They spray molasses on it." And contrary to what you may hear, fructose (found in some corn syrup) is not nutritionally superior to sucrose (table sugar), it just tastes sweeter. In fact, table sugar is a combination of fructose and glucose.

About the only difference between sugars is taste and calories. Honey, high-fructose corn syrup, and concentrated fruit juice, for instance, hold

POWER

COOKIES

BANANA-OATMEAL COOKIES

Don't let desserts be your downfall. Soft, chewy cookies like these are sweet and satisfying, yet low in fat and calories. Part of the trick is using mashed ripe bananas to mimic the creaminess of butter and the sweetness of sugar. Another is to get the flavor and crunch of nuts from toasted rolled oats—but not the fat. The bananas and oats have benefits sugar and fats don't: fiber and nutrients like potassium and the antioxidant selenium.

2	cups rolled oats
1	cup whole wheat flour
½	cup unbleached or all-purpose flour
1½	teaspoons baking powder
¾	teaspoon ground cinnamon
½	teaspoon salt
1	cup mashed very ripe bananas (2 large)
1	egg or ¼ cup liquid egg substitute
⅓	cup packed brown sugar
2	tablespoons canola oil
½	teaspoon vanilla extract
¾	cup raisins

more calories per teaspoon than table sugar. They're also stickier and thus potentially worse for your teeth. So if you're pouring on the sweetness, you might as well use plain old table sugar.

The Real Culprit Is Fat

While sugar displaces other, more nutritional foods in your diet, it won't necessarily make you fat, nor will it make you eat more.

That doesn't mean that you can eat all the sugar you want with no

Preheat the oven to 375°F. Spread the oats in a thin layer on a jelly-roll pan. Bake, stirring occasionally, for 10 minutes, or just until golden brown. Set aside to cool. Leave the oven turned on.

In a medium bowl, whisk together the whole wheat flour, unbleached or all-purpose flour, baking powder, cinnamon, and salt.

In a large bowl, combine the bananas, egg or egg substitute, brown sugar, oil, and vanilla. Beat with an electric mixer on medium speed until smooth.

Beat in the flour mixture. Stir in the oats and raisins.

Coat a baking sheet with cooking spray. Drop slightly rounded table-spoons of the dough about 1" apart on the sheet. Bake for 12 to 14 minutes, or until the bottoms are lightly browned around the edges. Remove to a wire rack and cool completely.

Makes 48

Per cookie: 50 calories, 1 g protein, 9 g carbohydrates, 1 g fat, 4 mg cholesterol, 1 g dietary fiber, 35 mg sodium

Note: Store the cookies in a covered container at room temperature for up to 2 days. After that, refrigerate or freeze them.

worry. But if you're trying to lose weight, limit all calories and fat, not just sugar calories.

Ah, but there's the rub. For where there's sugar, there's likely to be fat.

After all, think sweet and what comes to mind? Not carrots, but carrot cake. Not bananas, but banana split. Not apples, but apple pie.

Researchers theorize that we love candy and dessert not just for the sugar, not just for the fat, but for some amazing synergy that occurs when the two come together. Apparently, there's some switch in our brains that this calorically lethal combination triggers called the endogenous opioid peptide system (our pleasure center, in plain English). When scientists block these brain receptors in mice, for instance, the rodents eat less chocolate and fewer cookies, thus lowering their fat intake.

A Link to Heart Disease

Experts at the FDA say that sugar doesn't cause diabetes, heart disease, obesity, hypoglycemia, childhood hyperactivity, or nutrient deficiencies. But some scientists say that they're wrong.

"I've never found anything good about eating sugar," says Judith Hallfrisch, Ph.D., lead scientist in the diet and human performance laboratory of the USDA Beltsville Human Nutrition Research Center in Maryland. In numerous animal and human studies, she says, eating less starch and more sugar raised blood pressure, cholesterol, and triglycerides.

And for years, scientists have noticed in some studies that the higher the level of sucrose, the higher the levels of triglycerides. Triglycerides are tiny droplets of fat that the liver makes when metabolizing carbohydrates, fat, and protein. Eventually, they end up in your fat tissue (hips, thighs, and butt). The problem is, their means of transportation—called very low density lipoproteins, or VLDLs—keep roaming around, getting smaller and smaller after dropping off the triglycerides, eventually ending up as the kind of LDL particles that cause "bad" cholesterol. The smaller your LDL particles, the more dangerous they are. If they get oxidized—their version of a nervous breakdown—they can plug up your arteries and cause a heart attack. Fortunately, there are ways to lower your triglycerides, including exercising, losing weight, and adding more unsaturated fat into your diet in the form of nuts, seeds, avocados, and plant oils.

MASKED DISASTER

Sweetened Applesauce

Yes, applesauce counts as a serving of fruit. But just ½ cup has a sugary 97 calories. Buy unsweetened instead—it has just 52 calories.

High triglyceride levels are a risk factor for heart disease, particularly in postmenopausal women, who are just as likely to die from heart attacks as their husbands.

Dr. Hallfrisch saw women's triglyceride levels rise when she fed them diets with 18 percent of calories coming from sugar. "And that's what women are eating today, particularly young women," she says.

LOW-CALORIE SUGAR FIXES

To satisfy your sweet tooth and save calories, try these substitutes.

INSTEAD OF THIS . . .	HAVE THIS . . .	CALORIES SAVED	FAT SAVED (g)
1 cup caramel popcorn	7 Quaker Caramel Corn minicakes	100	2.5
3 Pepperidge Farm Milano cookies	2 Pims Orange or Raspberry chocolate-coated cookies	90	7.5
Small chocolate bar	3 small York peppermint patties	53	10.0
3 Rolo chocolate-covered caramels	3 Hershey's chocolate TasteTations candies	30	3.5

Other researchers have gotten differing results. Some studies show that triglyceride increase may be due to the amount of fat and calories in the diet and may not be directly linked to sugar intake. Another theory is that the reaction only occurs in some women who have Syndrome X: They respond to sugar with abnormally high secretions of insulin (a hormone that helps the body absorb sugar), which results in excess triglycerides.

What about Cavities?

"Unless you keep something with sugar in your mouth all day, sugar won't necessarily cause cavities—it's not that simple," says Clifford Whall, Ph.D., director of product evaluation in the Council of Scientific Affairs at the American Dental Association in Chicago.

Other key factors in determining your susceptibility to tooth decay include the amount of bacteria in your mouth, how sticky the foods are, the types and amounts of fluorides you're exposed to, and how effective your immune system is against decay-causing bacteria, Dr. Whall says. The bacteria use the carbohydrate as food, metabolizing the sugar. The by-product of their meal is the acid that causes tooth decay. The less time any carbohydrate-containing food—from candy or soft drinks to fruit or bread—stays in your mouth, the better off you will be.

To satisfy your sweet tooth while helping to minimize the possibility of getting cavities, here's what to do.

- Brush twice a day with a fluoride toothpaste and floss daily using products accepted by the American Dental Association.

- Swish water around in your mouth after eating any kind of sticky carbohydrate, like bread, cakes, or dried fruit.

- Chew unsugared gum. It increases the saliva flow, which washes out the bits of food that the bacteria could feast on, as well as washing out the decay-causing acids that the bacteria produce.

- Eat your sweets with meals. Again, the increased saliva flow that accompanies prolonged chewing tends to clear sugary foods out of the mouth faster. Also, if you only eat sweets with meals, the bacteria will only get three squares a day instead of being fed all day long.

Satisfy Your Sweet Tooth (without Committing Nutritional Suicide)

All things considered, you don't have to swear off sugar entirely. The key, says Tammy Baker, R.D., a Phoenix-based spokesperson for

STEVIA: NATURE'S SWEETENER

Want to skip the calories in sugar while avoiding artificial sweeteners? Consider stevia, an herbal sweetener sold in health food stores and derived from *Stevia rebaudiana*, a shrub native to Paraguay.

For centuries, people in Brazil and Argentina have used stevia leaves to sweeten food or tea. China has also been cultivating it, while Japan has added it to everything from soy sauce to pickles to diet cola. In this country, stevia is sold as a dietary supplement.

Stevia is 200 to 300 times sweeter than sugar, so a little goes a long way. Two teaspoons of sugar, for instance, equals the sweetness of ½ teaspoon of stevia blend, or ⅓ teaspoon of liquid stevia. It can be used in baking but is best as a sweetener for hot and cold drinks.

Waistline

If you cut your intake of added sugar by half and did nothing else, you'd lose a pound about every 3 weeks. In just 1 year, you'd have lost almost 17 pounds, which, for some women, is at least one dress size.

the American Dietetic Association, is to find a way to add some nutritional value to the empty calories of sugar. And stay away from the fat. Here's how.

If you want chocolate:

- Chomp dry chocolate cereals, like Count Chocula or Cocoa Puffs. They are sweet but are nearly fat-free and are fortified.

- Dip fruit in fat-free chocolate syrup.

- Drink a cup of reduced-fat hot chocolate or a glass of low-fat chocolate milk.

- Lick (don't bite) a low-fat frozen fudge pop. "The average craving disappears in less than 20 minutes," says Edward Abramson, Ph.D., professor of psychology at California State University in Chico. And it takes at least that long to lick a fudge pop into oblivion.

- Mix fat-free chocolate sauce with fat-free cream cheese for a sweet and creamy spread.

If you want something smooth and creamy:

- Spoon up sugar-free, fat-free or low-fat frozen yogurt.

- Feast on a yogurt parfait; Layer sugar-free, fat-free yogurt with sweet berries and top with fat-free whipped cream.

- Polish off a prepared pudding, preferably of the low-fat variety. "You're getting some sugar, but you're also getting calcium," Baker says.

For a sweet snack that's free of added sugar:

- Bake an apple sprinkled with cinnamon and raisins, then top with a dollop of low-fat vanilla yogurt.

- Add raisins to oatmeal, cereal, even stews—anything with liquid—to add sweetness. Just let them soak in the cooking liquid or even hot water for a few minutes until they plump up.

- Munch carrots. They're actually sweeter than pure sugar. Buy a bag of baby carrots or cut carrot coins and eat them like candy. Or dip them in a low-fat dip or dressing for added flavor.

- Smear all-fruit spread on toast, crackers, or rice cakes.

THE REAL SCOOP ON SUGAR SUBSTITUTES

Over the years, sugar substitutes have been blamed for ailments from migraines to bladder cancer. But how bad are they really? And what the heck are they made of, anyway?

They're basically a chemical sugar Scrabble, where the molecules of various substances are rearranged in the hope that the new, calorie-free substance will taste and act like the real thing.

But they don't.

"No one sweetener comes close to perfectly matching the taste of sugar," says Rosetta Newsome, Ph.D., director of science and communications at the Institute of Food Technologists in Chicago. Taste aside, the four FDA-approved artificial sweeteners don't seem to pose much of a health threat.

SACCHARIN. Sold as Sweet 'N Low in the pink packages, saccharin is about 300 percent sweeter than sugar and can be heated. Saccharin's bad rap comes from studies done on rats in the 1970s in which some male rats that were fed extremely high doses of saccharin developed bladder tumors. Not to worry, says Dr. Newsome. You would have to drink several hundred cans of diet soda _per day_ to equal those amounts. And new research indicates that the development of the bladder tumors was related to several variables, including the strain of rat and the high dose of the sodium component of this form of saccharin. Further, human studies do not support the association between saccharin and cancer in humans.

ASPARTAME. Sold under the brand names NutraSweet and Equal, aspartame is 180 percent sweeter than sugar. Unlike other sweeteners, aspartame

- Freeze grapes, then just pop them in your mouth like bonbons.
- Spritz bananas with lemon juice and sprinkle with cinnamon, then fry them in a nonstick skillet coated with cooking spray.

  To get some Power Foods with your sugar:

- Drizzle caramel sauce or honey over apples.
- Dip fresh strawberries in fat-free sour cream and then in brown sugar.

is metabolized by the body. But, at 4 calories per gram, it is essentially noncaloric. A cursory stroll on the Internet might convince you that aspartame is to blame for several evils, from overactive kids to brain cancer. Yet despite years of testing, no links between aspartame and illness have been found, even when humans consumed the equivalent of 70 cans of soft drinks in one sitting.

As for rumors that aspartame is degraded into methanol, which turns into formaldehyde in your body, the same could be said for other foods, including orange juice. Methanol is a normal part of digestion. The levels of methanol and formaldehyde formed in the body through the consumption of aspartame and citrus juices are well below the level of toxicity.

The only people who should avoid or restrict aspartame are those who have a rare hereditary disease in which they cannot metabolize phenylalanine, one of two amino acids that make up aspartame. Babies born to families with a history of phenylketonuria can be tested for it as soon as they are born.

ACESULFAME-K. This sweetener—the "K" stands for potassium—is about 200 times sweeter than sugar. It can withstand high cooking and baking temperatures and is not metabolized by the body at all. It's marketed as Sunett and is used in chewing gum, candy, desserts, and alcoholic beverages, among other foods.

SUCRALOSE. Approved in 1998, it is 600 times sweeter than sugar and is available as Splenda.

- Crush a candy cane and sprinkle it on fat-free yogurt.

- Slice nectarines or peaches, drizzle them with honey, then let them sit for ½ hour to bring out the full flavors.

- Favor figs. Naturally sweet fig bars are low in fat and have only 56 calories each.

- Substitute applesauce and pureed prunes (use baby food prunes) for half to all of the sugar in baked goods (use prunes in chocolate recipes, applesauce in the rest).

- Have your cake and eat it, too. Angel food cake with strawberries, that is. "At least you're getting the nutritional value of the strawberries," says Baker.

- Choose healthy ingredients. "An oatmeal-raisin cookie will do more for you than a sugar cookie," says Baker.

Watch for Hidden Sugar

Candy and desserts aren't the only sources of dietary sugar. A few surprising sources of added or natural sugar include:

- Prego pasta sauce (traditional): 4 teaspoons of sugar per ½-cup serving

- Hellmann's Fat-Free Honey Dijon dressing: 2½ teaspoons of sugar per 2-tablespoon serving

- Campbell's Old-Fashioned Beans: 3½ teaspoons of sugar per ½-cup serving

- Dannon coffee, lemon, or vanilla low-fat yogurt: 3 teaspoons of sugar per 1-cup serving

Sugar goes by numerous names. Look for corn syrup, dextrose, dextrin, sucrose, glucose, and fructose on labels.

PART 3

THE POWER OF VITAMINS, HERBS, AND SPECIALTY SUPPLEMENTS

Vitamins and Minerals: What Women Really Need

Power Maker #14: Supplement a diet high in fruits, vegetables, and calcium-rich sources with one multivitamin/mineral supplement, a calcium/magnesium supplement with at least 500 milligrams of calcium and up to 350 milligrams of magnesium, and a vitamin E supplement with 100 to 400 IU each day.

Squirrels don't take supplements. Neither do geese, rabbits, monkeys, or any other animal in the wild, for that matter. Because they don't need to.

Monkeys, for instance, get more nutrients from their plant-based diet of leaves, fruits, and flowers than we do from our highly processed omnivorous diet, says Katharine Milton, Ph.D., professor of biological anthropology at the University of California, Berkeley. Although she's not a nutritionist, over the years, much of Dr. Milton's research has come to center on not only what we eat but also what related mammals like apes, gorillas, chimpanzees, and orangutans eat. For instance, a 15-pound wild howler monkey consumes 600 milligrams of vitamin C a day—nearly seven times what the average American woman eats. The official recommendation for vitamin C is now 75 milligrams a day for women. Yet some experts

POWER

R I C E

BROWN RICE WITH SPINACH
AND FETA CHEESE

Jazz up plain old rice with the flavors of Greece. This main-dish casserole gets powerful antioxidants from the spinach and plenty of fiber from the brown rice.

1	teaspoon olive oil
1	large onion, finely chopped
1	cup brown rice
2½	cups water
1	box (10 ounces) frozen chopped spinach, thawed and well-drained
4	ounces reduced-fat feta cheese, finely crumbled
8	kalamata olives, pitted and finely chopped
4	eggs, lightly beaten, or 1 cup fat-free liquid egg substitute

In a large saucepan, warm the oil over medium heat. Add the onion and cook, stirring often, for 5 minutes. Stir in the rice and water. Bring to a boil. Cover, reduce the heat, and simmer for 45 minutes, or until all the water has been absorbed. Remove from the heat.

Preheat the oven to 350°F. Coat an 8" × 8" glass baking dish with cooking spray.

Stir the spinach, feta, and olives into the rice. Stir in the eggs or egg substitute. Spoon into the baking dish.

Bake for 25 to 30 minutes, or until a knife inserted in the center comes out clean. Let stand 5 minutes before serving.

Makes 4 servings

Per serving: 391 calories, 19 g protein, 49 g carbohydrates, 13.5 g fat, 213 mg cholesterol, 5 g dietary fiber, 677 mg sodium

Variation: To turn this into a hearty side dish, omit the eggs.

say that we should take in about 200 milligrams of C per day, two to three times what we get now. We're just not as good as the monkeys at figuring out how to get it.

We lean toward such foods as french fries smothered in cheese, fried mozzarella, doughnuts, and cheesecake, and eschew such healthful choices as whole grains, fruits, and vegetables.

"We've lost the ability other animals have of being able to judge what is good for us and what isn't," says Dr. Milton.

Nutritionists Say, "Supplement"

First christened "growth factors" in 1906, vitamins and minerals are now turning out to be critical elements in our overall health. Scientists are working to determine how much we need for optimal health, not just for preventing deficiencies. At one time, nutritionists said few men or women needed supplements of any kind. They've changed their tune.

"Most of the nutrition experts I know take supplements," says Gordon M. Wardlaw, R.D., Ph.D., associate professor of medical dietetics at Ohio State University in Columbus.

Try as they might, even nutritionists find it hard to figure out how to cover all the nutritional bases with food alone. Of 43 menus nutritionists designed to meet the benchmark Dietary Guidelines for Americans, only 11 met the Recommended Dietary Allowances for zinc, half were deficient in vitamin B_6, and one-third lacked enough iron.

WOMEN WHO TAKE VITAMINS ARE HEALTHIER ALL AROUND

Women who take supplements tend to be healthier in other ways. According to a study of almost 14,000 British women, they're less likely to smoke or to drink regularly, and more likely to follow a vegetarian eating pattern or at least eat more fruits and vegetables than those who don't take supplements.

And ironically, with the exception of vitamin B_{12}, women taking supplements get more of their necessary nutrients from food than nonusers of supplements.

Evidently, one healthful behavior begets others—all to the good.

"If even dietitians can't put together a good menu, how can we ever expect the typical American woman—who is out there juggling family, work, exercise, and everything else—to do it?" asks Elizabeth Somer, R.D., a nutritionist and author of *The Essential Guide to Vitamins and Minerals.*

The New Nutrition Paradigm

If women are going to reduce their risk of some chronic diseases and promote optimal health, he says, they are going to need to get more than the Daily Values of some nutrients, says Jeffrey Blumberg, Ph.D., chief of the antioxidants research laboratory at Tufts University in Boston. He calls it the new nutrition paradigm.

Take vitamin C, for instance. The current Daily Value is 60 milligrams, but that's the minimum amount required to prevent scurvy, notes Gerald F. Combs, Ph.D., professor of nutrition at Cornell University in Ithaca, New York. The official recommendation for women is 75 milligrams. "Almost no one in this country gets scurvy anymore," he says. "What we get, instead, is heart disease and cancer."

Women have other needs—like calcium, magnesium, iron, and various B vitamins—that we typically don't get enough of in our normal diets. "The point of view that if you're eating well, you don't need supplements is out of date," says Somer. "Ninety-nine percent of women aren't eating perfectly."

Even if you did eat ideal foods in ideal amounts, you just can't get certain nutrients from food. Experts recommend between 100 and 400 IU of vitamin E. To get, say, 200 IU, you would have to eat 6 cups of wheat germ or nearly 3 cups of corn oil. Or try 5 cups of peanut butter—with 658 grams of fat and a gargantuan 7,700 calories.

Even if the calories weren't exorbitant, your stomach couldn't physically hold that much food.

Not a Substitute for Food

The issue of vitamin/mineral supplements and food is not an either/or proposition. "You need to eat really well *and* supplement responsibly," stresses Somer. "That's the best way to cover your bases."

For instance, when researchers at the Harvard School of Public Health studied the diets of more than 83,000 women, they found that

POWER

BROCCOLI AND ORANGE SALAD

It's not your same old salad! Two big-time Power Foods—broccoli and or-anges—team up for a double dose of flavor and lots of antioxidants (like vitamin C) and the B vitamin folate. Turn ordinary meals into something special with this unique alternative to dressed lettuce.

4	cups bite-size broccoli florets
¼	cup orange juice
1	tablespoon white balsamic or white wine vinegar
1	tablespoon soy sauce
1	tablespoon olive oil
½	teaspoon Dijon mustard
2	large oranges, peeled and sectioned
⅓	cup finely chopped red onion

Steam the broccoli until crisp-tender.

In a large bowl, whisk together the orange juice, vinegar, soy sauce, oil, and mustard. Add the oranges and onion. Toss gently. Add the broc-coli and toss gently to combine. Serve at room temperature or chilled.

Makes 4 servings

Per serving: 100 calories, 4 g protein, 16 g carbohydrates, 4 g fat, 0 mg cholesterol, 4 g dietary fiber, 291 mg sodium

among premenopausal women with mothers or sisters with breast cancer, those who ate at least five servings of fruits or vegetables a day were 70 percent less likely to get breast cancer than those who ate less than two servings a day. Vitamin supplements (A, E, or multivitamins) offered no protection.

Consider, too, that less than 10 percent of us even get five fruits and vegetables a day. So first and foremost, enhance your diet with lots of fruits and vegetables—nine servings a day, on the Ultimate Power-Eating Plan. But to cover your bases, take a multivitamin/mineral supplement plus a few select single nutrient supplements.

Women already take more supplements than men. Still, only about one out of four women take some kind of vitamin once a day, mainly a multivitamin. What about the other three?

Here, you'll discover what nutrients you need and how to get them, based on the latest findings about these substances.

Antioxidants: the Pac-(Wo)men of Vitamins

Eating and breathing are basic life functions. Yet every time you take a breath or eat a meal, the by-products of the chemical reactions that occur create tiny yet devastating little devils called free radicals. They roam your body, latching onto normal cell molecules and damaging their DNA with the same glee a 2-year-old exhibits when smearing finger paint on a newly papered wall.

Unlike the mess on the wall, however, this damage can lead to more serious consequences, like cancer, heart disease, arthritis, and Alzheimer's disease, not to mention aging us even more than raising a 2-year-old does.

Holding your breath isn't an option. And we're not even going to consider a world without cheesecake. That's where antioxidants come in: vitamins C and E and vitamin A's precursor, beta-carotene. These powerful scavengers are to your body what a sponge and a bottle of spray cleaner are to that messy wall—seeking out and destroying free radicals before they can so much as glance covetously at your DNA. The benefits, science is discovering, are enormous.

Numerous studies over the past 20 years show how antioxidants play a role in protecting us against everything from skin cancer to high blood pressure.

"Antioxidants like vitamins C and E slow down the aging process of cells," says Michael Fossel, M.D., Ph.D., clinical professor of medicine at Michigan State University in East Lansing and author of *Reversing Human Aging*.

How they do that is still up for debate. A Japanese study, for instance, showed that vitamin C added to cells that line the arteries slowed the rate at which a cell's telomeres shortened. A telomere is at the end of the

FEEL TIRED? TRY A GLASS OF ORANGE JUICE

Don't feel like going to the gym and working out? A glass of orange juice just might give you the zest you need to get there. When Arizona State University researcher Carol Johnston, Ph.D., measured vitamin C levels in 350 mostly healthy women who went to a clinic for routine checkups, she found that 30 percent had levels low enough to be considered depleted. One of the first symptoms of scurvy is fatigue.

Dr. Johnston found giving vitamin C–depleted men and women 500 milligrams of the antioxidant improved not only their athletic performance but also their desire to exercise in the first place.

chromosome, like the plastic tip at the end of a shoelace. The telomeres shorten each time the cell divides. Telomeres act like a clock running down. As the telomeres get shorter, the cell runs down and dies. If new telomeres are added to the cell, the cell is capable of acting like a new cell. Figuring out how to keep them long—or even get them to grow again— would be the equivalent of finding the fountain of youth.

Various things effect telomere shortening, including ultraviolet light and those nasty free radicals, says Dr. Fossel, suggesting a role for antioxidants.

Vitamin C: A Valuable Partner

For years, you've heard that taking vitamin C can help relieve a cold. Here's why—along with a rundown of what else this famous nutrient can do.

You've had six deadlines at work, a major fight with hubby, and a call from the school principal, and just when things begin to settle down, you feel that scratchiness in the back of your throat that signals a cold. Vitamin C may strengthen your immune system for times like this.

"Certainly, people under stress have much higher incidences of illness and disease," says P. Samuel Campbell, Ph.D., professor and chairman of the biological sciences department at the University of Alabama in Huntsville. "Perhaps it's because they're not getting enough vitamin C."

Dr. Campbell and other researchers fed rats 200 milligrams of vitamin C daily, roughly the equivalent of several thousand milligrams in humans, then stressed the rodents. When they compared the levels of glucocorticoids—adrenal hormones both humans and animals release in response to stress, which can suppress the immune system—they found significantly lower levels in the supplement-popping rats than in the control group. As an added bonus, the rats getting the sunshine vitamin also had elevated levels of IgG antibody, one of the body's principal defenses against systemic infection.

The results fit with a human study in which levels of cortisol (a human stress hormone) also dropped in elderly women fed large doses of vitamin C, Dr. Campbell says. And it might explain earlier studies showing that ultramarathon runners who take vitamin C have a lower incidence of upper respiratory infections and that military recruits on vitamin C supplements have fewer cases of pneumonia when undergoing basic training.

"If nothing else, our study suggests that certainly under stress, people need more vitamin C," Dr. Campbell says.

Say the word *antioxidant*, and you might as well add "cancer preventive." More than 90 population studies examining the role of vitamin C–rich foods in cancer prevention found protective effects, particularly in esophageal, mouth, stomach, and pancreatic cancers. One overview article found that women getting 300 milligrams of vitamin C a day—the equivalent of about 4½ oranges or 3 cups of orange juice—had 30 percent less breast cancer risk than women who got less vitamin C.

Another study showed that women who took vitamin C supplements for at least 10 years were 77 percent less likely to develop cataracts than women who received the vitamin only through their diets.

In the eye, proteins are evenly distributed throughout the lens. But when proteins are damaged by free radicals, the proteins clump and the density of the lens changes. This change interferes with light refraction through the lens. Think of the ripples in old window glass—the density isn't uniform, and you can't see through it very well. Antioxidants like vitamin C can keep free-radical damage from occurring, says Paul F. Jacques, Sc.D., associate professor in the School of Nutrition Science and Policy at Tufts University, who conducted the vitamin C study.

In time, he expects to see a similar role for vitamins C and E in the prevention of another eye disease, age-related macular degeneration.

Vitamin C also plays a role in bone protection. You're old enough to

POWER

P U D D I N G

PUMPKIN FLAN

This is the best part of pumpkin pie (who needs that fatty, soggy crust?).
And it's so simple that it's ready for the oven in 5 minutes. You couldn't
ask for a more delicious way to get lots of beta-carotene.

4	eggs or 1 cup fat-free liquid egg substitute
1	can (15 ounces) pumpkin puree
1	can (12 ounces) fat-free evaporated milk
¾	cup sugar
1	teaspoon pumpkin pie spice
1	teaspoon grated orange rind

Preheat the oven to 325°F.

In a large bowl, whisk together the eggs or egg substitute, pumpkin,
milk, sugar, spice, and orange rind. Divide the mixture evenly among 10
custard cups (½-cup size).

Arrange the cups in a baking pan and place the pan in the center of
the oven. Carefully pour hot tap water into the pan to come halfway up
the sides of the cups.

Bake for 50 minutes, or until a toothpick inserted in the center of a
cup comes out clean. Carefully transfer the cups to a wire rack to cool
completely. Cover and chill.

Makes 10 servings

Per serving: 129 calories, 6 g protein, 23 g carbohydrates, 2.5 g fat, 87 mg cholesterol,
1 g dietary fiber, 72 mg sodium

know that you shouldn't smoke, so we'll spare you the lecture. But if you
haven't quit yet, you might want to pop a few vitamin C and E supplements. In a study of 66,651 women, Swedish researchers found that current smokers with a low vitamin C or vitamin E intake were three times

more likely to fracture their hips. Vitamin C is, after all, an essential ingredient in collagen formation—the main component of bone. Low intakes of *both* vitamins increased their risk twofold.

Additionally, Polish researchers gave 50 ulcer patients either antacids or 5 grams of vitamin C—admittedly, a massive dose—daily for 4 weeks. At the end of the trial, those taking antacids had no change in the number of *Helicobacter pylori* bacteria (a known cause of peptic ulcers and stomach cancer) in their guts, while 30 percent of those getting vitamin C got rid of the bacteria—with no negative side effects. This study and similar research suggests that vitamin C may play a role in the prevention of some stomach cancers and may explain why low intakes of vitamin C–rich foods are associated with increased risks of stomach cancer.

Other research suggests that vitamin C, applied in a cream, may reduce some signs of aging and wrinkles. For years, vitamin A, or retinoic acid, has been the belle of the dermatological ball. Now it's not dancing alone. There is evidence from several studies that vitamins C and E may protect against sun-induced skin damage.

When German researchers compared sunburns in men and women taking 200 milligrams a day of vitamin C and 1,000 milligrams a day of vitamin E for 8 days against those taking placebos, they found that those taking the vitamins could handle greater levels of ultraviolet radiation before burning than those who didn't.

We're not suggesting you that relinquish your sunscreen and just pop a few vitamins. But perhaps, the research suggests, getting enough of these vitamins might help protect against skin cancer.

Best food sources: Go for pineapple, broccoli, peppers, cantaloupe, strawberries, oranges, kiwifruit, and pink grapefruit.

MARKET LINE

Women buy more vitamin C than any other single vitamin. Last year, sales of C accounted for nearly 30 percent of all single vitamins sold. Vitamin E was a close second at 25.2 percent.

The top-selling mineral, as you might imagine, is calcium, with top billing at 37 percent of all single mineral sales.

WHEN TO AVOID VITAMIN C

Dosing yourself with massive amounts of vitamin C after a cancer diagnosis might not be a good idea.

Vitamin C may inhibit the action of chemotherapy, which works by generating free radicals to destroy cancer cells. What's more, malignant tumors seem to suck up vitamin C for much the same reasons we do: to prevent those nasty free radicals from harming them.

"It's been known that tumors tend to have higher concentrations of vitamin C than does normal tissue," says lead researcher David Golde, M.D., physician-in-chief at Memorial Sloan-Kettering Cancer Center in New York City. But showing how the tumors take up the vitamin C—through transporters that are typically used to take in glucose—suggests that the tumors *want* the vitamin C. You don't want to provide any extra protection to the tumor.

How much to aim for: The Daily Value for vitamin C is 60 milligrams a day. But vitamin C guru Mark Levine, M.D., chief of the molecular and clinical nutrition center at the National Institutes of Health in Washington, D.C., calls for a daily intake of about 200 milligrams. When he sequestered seven young, healthy men for 4 to 6 months, depleted them of vitamin C, and then slowly added the antioxidant back in varying amounts, their immune cells saturated with C at 200 milligrams a day. He expects similar results in women.

If you smoke, you need more C—more than 200 milligrams a day—to keep your blood levels even with nonsmokers taking 60 milligrams.

Vitamin E: The Xena Nutrient

If vitamins were people, E would be a female warrior because it is so powerful in so many ways.

When it comes to boosting immunity, vitamin E may beat out vitamin C, says Simin N. Meydani, Ph.D., chief of the nutritional immunology laboratory at the USDA Human Nutrition Research Center on Aging at Tufts University. In a study, older men and women were assigned to take 60, 200, or 800 milligrams alpha-TE (or about the equivalent of 90, 300, or 1,200 IU) a day of vitamin E for 235 days, while others took a placebo. After just 4 months, those supplementing with vitamin E had a greater immune response to a variety of vaccines.

In another study—in old mice—large doses of vitamin E also provided some protection against the flu.

Until recently, it was a common practice for doctors to put people with heart problems on vitamin E, says Dr. Wardlaw. Epidemiological studies showed that women who used vitamin E supplements of 100 IU or higher for 2 years or more had 41 percent lower risk of heart attack. That advice was welcomed by postmenopausal women, for whom heart disease is the number one cause of death.

But one well-designed study at the Canadian Cardiovascular Collaboration Project Office in Hamilton, Ontario, brings this practice into question. The study showed no benefit from taking vitamin E supplements in people at high risk of death from heart disease. Researchers speculate that vitamin E supplementation may work for younger people, however. After all, it's your total lifestyle that can help prevent heart disease, not just one supplement, Dr. Wardlaw says.

It's thought that vitamin E works to prevent the oxidation of that bad boy of the cholesterol world—low-density lipoprotein (LDL). Oxidized LDL helps cause artery walls to thicken, makes blood platelets stickier, and works in a host of ways to, bottom line, choke off blood supply to the heart.

The vitamin's benefits may extend to women already coping with heart disease. In the Cambridge Heart Antioxidant Study, for instance, 2,000 men and women with atherosclerosis were randomly assigned to receive either vitamin E—at 400 or 800 IU a day—or a placebo. The vitamin E groups reduced their risk of having a nonfatal heart attack 77 percent, although their risk of dying from a heart attack remained the same.

As for stroke, when researchers compared 342 men and women who had had strokes against 501 who hadn't, they found that those taking vitamin E supplements were nearly half as likely to have a stroke. Vitamin E from food had no influence.

Even though the answers to vitamin E's effects on heart disease aren't definitive, Dr. Blumberg urges us to keep the issue in context: "Twenty-seven percent of the population—including 41 percent of African-Americans—have vitamin E levels low enough to put them at a higher risk of heart disease."

POWER

CITRUS SALAD

AVOCADO, GRAPEFRUIT, AND PAPAYA SALAD

This Florida-fresh salad is overflowing with antioxidants like beta-carotene and vitamin C, thanks to the papaya and pink grapefruit. And the avocado is a wonderful source of heart-healthy monounsaturates. It's the perfect accompaniment to summer meals—and a great way to counteract the winter doldrums.

1   tablespoon olive oil
2   teaspoons lemon or lime juice
1   avocado, peeled and sliced
2   pink grapefruits, peeled and sectioned
1   small ripe papaya, peeled and sliced
2   scallions, thinly sliced
4   cups mixed baby greens
1   tablespoon finely chopped cilantro

In a medium bowl, whisk together the oil and lemon or lime juice. Add the avocado, grapefruit, papaya, and scallions. Toss gently to combine. Cover and refrigerate for 1 hour. Serve over a bed of the greens. Sprinkle with the cilantro.

Makes 4 servings

Per serving: 175 calories, 3 g protein, 20 g carbohydrates, 11.5 g fat, 0 mg cholesterol, 4 g dietary fiber, 12 mg sodium

Vitamin E may also play a role in controlling diabetes. When Finnish researchers compared the development of insulin-dependent diabetes between men with high and low vitamin E levels, they found that those with the highest levels were 88 percent less likely to develop the disease than those with lower levels. They suspect that it has to do with the vitamin's ability to scavenge free radicals that damage pancreatic beta cells, which make insulin. There's no reason to think the results won't be the same in women, says study author Paul Knekt, Ph.D., of the National Public Health Institute in Helsinki, Finland.

Vitamin E seems to also prevent memory loss. So don't forget to take it!

Researchers at the University of Indiana in Indianapolis found a connection between poor memory and low blood levels of vitamin E in an elderly, ethnically diverse population, linking it to E's ability to prevent and repair oxidative stress (those nasty free radicals again) implicated both in aging and in brain changes associated with Alzheimer's disease.

Among those with vitamin E levels lower than 4.8 per unit of cholesterol, 11 percent had poor memory. In contrast, just 4 percent of those with levels higher than 7.2 per unit had memory problems. These findings link vitamin E from diet, rather than from supplements, to memory.

Other research suggests that vitamin E supplements may reduce pain from rheumatoid arthritis—an autoimmune disease that affects primarily women—and decrease our risk of getting genital human papillomavirus, the precursor to cervical cancer. Some women even claim that it relieves menopausal hot flashes.

In the future, it may become easier to get more E from food: Scientists are working to genetically engineer certain plants, like soybeans, to produce more vitamin E.

Best food sources: Opt for vegetable and nut oils, including soybean, safflower, canola, and corn; sunflower seeds; whole grains; wheat germ; and spinach.

How much to aim for: The Daily Value for vitamin E is 30 IU—the max you'll get even from a healthy diet—including fortified breakfast cereals, says Dr. Blumberg. Women, on average, get one-third of that, which is why it's one of the few vitamins so many experts say should be taken in supplement form.

Optimum supplementation is 100 to 400 IU for most people, 800 to 1,000 IU for those with pre-existing conditions like diabetes and heart disease. If you can afford it, go for the natural version of vitamin E. It's absorbed at least 35 percent better than the synthetic form—maybe more. If the bottle doesn't say "natural," look for d-alpha tocopherol or mixed tocopherols on the ingredients list. The synthetic version is dl-alpha tocopherol.

Beta-Carotene: No Need for Supplements

It's already pretty easy to get enough of another antioxidant, beta-carotene: Eat your fruits and vegetables.

Beta-carotene is a carotenoid—one of more than 600 that give fruits and vegetables their bright colors. It's known as a pro-vitamin A, which, along with the carotenoids alpha-carotene and beta-cryptoxanthin, turns into vitamin A in the body. Because few foods provide preformed vitamin A (mainly animal products like meat and dairy), the best source is beta-carotene-rich fruits and vegetables. Get enough of the A precursors and you don't need to worry about how much preformed vitamin A you get, says John Erdman, Ph.D., professor of food science and human nutrition at the University of Illinois in Urbana–Champaign.

Generally, women get enough A. You don't need supplements.

That doesn't mean beta-carotene isn't important in its natural state. When researchers at Harvard School of Public Health looked at the diets of 83,000 nurses, they found that premenopausal women who ate foods high in pro-vitamin A's, including beta-carotene, as well as vitamin C and preformed vitamin A, had a lower risk of developing breast cancer even if they had a family history of breast cancer.

Best food sources: Help yourself to carrot juice, pumpkin, sweet potatoes, carrots, spinach, butternut squash, dandelion greens, cantaloupe, mangoes, turnip greens, and beet greens. Get five to nine servings a day—

TAKE YOUR VITAMINS AND . . . SMILE

Taking a multivitamin could be one of the best ways to prevent tooth decay and gum disease. When researchers at the State University of New York at Buffalo evaluated blood samples from 9,862 men and women, they found that those with the highest vitamin A and C levels had half the rate of gum disease compared to those with the lowest levels. And high selenium levels were linked to thirteenfold lower risk of gum disease. The reason? When the body fights bacterial invasion in dental plaque, it produces free radicals—substances looking to snatch an extra electron from other molecules in your cells—that can damage gum tissue. Antioxidant vitamins can help protect against this damage.

and eat them with a little fat to help you absorb this fat-soluble vitamin, or heat them slightly, which, Dr. Erdman says, increases your ability to absorb beta-carotene and other carotenoids.

How much to aim for: There's no Daily Value for beta-carotene—it's 5,000 IU (1,000 retinol equivalents) for vitamin A. Don't supplement above 10,000 IU, and if you're pregnant, don't go any higher than 5,000 IU. Too much preformed vitamin A can cause birth defects.

Selenium: One More Reason to Eat Plants

For decades, scientists puzzled over why residents in certain geographic areas had lower rates of some cancers. One piece of the puzzle, they now think, may be selenium.

A trace mineral in the soil, selenium is absorbed through plants and vegetables. Plants don't require it for growth, and the amount in fruits and vegetables varies extensively.

The theories came together in a 10-year study published in the prestigious *Journal of the American Medical Association.* The researchers found that the use of a selenium supplement was associated with reduced risk of lung and colorectal (and in men, prostate) cancers by as much as two-thirds. Overall, men and women who took selenium supplements were half as likely to die from any type of cancer and one-third as likely to get cancer as those not taking the supplement.

Although the supplement takers were mostly men, lead researcher Dr. Combs says that the effects should be the same for women (with, of course, the exception of prostate cancer).

Selenium may help check breast cancer. In test tube studies, selenium keeps breast cancer cells from growing and induces the death of these cells. In animal studies, selenium has been very effective in reducing breast cancer. It may also play a role in suppressing angiogenesis, the growth of blood vessels that feed tumors.

Best food sources: Although the foods highest in selenium are liver, kidney, and egg yolks, you won't be eating these foods often enough to suffice if you are on a cholesterol-lowering diet. Instead, opt for seafood, whole grains, lean red meats, chicken, and mushrooms.

How much to aim for: The Daily Value for this trace mineral is 70 micrograms a day. There is no need to consider taking more than 200 micrograms a day of selenium, the amount that studies showed was effective in reducing cancer risks. (Doses above 200 milligrams must be taken under medical supervision.)

Many multivitamins don't contain selenium, so check the ingredient label carefully.

Calcium: Head Cashier in the Bone Bank of Life

It would be so easy to get the calcium you need if you drank only milk. Yeah, and it would be so easy to quit your job and fly to Paris on the Concorde if you only won the lottery.

Reality check: Neither of these events are likely to happen.

"Women never eat or drink enough dietary sources of calcium," says Lorna Pascal, R.D., a nutrition consultant at the Dave Winfield Nutrition Center at Hackensack University Medical Center in New Jersey.

So if you are not fond of milk—and unless you're going to eat 6 ounces of tofu, plus a can of sardines with bones, 2 cups of black bean soup, and a pound of cooked spinach today and every day—you're not likely to get your recommended 1,000 to 1,500 milligrams of calcium a day from food alone. You need to supplement, or at least drink a lot of calcium-fortified orange, grapefruit, or citrus-blend juices.

The reasons are as numerous as the shoes in your closet.

For while it's bones we focus on when we talk about calcium, the reality is that this mineral is so important to the *rest* of your body that low blood levels switch on a veritable smorgasbord of hormones and enzymes to suck it out of your bones and feed it to your cells. This explains the growing body of research attributing to calcium (most often in the form of dairy products) everything from reducing your risk of stroke to protecting you against colon cancer to helping you lose body fat when you diet.

In partnership with vitamin D, calcium is also increasingly being considered as an important breast cancer preventive. In studies on mice, scientists at the Rockefeller University in New York City found that a Western-style diet—high in fat plus low in calcium and vitamin D—resulted in precancerous changes in breast, colon, and pancreatic tissues.

Epidemiological studies also link low calcium levels and increased fat to higher cancer rates in women. Thus, increasing calcium and vitamin D intake would do more than reduce our risk of osteoporosis—it may also reduce our risk of breast cancer, according to Martin Lipkin, M.D. of the Strang Cancer Research Laboratory at the Rockefeller University.

POWER

SHAKE

FROZEN BANANA-BERRY YOGURT

What a refreshing snack or dessert! And what a fun way to get vitamin C and a variety of B vitamins into your diet. Best of all, this frozen treat is so low in calories that you can enjoy it often. For best results, use very ripe—meaning, well-speckled—bananas.

 2 large ripe bananas, sliced
 1 pint strawberries
 16 ounces fat-free plain yogurt
   About 3 tablespoons superfine sugar

In a food processor, combine the bananas and strawberries. Process until smooth. Add the yogurt and sugar. (If your fruit is very sweet, cut back on the sugar. Taste the mixture before freezing to determine how much is needed.) Pulse just to blend. Pour the mixture into an 8" × 8" metal baking pan. Freeze for 3 to 4 hours, or until just firm.

Break the frozen yogurt into chunks and return the mixture to the food processor. Process until smooth. Transfer to a freezer container and freeze until solid.

Let the container stand at room temperature for 10 to 15 minutes to soften slightly before scooping.

Makes 5 cups

Per ½ cup: 63 calories, 3 g protein, 13 g carbohydrates, 0.5 g fat, 1 mg cholesterol, 1 g dietary fiber, 35 mg sodium

Best food sources: To get your calcium, eat dairy foods, collard greens, mustard greens, kale, canned salmon with bones, sardines with bones, corn tortillas processed with the mineral lime, tofu with calcium, and calcium-fortified citrus juice.

How much to aim for: The generic, one-size-fits-some-but-not-all

GET THE BIGGEST BANG
FOR YOUR CALCIUM BUCK

Supplements vary widely in the amount of calcium they contain and how they should be taken. Calcium carbonate is 40 percent calcium, whereas calcium gluconate is only 9 percent. What's more, calcium citrate is absorbed up to 2½ times better than calcium carbonate. To maximize absorption:

- Take calcium carbonate and other sources of calcium with meals.
- Take calcium citrate anytime.
- Split the dose. Don't take more than 500 milligrams of calcium at a time. The more calcium you take at one time, the less efficiently your body absorbs it.
- Buy quick-dissolving tablets. To test, place a tablet in white vinegar. It should dissolve within 30 minutes.

Daily Value for calcium is 1,000 milligrams. Women age 51 and older need 1,500 milligrams. If you're supplementing, don't take any more than 500 milligrams at a time. The more calcium you take at one time, the less efficiently you absorb it, explains calcium expert Connie Weaver, Ph.D., professor and director of the department of foods and nutrition at Purdue University in West Lafayette, Indiana. She recommends that women divide their calcium doses throughout the day.

The tastiest source is calcium "candy"—chocolate chews containing 500 milligrams of calcium, 100 IU of vitamin D, 40 micrograms of vitamin K, and just 20 calories. Look for them wherever vitamins are sold. (They also come in mocha and caramel.) Just remember that these aren't really candy. Aim for 1,000 to 1,500 milligrams of calcium. Too much calcium can cause constipation and kidney stones. Too much vitamin D can cause headache, nausea, calcium imbalance, and impaired kidney function.

Vitamin D: Needs Increase with Age

Unless you're swigging down the cod-liver oil or relishing a meal of fatty fish like sardines or salmon three or more times a week, you have to rely mainly on the sun for your vitamin D. Today, we keep 95 percent of our bodies covered and rarely leave the sterile environs of our offices or minivans. Just how much vitamin D do you think we're making from sunlight? Not nearly enough.

If you live in a northern climate—say, Boston; Chicago; Portland, Oregon; Edmonton, Canada; or anywhere north of Washington, D.C.— you're going to be hard-pressed to get enough in the winter, says Michael F. Holick, M.D., Ph.D., director of the General Clinical Research Center at Boston University Medical Center.

This may explain why researchers at Harvard Medical School found that 57 percent of patients on a general hospital ward in Boston were vitamin D deficient. Even among those already taking more than the recommended Daily Value, 37 percent still showed deficient blood levels of the vitamin.

And as you age, your ability to make vitamin D in your skin decreases 70 percent, says Dr. Holick. In its activated form, vitamin D turns into a hormone that tells the small intestine to crank up and increase calcium absorption. With it, you absorb about 30 percent of the calcium you eat; without it, 10 to 15 percent.

A child who doesn't get enough vitamin D gets rickets, which is why children used to get daily doses of cod-liver oil. But if you're an adult and you don't get enough vitamin D, you exacerbate your risk of osteoporosis and can develop a bone disease called osteomalacia, which Dr. Holick calls adult rickets.

"It's very subtle. Vitamin D deficiency results in a stealing of calcium from the bones and prevents calcium from being deposited in newly formed bones. So as you get older, you're at increased risk of fractures," he says. Many women complaining of bone pain, often diagnosed as arthritis, probably have osteomalacia, he says. "It's very misdiagnosed because few know about it." (If you're at risk, your doctor can test for the form of vitamin D made by the liver, called 25-hydroxyvitamin D.) But the benefits of vitamin D extend beyond the bone.

Research suggests that it may also inhibit breast and colon cancers. Both breast and colon cells have vitamin D receptors, Dr. Holick says, perhaps because they require a certain level of the vitamin to maintain good cell health and prevent rogue cells from turning cancerous.

His theory is borne out in studies showing greater rates of breast and colon cancer among women living in higher latitudes—areas where vitamin D synthesis from the sun is lowest.

POWER

SOUP

WHITE BEAN AND GREENS SOUP

The Italians know that beans and greens are a dynamic duo, in terms of both taste and health. Here they team up for a hearty soup that's overflowing with healing nutrients like folate and vitamins A and K.

1	tablespoon olive oil
1	large onion, finely chopped
1	carrot, finely chopped
1	tablespoon finely chopped garlic
1	teaspoon dried sage
2	cans (14½ ounces each) fat-free chicken broth
1	can (15½ ounces) small white beans, rinsed and drained
1	box (10 ounces) frozen chopped spinach, thawed and well-drained

In a large saucepan, warm the oil over medium heat. Add the onion and cook for 3 minutes, stirring often. Add the carrot, garlic, and sage and cook for 3 minutes longer. Stir in the broth, beans, and spinach. Bring to a boil. Reduce the heat to low and simmer for 10 minutes.

Makes 6 cups

Per cup: 120 calories, 8 g protein, 18 g carbohydrates, 3 g fat, 0 mg cholesterol, 2 g dietary fiber, 505 mg sodium

"We believe that there are two levels of vitamin D deficiency," Dr. Holick says. "Blood levels of 25-hydroxyvitamin D above 20 nanograms per milliliter is needed for maximum bone health. A level of 1½ to 2 times this amount may be necessary to have the most benefit on cellular health."

An added plus: Upping the D might improve your mood. According to one Australian study, supplementing with up to 800 IU daily improved mood in patients suffering from seasonal depression.

Best food sources: Vitamin D is found in herring, sardines, salmon, vitamin D–fortified milk, and fortified cereals, but it's difficult to get enough vitamin D from your diet, Dr. Holick says. And don't count on milk. He's done studies showing that upward of 50 percent of milk tested didn't contain even half the D touted on the label. Ten to 15 percent had none.

How much to aim for: The Daily Value for vitamin D is 400 IU, but men and women over age 70 should get 600 IU. Too much vitamin D can cause headache, nausea, calcium imbalance, and impaired kidney function.

Vitamin K Is for Kale—And More

You can get all the vitamin D you need, but if you're low on K, you're still likely to have an increased risk of hip fractures, suggesting that your bones are weak. Although vitamin D increases the amount of calcium your bones take in, vitamin K decreases the amount of calcium you lose in urine.

Historically, this fat-soluble vitamin's *raison d'être* was to clot our blood. And that's how the Daily Value of 80 micrograms was set. But newer research has shown that vitamin K is a powerful tool in building bone. It sets off a chemical reaction that refigures critical proteins that form the underpinnings of bone—the substructure that gets filled in with calcium, says Diane Feskanich, Sc.D., an instructor at Harvard Medical School.

In a 10-year prospective study of 120,000 women, Dr. Feskanich and other researchers found that women who got at least 109 micrograms of vitamin K in their diets had a 30 percent lower risk of hip fractures than women who got less vitamin K. That's more than the Daily Value.

Scientists are also looking at forms of the vitamin as a possible treatment—or prevention—for liver and other cancers. A special form of vitamin K—at least 2,000 times stronger than that occurring naturally—appears to kill breast, liver, and skin cancer cells in test tubes in the lab by blocking the activity of a group of enzymes, thus convincing the cells (biochemically at least) to shut down and die, says lead researcher Brian Carr, M.D., Ph.D., director of the Liver Cancer Center at the University of Pittsburgh Cancer Institute. In one small clinical trial in which liver cancer patients took 1,000 milligrams a day of the regular version of vitamin K, tumors shrank in about 20 percent of patients, Dr. Carr says.

Best food sources: Go for kale, mustard greens, spinach, brussels sprouts, collard greens, broccoli, parsley, and lettuce. Vitamin K is relatively easy to get from food: just ½ cup of cooked kale or mustard greens supplies about 715 micrograms, and collard greens have 374 micrograms. Women tend to get most of their vitamin K from lettuce, which contains 70 micrograms per cup, says Dr. Feskanich. Sprinkle a little olive oil on your spinach (or salad) to help your body absorb this fat-soluble vitamin.

How much to aim for: The Daily Value for vitamin K is 80 micrograms. If you're on blood thinners like warfarin (Coumadin), be careful about not overconsuming vitamin K. But there's no need to supplement with vitamin K unless prescribed. Just get a cup a day of some leafy green vegetable—even lettuce—and you'll more than meet the needs of your body—and bones.

Magnesium: Calcium's Pal

Bet you didn't know that magnesium is good for sore feet. Yet every time you soak your feet in Epsom salts, you're soaking them in magnesium sulfate, which works by drawing water from inflamed muscles and tissues.

Magnesium is easy to find in food. "It's in things like dark greens, soybeans, and whole grains," foods we should eat, but often don't, says Somer. As a result, most women get around 250 milligrams of magnesium from their diets—far below the recommended Daily Value of 400 milligrams.

Magnesium plays a role in muscle contraction and the way nerves transmit signals from cell to cell. Your body needs magnesium to use glucose.

Some studies have shown that magnesium can reduce bone loss in postmenopausal women. One even reported an increase in bone mass in 31 women after 1 year of dietary magnesium supplementation. But if you're postmenopausal, your body is probably getting rid of magnesium faster than you can take it in because as estrogen levels drop, you excrete more magnesium.

POWER

CHOWDER

MANHATTAN CLAM CHOWDER

When it comes to clam chowder, say "I'll take Manhattan!" It's much lower in fat than cream-based New England chowder, and the tomatoes contribute a superhelping of cancer-preventing lycopene. Of course, the clams pull their own weight, with more iron than even red meat.

1	tablespoon olive oil
1	onion, finely chopped
1	rib celery, finely chopped
2	medium potatoes, cut into ¼" cubes
1	can (14½ ounces) diced tomatoes (in juice)
1	can (14½ ounces) fat-free chicken broth
½	teaspoon dried thyme
¼	teaspoon salt
¼	teaspoon ground black pepper
1	can (6½ ounces) minced clams (in clam juice)

In a 3-quart saucepan, warm the oil over medium heat. Add the onion and celery and cook, stirring often, for 5 minutes. Add the potatoes and cook, stirring often, for 2 minutes.

Stir in the tomatoes (with juice), broth, thyme, salt, and pepper. Bring to a boil. Reduce the heat to low and simmer for 30 minutes, or until the potatoes are tender. Stir in the clams (with juice).

Makes 6 cups

Per cup: 100 calories, 6 g protein, 15 g carbohydrates, 3 g fat, 19 mg cholesterol, 3 g dietary fiber, 375 mg sodium

POWER

CASSEROLE

KALE-POTATO-TOMATO BAKE

Leafy greens like kale are big guns in the fight against stroke, cancer, macular degeneration, heart disease, and lots more. Here's a really luscious way to get them into your family's diet.

2   tablespoons olive oil

1   large onion, finely chopped

3   medium potatoes, peeled and cut into ¼" cubes

1   box (10 ounces) frozen chopped kale, thawed and well-drained

1   can (14½ ounces) diced tomatoes, drained

1   container (15 ounces) reduced-fat ricotta cheese

½   cup shredded reduced-fat Monterey Jack cheese

2   eggs, lightly beaten, or ½ cup fat-free liquid egg substitute

½   teaspoon salt

Preheat the oven to 350°F. Coat a 13" × 9" baking dish with cooking spray.

In a large nonstick skillet, warm the oil over medium heat. Add the onion and cook, stirring often, for 3 minutes. Add the potatoes and cook, stirring occasionally, for 15 minutes, or until tender. Add the kale and tomatoes. Cook for 1 minute.

In a large bowl, whisk together the ricotta cheese, Monterey Jack, eggs or egg substitute, and salt. Add the kale mixture and stir to combine. Spoon into the baking dish.

Bake for 40 minutes, or until a knife inserted in the center comes out clean. Let stand on a wire rack for 10 minutes before serving.

Makes 6 servings

Per serving: 284 calories, 17 g protein, 24 g carbohydrates, 14 g fat, 99 mg cholesterol, 3 g dietary fiber, 710 mg sodium

Variation: Replace the kale with collard greens or spinach.

The mineral is also being studied as a critical component in the prevention of heart disease. When researchers at the Centers for Disease Control and Prevention analyzed nutritional data and causes of death for nearly 13,000 men and women, they found that those who had the highest blood magnesium levels were 31 percent less likely to die from ischemic heart disease.

That's no big surprise: Magnesium is used extensively by the heart, where it relaxes the arteries and keeps the heart's electrical system working. Low levels are associated with abnormal heart rhythms and sudden-death heart disease, and intravenous magnesium given to heart patients reduces relapses and deaths.

There's also some evidence that magnesium might help with migraines. In a German trial, 81 migraine sufferers received either 600 milligrams of magnesium or a placebo daily for 12 weeks. By the 9th week, those getting magnesium had 41 percent fewer headaches, compared to the 15 percent drop in the placebo group. When the headaches did hit, they were less intense and didn't last as long.

Additionally, researchers are looking at magnesium's implications in PMS. In one study, 38 women took either 200 milligrams of magnesium or a placebo for 2 months. By the second month, those taking magnesium noticed fewer fluid-related PMS symptoms, including weight gain, swelling, breast tenderness, and abdominal bloating.

Best food sources: Choose seafood, legumes (especially soybeans), nuts, meats, whole grains, dark green vegetables, and fat-free milk products (milk, yogurt, and cheese).

How much to aim for: The Daily Value for magnesium is 400 milligrams. Neither Tums nor multiple vitamins have enough of this vital mineral, says Somer. But don't take any more than 350 milligrams from supplements. If you have heart or kidney problems check with your doctor before taking supplemental magnesium, and know that in some people excess magnesium may cause diarrhea.

A Woman's Guide to Iron

Elizabeth Somer knew something was wrong when she was pregnant with her second child. She was exhausted, but when she complained to her doctor, he reassured her that her anemia test was negative, figuratively patted her on the head, and blamed it on the pregnancy.

As a nutritionist, however, Somer knew better. She went for a serum ferritin test—a more sensitive blood test which measures iron deficiency before it becomes anemia. A normal score is 20; hers was 4.

Hence her philosophy: "I recommend that every woman of child-bearing age have a serum ferritin test done. And be feisty about it. Find out what your value is. Because every single woman that has come to me complaining of tiredness who had the test done was iron deficient."

Overall, studies show that between 30 and 80 percent of us are iron deficient. Not anemic, just low. The symptoms are similar, says Somer: fatigue, breathlessness from walking up a flight of stairs, increased susceptibility to colds and infections, and muddled thinking.

Another possible sign is restless leg syndrome, when your legs feel jumpy at night. Some studies found low iron levels in sufferers of restless leg syndrome, and that their symptoms were relieved by iron supplements. Why is still a question, but it may have something to do with iron's effects on the brain chemical dopamine, which plays a role in nerve transmission.

Best food sources: You can get iron from red meats, poultry, eggs, legumes, Cream of Wheat cereal, baked potatoes, soybeans, pumpkin seeds, and clams.

How much to aim for: The Daily Value for iron is 18 milligrams. Women who menstruate heavily or use an IUD should get more, up to 25 milligrams, says Somer.

FORTIFIED CEREALS: A GOOD START— BUT NOT ENOUGH

Think you're getting everything you need in your breakfast cereal? Probably not, says Elizabeth Somer, R.D., a nutritionist and author of *The Essential Guide to Vitamins and Minerals.*

"Check the package label," she says. "Do you find chromium? Selenium? Molybdenum? Manganese? Copper? If all of those plus the regulars: at least eight of the B vitamins; vitamins A, C, D, E, and K; calcium; iron; magnesium; zinc; and more, are in there at 100 percent of Daily Value levels, and you eat that cereal every day, you probably don't need to supplement." But chances are, they aren't.

"It's one reason to take a multivitamin/mineral supplement—most have 18 milligrams of iron," says Somer. If you're at the point that you're actually iron deficient, she says, your physician probably will prescribe prescription-strength iron for a few months to get your levels back to baseline.

And watch your iron levels if you're dieting. When 14 obese, premenopausal women went on diets of 1,000 to 1,200 calories (half of what they usually ate) for 15 weeks, seven of the women's iron levels dropped—despite the fact that they were getting about twice the recommended amount of iron in their diets. They also scored 50 percent lower on a concentration test than women with adequate levels. The study suggests that your body may not use iron as effectively when you restrict calories, says study author Molly Kretsch, Ph.D., a research nutrition scientist at the USDA Western Human Nutrition Research Center in Davis, California.

But don't load up on extra iron, thinking that it will equate to extra energy. Some women have a gene that causes them to absorb too much iron, causing a disease called hemochromatosis. One out of every 250 Americans is at high risk for this condition. Because women menstruate and have babies, if they have the gene, symptoms of the disease usually don't show up until after menopause. Postmenopausal women, whose iron requirements are relatively low, are susceptible to it (as are men). And some research suggests that taking too much iron may raise the risk of heart disease and colon cancer. If you're postmenopausal, don't take any extra iron unless directed to by your doctor, says Somer.

B Vitamins You Can't Do Without

Back in the 1940s, some advertising executive came up with a health drink called V. V. Vitawater—sparkling tonic water containing "the necessary vitamin B factor that helps to make you feel better."

We now know that there is no one "factor," but a whole family of B vitamins: B_6, B_{12}, folate, thiamin, riboflavin, niacin, pantothenic acid, and biotin. They are particularly important to women for a variety of reasons—not the least of which is that they help our bodies break down food for energy. Without them, we'd be even more exhausted.

The three B vitamins women need most are folate and vitamins B_6 and B_{12}. Together, they control levels of homocysteine, an amino acid that

ON BIRTH CONTROL PILLS? MIND YOUR ABC'S

Women taking oral contraceptives generally have lower blood levels of folate, the other B vitamins, and vitamin C, and slightly higher levels of vitamin A," says Jeffrey Blumberg, Ph.D., chief of the antioxidants research laboratory at Tufts University in Boston. Additionally, they usually have lower tissue levels of antioxidant enzymes. Although the reasons for this are not well-understood, he says, "in my view, supplementing with vitamins for women using oral contraceptives, while not definitively established through extensive clinical trials, is a reasonable, safe, inexpensive, and proactive health behavior."

has been linked to an increased risk of heart disease and stroke. Several studies have shown that diets lacking in these B vitamins lead to high blood levels of homocysteine, and at least one major study, the Nurses' Health Study, shows that women who consume high amounts of folate and vitamin B_6, from either food or supplements, have a risk of developing heart disease that's nearly half that of women who get lower amounts.

Even within normal ranges, lower levels of these three Bs may affect your memory. In several studies, men and women with either high-normal levels of homocysteine or low-normal levels of these three B vitamins scored worse on tests of mental acuity than those with higher levels. Preliminary evidence suggests that those with low levels are more likely to develop Alzheimer's disease.

So you know how when you're really stressed and tired you have trouble remembering your own name? A nap might help—but so could a balanced B supplement.

Folate: You Can't Afford to Take It for Granted

Maybe you're no longer dealing with diapers, baby bottles, and all of the other trappings of new motherhood. But that doesn't mean you're done with folate—which might be called the baby vitamin.

Folate, or folic acid as it's called when it's in supplement form, took center stage in the vitamin arena when numerous studies showed women could halve their risk of having babies with neural-tube defects (a birth defect of the spinal cord or brain) if they got 400 micrograms of folate daily before pregnancy and 600 micrograms during.

Next came a strong connection between folate and lowered risk of heart disease, based on observational studies. If this association is true, Shirley A. A. Beresford, Ph.D., professor of epidemiology at the University of Washington in Seattle, estimates that if just 10 percent of the women not getting enough folate—more than half of all women—began supplementing, about 5 per 1,000 heart disease deaths in women could be prevented each year. That's 1,500 women a year who might still be alive today.

Folate may also help lift depression. "Between 15 and 40 percent of adults diagnosed with major depression also have low or borderline levels of folate," says Jonathan E. Alpert, M.D., Ph.D., assistant professor of psychiatry at Harvard Medical School. In some studies, the lower the levels, the higher their ratings on the depression scales.

In some studies, depressed men and women treated with daily doses of folic acid alone or in conjunction with standard antidepressants showed significant improvement. Similarly, when Dr. Alpert tested B levels in healthy, albeit depressed, volunteers just before they began taking the antidepressant fluoxetine (Prozac), he found that those with the lowest folate levels had a poorer response to the drug. "It's as if those low levels blunted their responses to antidepressants," he said.

"We don't know where the connection comes in," says Dr. Alpert. The low folate and B_{12} levels could be the cause of the depression, or, conversely, depression itself, often accompanied by poor eating habits, could trigger the low levels.

You don't want to escape a heart attack and depression only to succumb to cancer. Here, too, folate can help. Two studies found that taking up to 1,000 micrograms a day of folic acid could possibly reduce the risk of cancerous cells or full-blown colorectal cancer in men and women with chronic ulcerative colitis. Another study has shown protective effects against cervical cancer.

Last, taking folic acid as part of a multivitamin may cancel out the link between alcohol and breast cancer, according to researchers working on the Nurses' Health Study.

Best food sources: For folate, eat fortified cereals, pinto beans, navy beans, asparagus, spinach, broccoli, okra, and brussels sprouts. (By law, all enriched products, including flour, bread, rolls, grits, cornmeal, and pasta

POWER

STIR-FRY

BEEF, BROCCOLI, AND ONION STIR-FRY

Stir-fries are the ideal way to serve meat. You can take a modest amount of beef and turn it into a filling dinner with the addition of rice and vegetables. We've used broccoli (that mighty cancer-preventing crucifer), but you can try other super veggies like carrots, cabbage, snap peas, or a combination.

1	cup cooked brown rice
1	tablespoon canola oil
¾	pound top round, thinly sliced
1	bunch scallions, cut into 1" pieces
2	cups broccoli florets
½	cup water
3	tablespoons reduced-sodium soy sauce
1½	teaspoons sesame oil

In a large nonstick skillet, warm the canola oil over medium-high heat. Add the beef and cook, stirring constantly, for 1 minute, or until browned on all sides. Remove from the pan and set aside.

Add the scallions to the pan. Cook, stirring, for 1 minute. Add the broccoli. Cook, stirring, for 1 minute. Add the water, soy sauce, and sesame oil. Cook, stirring often, for 5 minutes, or until the broccoli and scallions are tender. Stir in the beef and heat through. Serve over the rice.

Makes 4 servings

Per serving: 385 calories, 26 g protein, 47 g carbohydrates, 10.5 g fat, 40 mg cholesterol, 3 g dietary fiber, 464 mg sodium

and noodles, must include folate. So be aware that if you eat whole wheat products—which you should—they aren't enriched and you aren't getting any extra. Also, more than half the folate in foods can be lost in cooking and processing since folate is destroyed by heat and ultraviolet light.)

How much to aim for: The Daily Value for nonpregnant women is 400 micrograms a day. For women trying to conceive or who are already pregnant, it's 600 micrograms a day. Dr. Jeffrey Blumberg of Tufts University has reason to believe that perhaps 600 or even 800 micrograms a day would be a better Daily Value. But too much folate (over 1,000 micrograms) can mask signs of a B_{12} deficiency, so you don't want to aim higher than that. For all-purpose nutritional insurance, Somer recommends a multivitamin, which typically contains 400 micrograms.

Vitamin B_6: More Is Not Necessarily Better

Getting the Daily Value for this vitamin from your diet alone could force you into a weight-loss program. You could eat six slices of whole wheat bread, 3 cups of whole milk, and 1 pound of broiled lean ground beef and still not be getting enough. This may explain why nearly half of all women in this country get less than the recommended Daily Value of 2 milligrams.

And if you want your B_6 levels high enough for some of its protective effects, you'll need daily amounts of 50 milligrams, says John M. Ellis, M.D., author of *Vitamin B_6 Therapy: Nature's Versatile Healer.*

Vitamin B_6 is particularly important for women, says Dr. Ellis. "The movement of female hormones in and out of tissues, particularly the breast and uterus, is, to a degree, regulated by B_6," he says.

Thus the vitamin's potential for relieving PMS symptoms. When British researchers evaluated four controlled trials, they found vitamin B_6 more effective than a placebo, particularly when it came to premenstrual depression. There was no benefit in taking more than 50 milligrams a day for PMS symptoms.

Yet another study suggests that there may be some link between low B_6 levels and chronic fatigue syndrome, a debilitating autoimmune disorder more prevalent in women than in men.

The vitamin also shows up as a preventive for kidney stones. Researchers at Harvard Medical School evaluated the diets of 85,557 women with no history of kidney stones and found that those getting 40 milligrams of B_6 or more a day from diet and supplements were one-third less likely to develop kidney stones than those getting only 3 milligrams. The researchers theorize that B_6 may decrease oxalate production, a risk factor for stones.

Then there is the connection between B_6 and carpal tunnel syndrome.

WHAT TO LOOK FOR IN A MULTI

Confused? Here's what to look for the next time you shop for a multivitamin/mineral supplement.

- Vitamin A/Beta-carotene: 5,000 IU
- Vitamin D: 400 IU
- Vitamin K: 25 micrograms
- Thiamin: 1.5 milligrams
- Riboflavin: 1.7 milligrams
- Niacin: 20 milligrams
- Vitamin B_6: 2 milligrams
- Folic acid or folate: 400 micrograms
- Vitamin B_{12}: 6 micrograms, especially if you're over age 50
- Iron: At least 18 milligrams if you're premenopausal, 0 to 9 milligrams if you're postmenopausal.
- Magnesium: 100 milligrams; although it's only 25 percent of the Daily Value, more would make the pills too large. In a divided-dose multi, look for up to 350 milligrams.
- Zinc: 15 milligrams
- Selenium: 10 micrograms
- Copper: 2 milligrams
- Chromium: 120 micrograms

You won't find optimal doses of the following nutrients in any multi, so take them separately.

- Vitamin C: 100 to 500 milligrams a day, but you'll keep your blood better saturated if you take two 250-milligram doses 12 hours apart
- Vitamin E: 100 to 400 IU
- Calcium: 500 to 1,000 milligrams in divided doses of no more than 500 milligrams at a time

Dr. Ellis has published numerous studies showing its effectiveness in treating carpal tunnel syndrome and linking low levels of the vitamin to the malady. The vitamin supposedly works by improving the function of the synovium, the sheath that surrounds the tendons, he says. It also helps stimulate the body's production of cortisone, which, in turn, reduces swelling in the tendons compressing the median nerve.

"When you see those signs and symptoms of carpal tunnel syndrome appearing in a woman," he says, "in my opinion, her body is crying out for the vitamin." If taking 100 to 200 milligrams of vitamin B_6 for 3 months doesn't relieve the numbness, tingling, and pain, work with your physician to consider the next step.

Best food sources: Go for potatoes, bananas, avocados, chicken, beef, fish, brown rice, and peanuts.

How much to aim for: The Daily Value for vitamin B_6 is 2 milligrams. Dr. Ellis recommends between 50 to 100 milligrams for most adults. Don't take more than 100 milligrams of B_6 a day without your doctor's supervision. At high doses, vitamin B_6 can cause nerve damage. Although the damage is reversible, it's better to take the lowest amount of the vitamin you need to get the job done, not the highest. And if you take 50 milligrams a day or more, be sure to taper supplements over several days, rather than discontinue abruptly, to avoid a rebound deficiency.

SIZING UP SUPPLEMENT ADDITIVES

In addition to the vitamins and minerals in your daily multi, you may be getting a dose of sugar, dyes, and other fillers.

These additives are also used in many drugs and aren't of concern unless you have certain food sensitivities, says V. Srini Srinivasan, Ph.D., director of dietary supplements for the United States Pharmacopeia in Rockville, Maryland, a nonprofit organization that develops and establishes standards for drugs and dietary supplements. Sugar, for instance, is required to mask the bitter taste of the ingredients. Talc or talcum powder is often added so that the pills don't stick to the machines that shape them. Starch ensures that the tablet disintegrates and dissolves once it's swallowed.

"These additives are all safe," says Dr. Srinivasan. Other additives you might see include lactose and food dyes. If you have food allergies, read the labels carefully—there are vitamin brands that don't contain any such substances.

Vitamin B$_{12}$: Folate's Pal

When it comes to vitamin B$_{12}$, scientists recommend its crystalline form over the form found naturally in food.

One reason you don't see too many foods supplemented with high amounts of vitamin B$_{12}$, says Dr. Wardlaw, is that B$_{12}$ is bright red. It turns food pink. And who wants to cook with pink flour?

But you need to get enough. If you get too little, you run the risk of irreversible neurological problems, like dementia. One study out of the University of Georgia in Athens connected relatively low levels of B$_{12}$ and folate to hearing loss. When researchers there examined the amounts of folate and B$_{12}$ in 55 healthy women ages 60 to 71, they found that women with hearing loss had B$_{12}$ levels 38 percent lower than women with normal hearing, and folate levels 31 percent lower.

And, although folate seems to be more closely related to depression than vitamin B$_{12}$, for some people, depression may be linked to low levels of B$_{12}$ as well. Dr. Alpert says that studies show 12 to 14 percent of clinically depressed people have low B$_{12}$ levels.

Best food sources: Vitamin B$_{12}$ is available from meat, seafood, and dairy products, and breakfast cereals and soy products are often fortified with it.

NATURAL OR SYNTHETIC: WHICH IS BETTER?

Natural supplements—vitamins extracted from food—are no more potent than compounds synthesized in factories. Each vitamin and mineral—from vitamin C to calcium—has a specific chemical composition. Your body can't tell the difference between compounds that occur naturally in food and those that are manufactured. So, in general, there's no need to scout out natural vitamins. "There is no scientific evidence that says one is better than the other," says V. Srini Srinivasan, Ph.D., director of dietary supplements for the United States Pharmacopeia in Rockville, Maryland. In fact, synthetic folic acid is better absorbed by your body than the natural type, he says, because of its composition.

The one exception is vitamin E. Natural forms are more readily absorbed.

BUYING VITAMINS

When shopping for a multivitamin/mineral tablet:

- Check the expiration date. Don't buy more than you can use by that date.
- Look for "USP". This seal of approval from the nongovernmental United States Pharmacopeia means the supplement should dissolve inside you.
- If you find that multis are too big to swallow, try chewables. Children's multivitamins can be complete for adult needs. Check the label. Or grind up your multi with a mortar and pestle and drink it down with some juice. Some multis come in liquid form, but tend not to be complete.
- You don't need divided-dose multis or timed-release multis. Unlike prescription drugs such as antibiotics or birth control pills, which require constant levels in the blood for optimal effectiveness, maintaining a constant level of vitamins and minerals in the body isn't necessary.

When you get them home:

- Store them in a cool, dry place like the cupboard where you keep dried spices—not above the stove.
- Take them with meals. You need a little fat—about the amount in ½ to 1 teaspoon of oil—to help you absorb vitamins A, D, E, and K.
- Don't take multis with iron at the same time as you take calcium supplements—the calcium may interfere with the iron's absorption.

How much to aim for: The Daily Value for vitamin B_{12} is 6 micrograms. If you're 50 or older, chances are that you may have trouble absorbing it from food. So the Institute of Medicine at the National Academy of Sciences says that people 50 and older should get their B_{12} in crystalline form. A multivitamin should more than meet your needs. Some researchers have raised the bar on B_{12} and now recommend 25 micrograms, and some manufacturers are adding this amount to their "senior" supplements.

Phytonutrients: The Latest on Nature's Healing Agents

Power Maker #15: Make a point of choosing foods from the 10 "New Food Groups": onions and garlic; cabbage and its cousins; nuts and seeds; whole grains and flax; soy and other beans; fruit; cooked tomatoes; greens; carrots and savory herbs; and dairy and lean meats.

Once upon a time, buying produce was as simple as identifying colors. A couple of green vegetables, a yellow and an orange, maybe a red if sweet peppers were on sale. Hit the fruit aisle and buy what's in season, along with the ubiquitous apples and bananas—all great choices. But they're just the beginning. In recent years, scientists have unearthed thousands of vitamin-like compounds, called phytonutrients, in plant foods. These, they say, are nature's way of protecting us against cancer and a variety of chronic diseases.

The amazing thing is the speed with which these discoveries occurred. In the early 1990s, hardly anyone had heard of phytonutrients. Yet by the end of the 20th century, scientists had identified more than 10,000 of these compounds from fruits and veggies, including more than 600 related to beta-carotene (called carotenoids) and 4,000 others known as flavonoids. In just 5 years, the National Cancer Institute spent over $20 million researching the anti-cancer potential of phytonutrient-containing plant foods.

Phytonutrients have tongue-twisting names like lutein and lycopene, diallyl sulfide and daidzein, and caffeic and ferulic acids. But they make headlines every day.

"You can't get these compounds in anything but food," says J. Robert Hatherill, Ph.D., professor of toxicology at the University of California, Santa Barbara, and author of *Eat to Beat Cancer*. They are what make the tomato red, the onion pungent, and the walnut rough and leathery. They repel insects and other predators, enable sunshine to be turned into food, and prevent plant "sunburns."

POWER-EATING TIP

Buy green tea in bulk. It's generally much higher in antioxidants than the tea in tea bags. Usually the best-quality tea can be found at Asian specialty food stores. If you're overwhelmed by the varieties of tea, try sencha, which is a variety popular in Japan. Never boil green tea. Instead, steep it for 5 to 8 minutes in water that is about 192°F. If you prefer black tea, drink it without milk. A British study showed that tea with milk did not lower heart disease risk; researchers theorize that the milk interferes with the activity of the phytonutrients.

From Photosynthesis to Cancer Prevention

To plants, phytonutrients are protective clothing—a suit of armor against disease. For us, they provide a long list of health benefits.

"Think about it: Plants don't get cancer," says Michele L. Trankina, Ph.D., professor of biological sciences at St. Mary's University in San Antonio, where she is also a nutrition consultant.

In fact, phytonutrients seem to impact cancer and heart disease more than any other illnesses, says Winston Craig, Ph.D., professor of nutrition at Andrews University in Berrien Springs, Michigan. Although modern medicine attributes a variety of causes to these diseases, he says, perhaps the single common thread among them is the activity of unwanted by-products called free radicals, "handicapped" molecules missing one electron. Like a duped lover out for revenge, they roam around our cells snatching electrons from other molecules, creating more free radicals. As this cascading effect continues, it damages cells, which malfunction and, in turn, damage body systems and cause diseases like atherosclerosis, heart disease, diabetes, arthritis, and dementia.

Just the simple consumption of oxygen during activities of daily living such as eating, breathing, and even walking around in the sun creates free radicals. Antioxidants, however, trap and destroy these free radicals. And phytonutrients—those thousands of healing substances in plants—are powerful antioxidant substances.

In the prevention of heart disease, for instance, antioxidants prevent LDL cholesterol from being oxidized—the process by which these fat particles are altered so that the body cannot effectively remove them out of the blood, clogging our arteries. When it comes to cancer, antioxidants prevent free radicals from damaging cell membranes and DNA.

"If our antioxidant levels are high enough and the antioxidants are mobilized in the cells at the right parts of the cell at the right time, they keep these chronic diseases in check," says Dr. Craig. With each new discovery, shopping for produce takes on a whole new dimension. It's like going to a phytonutrient pharmacy.

"The point is to get to know that in those berries, melons, and dark green, leafy things, you have these powerful, wonderful nutrients working in combination to help you stave off disease, have fewer aches and pains, keep your hormones in balance, reduce your risk of cancer, and stave off some of the perils of perimeno-

---

MASKED DISASTER

Souped-Up Snack Foods

Chewing gum with phosphatidylserine, a fatty acid that can improve memory. Chocolate drink mixes laced with kava kava, an antianxiety herb. Tortilla chips baked with the antidepressant herb St. John's wort.

Foods enhanced with herbs or nutrients lead you to believe that they will magically solve your health problems. But they're not worth the money.

"For one thing, we don't even know if some of these added ingredients work," says Barbara Gollman, R.D., a spokesperson for the American Dietetic Association. Second, you'd have to drink four to five bottles a day of one kava kava–containing tea to feel less anxious (adding about 500 calories to your diet).

pause," says Stephanie Beling, M.D., a physician at Canyon Ranch, a health and fitness resort in Lenox, Massachusetts. Here's how they do it.

I. Onions and Garlic

Onions, garlic, leeks, chives, shallots, and scallions contain organosulfur compounds—aromatic phytonutrients that make your eyes water. These powerful phytonutrients can reduce cancer and coronary heart disease risk and control high blood pressure.

In one study of more than 40,000 postmenopausal women, for instance, eating garlic cut the women's risk of colon cancer nearly in half.

One organosulfur, allicin, blocks cancer-causing agents, stops the process that creates cholesterol, boosts immunity, and prevents infection. Other compounds produce a freight train of enzymes that literally push carcinogens out of your body, decrease tumor cell division, and stop chemical compounds associated with stomach cancer from forming.

These vegetables also contain another major class of phytonutrients: flavonoids. Onions are particularly high in the flavonoid quercetin, a powerful antioxidant. Experts tout this natural chemical as preventing tumors and slowing their growth once they've formed, protecting blood vessels, and treating asthma. In German experiments, onion extract given to bronchial asthma sufferers provided relief; applied directly to the skin, it helped allergic patients ward off reactions to various substances.

Quercetin also helps prevent heart disease in two ways. It helps prevent the oxidation of LDL cholesterol—the kind that sticks to artery walls—and also helps prevent blood cells from sticking together and forming harmful clots.

POWER-EATING TIP

Choose red or yellow onions instead of white onions because they are a better source of quercetin.

2. Cabbage and Its Cousins

Broccoli, brussels sprouts, cabbage, cauliflower, radishes, turnips, and watercress are called cruciferous vegetables because their flowers are shaped like crosses (*crucis* is Latin for cross).

One of their claims to fame is indole-3-carbinol compounds, or I3C, a phytonutrient that gives crucifers their pungent taste. I3Cs may also protect against breast cancer by lowering levels of a certain cancer-causing estrogen. This antiestrogenic effect was also demonstrated in a study in which mice prone to cervical cancer were given high doses of estrogen. Only 2 of 24 mice fed I3C got cervical cancer, compared to 19 of 25 in a control group.

The crucifers are also rich sources of sulforaphane. In yet another study, rats fed sulforaphane extracted from broccoli developed 60 percent fewer tumors than rats that didn't eat it. The tumors that did develop in the sulforaphane group were 75 percent smaller than tumors in the placebo group, and they also grew more slowly.

Don't like broccoli? Try broccoli sprouts, tiny 3-day-old plants grown from seeds. They're 20 to 50 times richer in sulforaphane than an equal weight of mature broccoli. That's because each broccoli plant is born with a certain amount of sulforaphane; as the plant grows, it maintains that same amount, which gets spread throughout the entire plant. You'd have to eat an entire broccoli plant to get the full amount of sulforaphane found in just a tablespoon of broccoli sprouts.

POWER-EATING TIP

Cook cruciferous vegetables lightly, if at all. Studies suggest that the phytonutrients are most powerful when the vegetable is eaten raw or lightly steamed.

3. Nuts and Seeds

Although nearly 79 percent of the calories in nuts may come from fat, it's "good" unsaturated fat, not artery-clogging saturated fat. In fact, an analysis of nine studies using nuts showed that the crunchy snacks lowered both LDL cholesterol and total cholesterol levels.

It could be due to the unsaturated fat or to the phytonutrients in nuts. Nuts are rich in antioxidants like luteolin and flavonoids, which work as antioxidants to suppress the process that makes LDL molecules stick to arteries; and tocotrienol, a form of vitamin E known to lower cholesterol and reduce heart disease risk.

POWER
SOUP

CREAMED CARROT SOUP

Carrots are one of the best sources of cancer-fighting beta-carotene. You'd be smart to have some every day, and this soup is a great way to expand your carrot repertoire. It's smooth, creamy, subtly spiced, and super easy to prepare. Make a batch on Sunday and enjoy it all week.

2	tablespoons olive oil
1	large onion, finely chopped
1	rib celery, finely chopped
4	large carrots, finely chopped
1	parsnip, finely chopped
½	cup basmati or other aromatic rice
1	teaspoon ground cumin
¼	teaspoon ground coriander
6	cups vegetable stock
½	cup 2% milk
2	tablespoons lemon juice
¼	teaspoon salt
	Pinch of ground black pepper

In a large saucepan, warm the oil over medium heat. Add the onion and celery. Cook for 5 minutes. Add the carrots, parsnip, and rice. Cook, stirring often, for 5 minutes, or until the carrots soften. Stir in the cumin and coriander.

Add the stock and bring to a boil. Reduce the heat to medium-low and simmer for 20 minutes, or until the rice is tender. Stir in the milk, lemon juice, salt, and pepper.

Working in batches, puree the soup in a blender.

Makes 8 cups

Per cup: 172 calories, 4 g protein, 28 g carbohydrates, 5.5 g fat, 2 mg cholesterol, 4 g dietary fiber, 416 mg sodium

EAT FOOD, NOT PILLS

It seems that no sooner is a phytonutrient identified than a pill bearing its name shows up on health food store shelves. Quercetin, genistein, lutein—and the list goes on.

Save your money. The best sources of phytonutrients are food, not pills. What's more, studies suggest that some phytonutrients taken in isolation and in high doses may be toxic and actually turn *pro*-oxidant, instead of behaving as an antioxidant.

"Nutritionists have known for years that many of the standard vitamins and minerals become toxic at high levels," says Winston Craig, Ph.D., professor of nutrition at Andrews University in Berrien Springs, Michigan. "So it shouldn't be any surprise that if we extract and concentrate these small amounts of phytonutrients and take whopping doses, it may actually reverse their activity."

There are also too many unanswered questions about phytonutrients, he says. How do they work together? How does the fiber in the fruit or vegetable affect their action? Which phytonutrient is responsible for which health effect? What factors affect their absorption in the body? What are the levels that you need for optimal health?

Your best bet is to "just eat naturally," he says. One bite into a carrot, for example, and you get dozens of health-bestowing carotenoids that protect against heart disease, cancer, and other diseases.

Then there's resveratrol, prominent in peanuts (technically a legume). Also found in red wine and grape juice, experts credit this phytonutrient as a factor in the low rate of heart disease in the French (despite their artery-clogging diets).

Nuts and seeds also have strong cancer-crushing abilities thanks to a variety of other phytonutrients. There are phytosterols, which inhibit cancer-causing hormones, and ellagic acid, which neutralizes cancer-causing chemicals found in tobacco smoke, processed foods, and barbecued meats. Ellagic acid from walnuts, for instance, inhibited cancer in lung, liver, skin, and esophagus cells in rodents by protecting them against DNA damage—the starting gate of cancer.

Also at work are protease inhibitors. Protease is like a shuttle service for tumor cells—they use it to invade distant sites and increase blood vessel production and cell division. So anything that knocks out protease helps prevent cancer and slow tumor growth.

Nuts, particularly walnuts, are also one of the few sources of linolenic acid other than fatty fish, which can be converted in the body to omega-3 fatty acids, helping fight a variety of diseases, including arthritis.

POWER-EATING TIP

Help yourself to almonds, peanuts, walnuts, Brazil nuts, pumpkin seeds, and sunflower seeds. But take it easy on pecans and macadamias—both are low in nutrients and superhigh in fat.

4. Whole Grains and Flax

A nutrition teacher brought a loaf of white bread into class one day and balled it up in his hand, recalls Dr. Craig. The result looked nothing like a Power Food. White bread—along with white rice, white pasta, and white flour—is so stripped of fiber and phytonutrients that it's a wonder it has any nutrition at all.

One critical phytonutrient that's missing is lignan, which gives all plant cells their structure. They also provide major antitumor and antiviral activities.

"Lignans stop cell division," says Kenneth D. R. Setchell, Ph.D., director of clinical mass spectrometry and professor of pediatrics at Children's Hospital Medical Center in Cincinnati. And if you're trying to prevent cancer, that's a first step because the more cells divide, the more likely it is that their "off" switches can break. When that happens, you get cancer.

Dr. Setchell first discovered lignans 20 years ago. They're so ubiquitous in plant-based foods, he suspects that they may be responsible for some of the colon cancer protection attributed to fiber. "The more fiber you take in, the more lignans you'll have," he says. And studies have found that women with the greatest amount of lignans in their urine—an indication of how many whole grain products they consume—are less likely to develop breast cancer than those with lower levels.

The greatest source of lignans is the flax plant, and flaxseed is often baked into breads. In rodents, flaxseed shrank colon, breast and lung cancers; lowered LDL and total cholesterol; made blood platelets less sticky; and elicited several hormonal changes, suggesting reduced breast cancer risk.

It may also help prevent postmenopausal osteoporosis. In a 6-week study of 38 postmenopausal women who were not taking replacement hormones, those who ate about 1½ ounces of flaxseed a day had less bone loss than those who ate sunflower seeds. Researchers aren't sure just how flax works on the bone, but it may reduce calcium lost through the urine as well as provide an antioxidant effect.

Whole grains are also flavonoid powerhouses, chock-full of these phytonutrients that not only have their own individual health-promoting benefits but also boost the power of vitamin C.

Oats, for instance, contain beta-glucan, which studies show lowers total and LDL cholesterol, reducing the risk of heart disease. Wheat and other whole grains are rich in phenols, which muzzle enzymes that could turn genes in our cells into cancer-causing triggers.

Other phytonutrients in whole grains include plant sterols, vitamin E–like tocotrienols, ellagic acid, and saponins, thought to bind up cholesterol and escort it out of the body unabsorbed. All of these substances, however, are concentrated in the bran and germ of grains, and refining wheat causes a two- to three-hundredfold loss in phytonutrients.

POWER-EATING TIP

For the biggest nutritional and phytonutrient punch, choose old-fashioned rolled oats, which are whole oats, not instant oatmeal.

5. Soy and Other Beans

When it comes to legumes, soybeans are phytonutrient powerhouses. Soy is the primary source of isoflavones, phytoestrogens that weakly mimic our own natural estrogen. The best part, however, is that phytoestrogens also act as an antiestrogen, blocking natural estrogen's path in the body, thus preventing many of the hormone's cancer-causing effects.

HEALTH BY THE TEACUPFUL

Call it the Japanese paradox: They smoke more than anyone else in the Western world, yet they get less lung cancer than anyone else.

It could be the gallons of green tea they drink, says J. Robert Hatherill, Ph.D., professor of toxicology at the University of California, Santa Barbara, and author of *Eat to Beat Cancer.* When Japanese scientists surveyed 8,552 men and women over age 40 about their living habits, including tea consumption, they found that women who drank 10 or more cups of green tea per day reduced their overall cancer risk 43 percent compared to women who drank less.

Green tea contains a variety of phytonutrients, including flavonoids called catechins, which have been shown to neutralize free radicals and possibly reduce cancer risk. If you like black tea, though, you're out of luck when it comes to catechins. The fermentation process that makes black tea also breaks down the catechins and changes them into different substances. So stick with green tea, which is produced by just steaming tea leaves, not fermenting them. Experiments show that green tea is 100 times more effective than vitamin C and 25 times better than vitamin E at protecting cells from damage linked to cancer, heart disease, and other illnesses. It's also been shown to be 10 times as powerful as black tea at arresting cancer cell growth, according to Dr. Hatherill.

An added bonus: Preliminary research suggests that green tea extract may speed up the metabolism and assist in weight loss.

One isoflavone, genistein, appears to thwart cancer at every stage of its development; interfering with the enzymes that breed cancer genes, cutting off the blood vessels that act as supply lines to developing cancers, and stunting the growth of cancer cells. It also stops the growth of cells that can clog arteries, those scavenging free radicals that oxidize LDL cholesterol and make it sticky.

Soybeans and other legumes like chickpeas also contain saponins, which bind with and flush out cholesterol, stimulate our immune systems, and prevent heart disease and certain cancers. What's more, soybeans are tops when it comes to protease inhibitors, a powerful antioxidant against aging, various cancers, and other diseases. Beans in

POWER

CAULIFLOWER AND WATERCRESS SALAD

Cauliflower and watercress both contain cancer-preventing sulforaphane as well as other phytonutrients. (One compound in watercress has even been found to render a noxious tobacco carcinogen harmless.)

1	head cauliflower, cut into bite-size florets
	Juice of ½ lemon
2	tablespoons canola oil
2	tablespoons white wine vinegar
½	teaspoon curry powder
½	teaspoon salt
¼	teaspoon ground black pepper
1	bunch watercress, torn into bite-size pieces
2	tomatoes, chopped

Place the cauliflower in a steamer basket. Sprinkle with the lemon juice. Steam for 6 to 8 minutes, or until tender. Let cool for 10 minutes.

In a large bowl, whisk together the oil, vinegar, curry powder, salt, and pepper. Add the cauliflower and the watercress. Toss to coat. Add the tomatoes and toss gently.

Makes 6 servings

Per serving: 77 calories, 3 g protein, 8 g carbohydrates, 5 g fat, 0 mg cholesterol, 3 g dietary fiber, 202 mg sodium

Variation: For a slightly different taste treat, replace the watercress with broccoli sprouts; they're also loaded with sulforaphane—over 20 times more than what's in broccoli.

general also have other phytonutrients—such as sterols and phytates—that seem to hinder cancer cell growth and keep normal cells from turning cancerous.

Even the pigment isolated from the common bean, a form of anthocyanin, exhibits strong antioxidative activity, protecting against cell membrane damage and supplementing the work of vitamins C and E.

POWER-EATING TIP

A pinch of summer savory or a teaspoon of ground ginger is a delicious addition to bean dishes (and may also reduce their gas-producing effects, according to some studies).

6. Fruit

What phytonutrient *doesn't* fruit contain?

Take berries. Not only are they high in ellagic acid and lignans but also they are tiny treasure troves of the flavonoid anthocyanin, the red, blue, and purple pigment that gives fruits their color. It also neutralizes free radicals and may reduce the risk of cancer.

At the Jean Mayer USDA Human Nutrition Research Center on Aging at Tufts University in Boston, researchers fed rats a diet laced with blueberry extract as well as other plant extracts with high antioxidant activity. After 8 weeks of supplementation, the rats with the blueberry-stained whiskers did better on memory and motor behavior performance tests than they did before the supplementation. This led researchers to theorize that the phytonutrients in antioxidant-rich foods such as blueberries may also be helpful in reversing the course of neuronal and behavioral aging.

Proanthocyanidins are one reason for red wine's health-enhancing effects. They inhibit cholesterol synthesis, providing protection against heart disease. They also block carcinogens, suppress malignant changes in cells, and keep collagen healthy. Collagen, which gives tissue its structure, keeps our skin from wrinkling and our bones from crumbling.

There are thousands of flavonoids, many of which appear in fruit. For instance, in a Finnish study of nearly 10,000 men and women over a period of 24 years, researchers found that those getting the most flavonoids by eating apples were 58 percent less likely to develop lung cancer than those eating less of these fruits.

There is also some evidence that flavonoids can help manage a variety of health problems associated with aging, including hardening of the arteries and weakened capillaries, which can lead to easy bruising. They may also lower your risk of stroke. Flavonoids may help prevent heart disease by scavenging LDL-damaging free radicals.

You can even drink your fruit. Oranges are particularly high in compounds called limonoids, found in the peel and white membrane, which wind up in commercial juice. They have been shown to inhibit cancer in test tube studies. And another orange juice flavonoid, hesperidin, may be one reason the juice seems to increase levels of "good" HDL cholesterol. In one study, researchers asked 16 men and 9 women with high cholesterol levels to drink one glass of orange juice a day for 4 weeks, then two glasses a day for 4 weeks, then three glasses a day for 4 weeks. When drinking three glasses a day, their HDL cholesterol levels increased 21 percent and their LDL/HDL cholesterol ratio dropped 16 percent.

Then there are terpines, found in oranges, lemons, and grapefruits. These chemicals give a jump start to protective enzymes in our bodies that interfere with the actions of carcinogens like environmental poisons, prevent dental decay, and have some antiulcer activity.

If you're into popping grapes or drinking grape juice, then you're getting great doses of resveratrol, a flavonoid that appears to suppress the effects of the carcinogen benzopyrene in animal experiments. This cancer-causing chemical occurs in soot, engine exhausts, charred meats, and cigarette smoke—things you are exposed to on a daily basis. Salicylates in fruit may also boost blood levels of salicylic acid, the cardio-protective substance in aspirin, according to a British study.

POWER-EATING TIP

When you eat grapes, eat the skins and seeds—that's where the bulk of the phytonutrients lie.

7. Cooked Tomatoes

You may have heard about studies suggesting that tomato-based products reduce the risk of prostate cancer. Since you don't have a prostate, you probably ignored them. But women still need tomatoes.

The active ingredient thought to provide most of tomato's health-promoting effects is lycopene, a powerful carotenoid. Carotenoids give plants

FUNCTIONAL FOODS WORTH CONSIDERING

In the future, expect to see more foods engineered to improve health, like the eggs fortified with omega-3 fatty acids (from chickens fed more of the nutrient in their feed), cholesterol-lowering margarines that are FDA approved, and calcium-fortified orange juice that are already staples on grocery store shelves.

"These are perfect examples of the health potential for foods of the future," says Barbara Gollman, R.D., a nutrition educator from Dallas, a spokesperson for the American Dietetic Association, and author of *The Phytopia Cookbook*.

their yellow and orange color, with more than 600 found in nature, about 80 identified so far in our food supply.

In a study at the University of North Carolina in Chapel Hill, researchers drew fat samples from both men and women who'd had heart attacks and those who had not and analyzed them for the presence of lycopene and other carotenoids. They found significantly more lycopene in the fat of the control group than in those who'd had heart attacks. The control group also had diets higher in tomato products, suggesting that a lycopene-rich diet may have protected them against heart disease.

Another study found a connection between lycopene levels in women's blood and risk of breast cancer. Overall, a review of numerous population-based studies found that high intake of this phytonutrient is strongly associated with reduced prostate, lung, and stomach cancers, and may have some effect on pancreatic, colon and rectal, esophageal, oral, breast, and cervical cancers.

POWER-EATING TIP

Cook tomatoes and other carotenoids to release lycopene. You should also sprinkle a little olive oil on them; carotenoids need to hitch a ride on fat molecules to make it out of your intestine and into your bloodstream, where they can go to work.

A LITTLE WINE GOES A LONG WAY

You don't have to polish off half a bottle of cabernet to reap the benefits of the antioxidants it bestows. One glass of red wine (a little more than ½ cup) has the antioxidant equivalent of any of these.

- 12 glasses of white wine
- 7 glasses of orange juice
- 2 cups of tea
- 4 apples
- 1 ¼ cups of onion
- 2 ⅓ cups of eggplant
- 3 ½ glasses of black currant juice
- 3 ½ glasses of beer
- 20 glasses of apple juice

8. Greens

If iceberg lettuce is a staple at your house, you are missing out on valuable phytonutrients found only in darker greens (the darker, the better). So instead, feast on the darkest green veggies you can find. Kale and spinach. Mustard greens and arugula. Radicchio and romaine.

Need to squint a bit? Maybe you need more dark greens. Research shows that these veggies, rich in the carotenoids lutein and zeaxanthin, may protect against age-related macular degeneration, the leading cause of irreversible blindness among Americans over 65. A Chicago ophthalmologist found that eating 5 ounces of sautéed spinach four to seven times a week improved vision in his macular degeneration patients in as little as 3 months.

POWER-EATING TIP

To speed cooking and retain nutrients in cooked greens, microwave cook them with as little water as possible. For convenience, look for canned chopped kale, available out of season.

9. Carrots and Savory Herbs

Collectively known as umbelliferous herbs and vegetables, carrots, celery, celeriac, parsnips, lovage, angelica root, anise, cumin, chervil, dill, fennel, caraway, and coriander have one thing in common: umbrella-shaped flowers. Think of them as the kinds of ingredients you throw into chicken soup.

Together and individually, they protect against a variety of cancers, including uterine lining, bladder, colon, and lung. These vegetables and herbs are packed with a variety of carotenoids, including lutein, which reduces the risk of macular degeneration, and beta-carotene, which stimulates the immune system and protects cells from free-radical attacks.

Carrots are a great source of beta-carotene in our repertoire, and, in an Italian study, eating them was related to a decreased risk of breast cancer.

Best known as a handy vehicle for transporting peanut butter or cream cheese to your mouth, pale green, crunchy sticks of celery make up for their lack of tastebud pizzazz with a plethora of phytonutrients. One is 3-n-butyl phthalide. When researchers injected test animals with a small amount of this phytonutrient, the animals' blood pressures dropped 12 to 14 percent within 1 week. It works by relaxing the muscles of the arteries that regulate blood pressure, enabling them to dilate. Phthalides also reduce stress hormones in the blood, which typically cause pressure to rise by constricting vessels.

Phthalides also stimulate glutathione S-transferase (GST), an enzyme that acts as a catalyst, turning toxic substances into less harmful ones. Another celery compound, polyacetylenes, detoxifies carcinogens like those

Waistline

A national survey indicated that only 23 percent of adults ate the minimum recommended five servings of fruits and vegetables per day. Women are more likely than men to eat less than a single serving of vegetables per day.

found in cigarette smoke, while acetylenics, also in celery, put the brakes on the growth of any tumor cells that managed to avoid the other roadblocks.

Eat the celery leaves—they're concentrated sources of phytonutrients.

10. Dairy and Lean Meats

You already know that milk and meat are primary sources of calcium and protein. What you probably didn't know is that they're also rich in a phytonutrient known as conjugated linoleic acid, or CLA, and it's—surprise!—a fat.

First isolated from grilled beef in 1987, CLA has been shown to be effective in suppressing stomach tumors in mice, and colon and breast cancer in rats. It is also found in dairy products, particularly whole milk and cheese.

A Finnish population study showed that women who drank about 3 cups of whole milk a day reduced their risk of breast cancer nearly 60 percent compared to women who drank less than 1½ cups.

Another study, at the University of Wisconsin in Madison, found that CLA burns fat at 5 to 10 times the normal rate, while increasing muscle tissue in mice.

POWER-EATING TIP

Drink organic milk, and try to get 2 to 3 cups of milk a day. The highest CLA levels were found in milk from animals that were fed pasture grass.

Female-Friendly Herbs: From Heart Savers to Mood Menders

BY LINDA B. WHITE, M.D. We use herbs to flavor soups or stews, scent rooms, or line garden paths. And a growing number of us turn to herbs for yet another centuries-old purpose—healing. Used properly, these simple plants can calm us down, protect us against winter's germs, and nourish our spirits in the midst of the maelstrom that is all too often our daily lives.

Medicinal herbs enable us to take charge of our own health, rather than simply turning to a doctor to "fix" us; and they bring us back in touch with the natural world. By learning how and when to use nature's medicines, you can find the power to replenish, rejuvenate, and refresh yourself.

Before you head out to pick wild fresh herbs, learn as much as you can about the identification and safe harvest of local plants. Contact your local botanical garden, university, museum, or hiking club and ask about classes or programs in your area.

Effective herbal dosages may vary from person to person and condition to condition. When a remedy or product label recommends a dosage range, start with the lowest amount. If you aren't experiencing a benefit and haven't noticed any side effects from the herb, only then should you attempt to increase the dose within the recommended range. Please note the cautions for appropriate use stated here. Unless otherwise noted, the herbs discussed are generally recognized as safe.

219

Turbocharge Your Immunity

As winter approaches, it seems like the microbes grow stronger. Particularly the ones your kids bring home from school and your coworkers pass on with every handshake. Add to that the stress of daily life—too little sleep, too many deadlines, worries over money, relationships, work—and it's no wonder that we're as likely to fall victim to a cold or flu as we are to be the one making chicken soup.

That's when it is time to turn to herbs.

Echinacea (*Echinacea angustifolia, E. purpurea,* and *E. pallida*)

Native Americans used echinacea against more illnesses than any other plant. But it has only been in the past few years, as studies touting its immune-enhancing benefits multiplied, that the purple coneflower leapt beyond health food store shelves onto aisles of mainstream supermarkets and mass market retail stores and drugstores.

Although the earliest Americans used it for everything from burns to insect bites, even as an antidote for snakebites, we best know echinacea as a way to short-circuit a cold or flu. It stimulates our white blood cells, the foot soldiers of the immune system, supercharging them to action. The herb also increases production of antibodies and an antiviral and antitumor substance called interferon.

But you must know your own body to use echinacea effectively. Take it at the first sign of a cold or other respiratory infection, says Varro E. Tyler, Ph.D., distinguished professor emeritus of pharmacognosy at Purdue University in West Lafayette, Indiana, and author of *Tyler's Herbs of Choice* and other books on the medicinal uses of plants. Some, but not all, studies show that it prevents the common cold, but several show that it can shorten the duration and severity of colds.

Echinacea has a folk reputation for quelling inflammation and, when applied to the skin, promoting wound healing, which explains all those uses the Native Americans found for it.

If you don't take enough, however, it won't work. A German study found that 180 drops (900 milligrams) a day of an alcohol extract of *Echinacea purpurea* root significantly reduced flu symptoms compared to a placebo or half the dose. Discontinue its use once your symptoms clear.

Forms and dosages: You can find echinacea in capsules, tinctures, fresh-pressed juice, and teas. Scientists who've studied echinacea aren't sure which plant parts or preparations work best in what amounts. Experts who've reviewed the evidence recommend the following daily total doses:

- Tincture: 1 to 1½ teaspoons each day for 3 days, then just under 1 teaspoon daily
- Dry powdered plant in capsules: 1,500 to 2,500 milligrams a day
- Fresh-pressed juice: 2½ teaspoons for the first couple of days; then 1 to 1½ teaspoons daily

During the first couple of days of the illness, divide the total daily amount into five or six doses. Afterward, you can go to three or four daily doses until the cold or flu symptoms abate.

Caution: Rarely, people with allergies to other members of the daisy family are also allergic to echinacea. And until more is known about echinacea's interaction with the immune system, many experts don't recommend taking it if you have multiple sclerosis, HIV infection, or other immune system diseases.

Astragalus (*Astragalus membranaceus*)

Also known as huang qi, astragalus root has been used by Chinese healers for more than 2,000 years to improve resistance. According to Asian studies, it has immunostimulating, antiviral, liver-protecting, and anti-inflammatory effects. Astragalus is also used as a tonic, an herbal product that strengthens various organs and systems.

"It is one of the preeminent Chinese herbs for strengthening the whole body," says Efrem Korngold, L.Ac., O.M.D., licensed acupuncturist, doctor of oriental medicine, faculty member of the American College of Traditional Chinese Medicine in San Francisco, and coauthor of *Between Heaven and Earth: A Guide to Chinese Medicine*. "It's particularly good for people who have low resistance and get sick easily with colds, flus, or any kind of infection." Chinese physicians also use it to support immune-compromised people, including patients with cancer or those undergoing chemotherapy or radiation therapy.

Forms and dosages: You can buy sliced astragalus root from the bulk herb sections in health food stores. During cold and flu season, add a long slice of the root—about 6 inches—to soup stock (along with plenty of garlic, onions, shiitake mushrooms, and beta-carotene-rich orange root veggies). Remove the tough, fibrous root before serving.

You can also take one to two cups of tea, four to six 400- to 500-mil-

TEA FOR THE CHANGE

To nourish your body, balance hormones, and reduce menopausal symptoms, try this tea, recommended by herbalist Betzy Bancroft, a professional member of the American Herbalists Guild and manager of Herbalist and Alchemist, an herbal medicine company in Washington, New Jersey. The proportions in this recipe are based on weight, so when you purchase herbs, have each type of herb weighed and packaged in equal quantities, or use a kitchen scale. Make a large batch and use as needed.

- Two parts oat seed (*Avena sativa*)
- One part cut and sifted licorice root (*Glycyrrhiza glabra*)
- Two parts red clover blossom (*Trifolium pratense*)
- Two parts lemon balm leaf (*Melissa officinalis*)

To make tea, pour boiling water over the herbs (1 heaping or 2 level teaspoons per 4-ounce cup). Cover and steep for ½ to 1 hour. Drink three to four cups a day.

Caution: Oat seed contains gluten, a grain protein—don't use it if you have celiac disease (gluten intolerance). Don't use licorice if you have diabetes, high blood pressure, liver or kidney disorders, or low potassium levels. Do not use licorice daily for more than 4 to 6 weeks because overuse can lead to water retention, high blood pressure caused by potassium loss, or impaired heart and kidney function. Do not use it while pregnant or breastfeeding. Don't use red clover blossom if you're pregnant.

ligram capsules, or 30 to 60 drops of tincture a day, divided into two or three doses. Since it's a tonic herb, you usually take it preventively. You can use it long-term, as do many people with weakened immune systems.

Energy-Enhancing Herbs

Some days, maybe more than you'd like, the honest answer to the question "How are you?" is "Tired." It's a rare woman who doesn't fantasize about a day to do nothing but sleep and maybe recapture some of that energy she had in her twenties.

If you always feel tired, you're probably doing too much. Slow down. Learn to say no. Let the answering machine take your calls. Nap. Eat better. If a commitment to a healthier diet and sufficient rest doesn't restore your energy, consider one of the tonic herbs below.

Asian ginseng (*Panax ginseng*) and American ginseng (*Panax quinquefolius*)

Asian ginseng comes in two main types: White ginseng has been dried; red ginseng has been steamed, then dried. According to traditional Chinese medicine, the latter produces more "heat" and stimulation (which could be a problem for highly strung folks or women with hot flashes). American ginseng is generally cooler (less heating and stimulating) than Asian ginseng.

Studies show that ginseng enhances both mental and physical performance under stress, and limited evidence suggests that it boosts immune function in healthy people as well as those with immune-related illnesses like AIDS and chronic fatigue syndrome.

Those and other studies convinced Commission E, an expert committee that advises the German government on the safety and efficacy of herbal remedies, to approve Asian ginseng as a tonic for "invigoration and fortification in times of fatigue and debility, for declining capacity for work and concentration, also during convalescence."

If you're always complaining that you're cold, either ginseng might help.

However, "a woman with hot flashes might not want to take Asian ginseng, as it could make the condition worse," says Dr. Korngold. American ginseng, considered the "cooler" herb, might be more appropriate.

Forms and dosages: Up to four 500- to 600-milligram capsules a day. For products standardized to 5 to 7 percent ginsenosides, the dosage drops to 100 milligrams one or two times a day. Do not exceed recommended dosages.

Take the herb for 2 to 3 weeks at a time, followed by a 1- to 2-week rest, recommends Donald J. Brown, N.D., a naturopathic physician, director of Natural Products Research Consultants in Maplewood, New Jersey, author of *Herbal Prescriptions for Better Health*, and editor of *Healthnotes Review of Complementary and Integrative Medicine*.

But don't take Asian ginseng every day if you're under 40, says Dr. Korngold, "unless you're in a stressful occupation or environment. After age

40, our core energies begin to decline anyway, so it's safe to supplement because we no longer have a surplus and it's less likely to overstimulate us."

Caution: Stop using Asian or American ginseng if your blood pressure rises, or if you have hot flashes, insomnia, nervousness, or irritability. Combining ginseng with caffeine or other stimulants increases the risk of side effects. In some women, Dr. Brown says, long-term use of Asian ginseng may cause menstrual abnormalities and breast tenderness. While this is rare, you should discontinue use if you experience either problem.

Eleuthero or Siberian ginseng (*Eleutherococcus senticosus*)

Although not a true ginseng, eleuthero possesses similar properties. For over 2,000 years, the Chinese have used it to strengthen vital energy (*chi*), prevent respiratory tract infections, and improve overall health. Studies show that it enhances immune function, athletic performance, physical endurance, mental alertness, and our ability to cope with stress.

In his practice, Dr. Korngold frequently recommends Siberian ginseng as a tonic—that is, an all-purpose maintenance herb. "You can use it for any condition, and it won't aggravate symptoms like hot flashes," he says. Whereas the true ginsengs are weighted with cautions, most women can safely take Siberian ginseng.

Forms and dosages: Two to 3 grams a day of dried root in capsule form divided into two or three doses, or 20 to 40 drops of tincture up to three times a day.

Elixirs to Soothe the Nerves

Ever feel as if there's a nonstop rock concert inside your head? Between career, kids, husband, volunteer work, and the dog that just threw up on the back steps, it can be nearly impossible to turn off life and get the rest we deserve. But a raft of herbs can help in our struggle for sanity.

Herbs that gently smooth frayed nerves include catnip, chamomile, linden flowers (*Tilia* species), and lemon balm (*Melissa officinalis*). More strongly sedating herbs include valerian, kava kava, passionflower, and skullcap. Reishi mushroom also eases anxiety and insomnia.

These herbs blend nicely. Not that you'd take all nine at once. Try two or three blended—perhaps passionflower and valerian, or chamomile and skullcap—the sort of combinations often found in widely sold soothing tea blends. In general, lower doses calm the nerves by day; higher doses grease the sleep wheels at bedtime. (If you regularly feel anxious by day or sleep-less by night, don't rely on herbs indefinitely. Instead, talk to your doctor.)

Valerian (*Valeriana officinalis*)

This showy plant with feathery pink blooms smells so awful that the ancient Greeks nicknamed it "phu." But don't let a little stink keep you from it. Valerian is widely used as an insomnia aid in Europe and else-where. Extracts of the root both shorten the time it takes to fall asleep and improve your sleep without side effects.

Valerian root also has antispasmodic activity, meaning it can relax tight muscles. That's why it's useful for relieving menstrual cramps, says Tori Hudson, N.D., a naturopathic physician, professor of gynecology at the College of Naturopathic Medicine in Portland, Oregon, and author of *Women's Encyclopedia of Natural Medicine.*

Forms and dosages: To counter insomnia, take 20 to 60 drops of tinc-ture or 300 to 500 milligrams of a capsule of concentrated extract stan-dardized to contain at least 0.5 percent valerenic acid ½ hour before bed each day.

To reduce menstrual cramps, Dr. Hudson recommends 1 teaspoon of tincture or one to two capsules every 3 to 4 hours as needed for pain.

Caution: Because valerian has such a sedative effect, don't use it during the day for anxiety or menstrual cramps unless you're able to stay home and sleep. Do not use valerian with sleep-enhancing or mood-reg-ulating medications because it may intensify their effects.

Some sensitive people find that valerian stimulates, rather than se-dates, says David Hoffmann, a fellow of the National Institute of Med-ical Herbalists in Great Britain, founding and professional member of the American Herbalists Guild, and author of *An Herbal Guide to Stress Re-lief.* It may even cause heart palpitations and nervousness. If this happens to you, give up on valerian and try another sedative herb or reishi mush-room. Beyond these special considerations, valerian is nonaddictive and generally considered safe when taken at recommended dosages.

Passionflower (*Passiflora incarnata*)

"This is an important herb for anxiety, insomnia caused by mental worry, and nightmares," says Christopher Hobbs, L.Ac., a licensed acupuncturist and herbalist in Santa Rosa, California, and author of *Stress and Natural Healing.* Along with valerian and chamomile, the active ingredients in passionflower have an affinity for the same brain receptors that bind to prescription benzodiazepine medications.

Forms and dosages: Before bed, drink a cup of tea or take 20 to 40 drops of tincture in water. To relieve anxiety, take the same amount of tincture up to four times a day. Take a dose before bed to help overcome insomnia, and more doses by day if you have anxiety. Hobbs says that you can do this without inducing sleep, in much the same way people use the benzodiazepines for both conditions.

Skullcap (*Scutellaria lateriflora*)

"This herb acts as a nerve tonic in women," says Hoffmann. It is particularly helpful in alleviating the dark cloud that can accompany PMS as well as other hormone-induced emotional upheavals.

Forms and dosages: To banish insomnia, drink a cup of tea before bed. For stress and anxiety, drink ½ cup three or four times a day or take 30 drops of tincture three times a day.

Skullcap blends well with other calming herbs such as lemon balm, catnip, chamomile, and linden flowers.

Catnip (*Nepeta cataria*)

This herb acts like a good massage, quieting your nervous system and relaxing your muscles. It's a traditional remedy for intestinal cramps, flatulence, and fevers. And catnip contains nepetalactone, a mild sedative, making it useful as an antidote for insomnia. A blend of catnip, chamomile, and skullcap can also help ease nicotine withdrawal.

Forms and dosages: Steep 1 heaping teaspoon of dried herb per cup of hot water and drink two to three cups a day as needed, or take 30 to 40 drops of tincture two or three times a day. Combining it with lemon balm and chamomile improves catnip's somewhat musty taste.

Chamomile (*Matricaria recutita*)

A member of the daisy family, this herb has an age-old reputation for calming the nerves. Animal studies help explain that reputation by showing that chamomile binds to the same receptors in brain cells as antianxiety drugs like diazepam (Valium).

Studies on the chemical constituents of chamomile show that it also has anti-inflammatory and antispasmodic properties. Along with valerian and catnip, this gentle herb can help when intestinal cramps make you edgy or sleepless. And no matter where you go, you can usually find tea packets of this pleasant-tasting herb.

Forms and dosages: Take one cup of tea two or three times daily, or 30 drops of tincture three times daily.

Caution: It's quite rare, but if you're allergic to other members of the daisy family, such as ragweed and chrysanthemum, you might also be allergic to chamomile and should drink the tea with caution. Chamomile isn't recommended for use during pregnancy. According to Hobbs, very strong chamomile tea can cause vomiting. And you should keep the tea away from your eyes, as it can cause irritation.

Enhancing Emotional Health

Some women cope with stress in an almost Buddha-like fashion, letting the insanity of their lives wash over them with a joke or a laugh. For others, however, stress may lead to anxiety or depression. Although there

REGULATE YOUR MENSTRUAL CYCLE

This tincture helps regulate menstrual cycles at either end of your reproductive years, says herbalist Shelley Torgove, owner of Apothecary Tinctura, an herb store in Denver.

Blend the following tinctures.

- Two parts chasteberry (*Vitex agnus-castus*)
- Two parts dandelion root (*Taraxacum officinale*)
- One part dang gui (*Angelica sinensis*)
- One part lemon balm leaf (*Melissa officinalis*)
- One part oat seed (*Avena sativa*)

Pour into a darkly tinted bottle, shake, and cap tightly. Take 60 drops three times a day. During your periods, take a break from this tincture, Torgove says.

Caution: If you suffer from a condition that may involve heavy menstrual bleeding, such as endometriosis, do not use dang gui without the guidance of a qualified practitioner. Do not use this tea during pregnancy. Don't use oat seed if you have celiac disease (gluten intolerance) as it contains gluten, a grain protein.

are numerous new medications on the market these days to treat these disorders, natural remedies can be just as effective.

"Among the most promising herbal substitutes for antidepressants and antianxiety agents are St. John's wort and kava kava," says Hyla Cass, M.D., assistant clinical professor of psychiatry at UCLA and author of *St. John's Wort: Nature's Blues Buster* and *Kava: Nature's Answer to Stress, Anxiety, and Insomnia.*

Other herbs that stabilize our emotions include Asian and American ginsengs, Siberian ginseng, ginkgo, valerian, licorice, and reishi mushroom. But if your anxiety persists, seek professional help.

St. John's wort (*Hypericum perforatum*)

This herb eases depression and anxiety, stabilizes premenstrual and menopausal mood swings, and brightens seasonal affective disorder, the sad mood some women experience with winter's reduced sunlight. Applied to the skin as an oil, St. John's wort also has antiviral and antibacterial properties, decreases inflammation and pain, and speeds wound and burn healing. When researchers analyzed data from 23 studies, they concluded that St. John's wort performed significantly better than placebos for treating mild-to-moderate depression and may be as effective as some standard antidepressants with fewer side effects. And a German study of men and women with severe depression demonstrated that a double dose of St. John's wort extract (1,800 milligrams over the course of the day) was as effective as the tricyclic antidepressant imipramine (Tofranil), but with far fewer side effects.

"I've seen it work wonders in people with mild to moderate depression," says Alan Miller, N.D., a naturopathic physician and senior editor of *Alternative Medical Review.* For severe depression, however, you should be under the care of a physician.

Forms and dosages: Dr. Miller reports success using an extract standardized to 0.3 percent hypericin at a dosage of 300 milligrams in capsule form three times a day—the same form and strength used in many clinical studies. He has found 15 to 40 drops of tincture three times a day to be successful as well. Although some women notice results immediately, it can take anywhere between 1 and 6 weeks to detect benefits.

Caution: Do not use St. John's wort with antidepressants without medical approval. This herb may cause photosensitivity, so avoid overexposure to direct sunlight when taking it. Fair-skinned people, particularly those on higher doses of St. John's wort, may sunburn more easily than others.

No one yet knows if this herb can safely be used during pregnancy or nursing. Nor have scientists precisely worked out how St. John's wort influences brain chemistry, though it appears to influence feel-good neurotransmitters, including serotonin and norepinephrine. In the meantime, if you're on prescription antidepressants, don't take St. John's wort without your doctor's approval.

Kava kava (*Piper methysticum*)

Also called kava, this South Seas native plant has long been consumed as a social or ceremonial beverage. It relaxes muscles, decreases pain, and produces a heightened sense of tranquillity and sociability without clouded judgment, mental fog, or morning hangover. At higher dosages, however, it may make you sleepy.

German trials comparing kava kava to a placebo and conventional drugs such as oxazepam (Serax) found that it safely and effectively reduces anxiety. The German Commission E approved kava kava for "conditions of nervous anxiety, stress, and restlessness."

It also serves as a good alternative to antianxiety medications without some of the side effects associated with these drugs, such as drowsiness, clumsiness, dizziness, and the potential of addiction or dependency. In a study of 20 menopausal women, kava reduced associated anxiety and depression. Dr. Cass also finds kava useful for quelling premenstrual nervous tension.

Forms and dosages: The usual dosage for reducing anxiety is 70 milligrams of kavalactones two or three times daily. Read labels for kavalactone content: Specifically, look for kava kava capsules standardized to 30 percent kavalactones. To counter insomnia, take 70 to 210 milligrams of kavalactones an hour before bed. For a tincture, take 15 to 40 drops in water up to three times a day to reduce anxiety, 1 to 2 dropperfuls (about 30 drops per dropperful) at bedtime.

Caution: Most experts don't recommend kava for pregnant women, nor in combination with alcohol or sedatives, including prescription antianxiety medication. Since kava is a muscle relaxant, it's best to avoid using it if you're going to be driving a car or operating any kind of machinery that requires concentration and alertness. And never take more

MUSHROOMS THAT HEAL

Mushrooms are fungi, not herbs. But like herbs, they're botanical healers, says Christopher Hobbs, L.Ac., a licensed acupuncturist and herbalist in Santa Rosa, California, and author of *Medicinal Mushrooms* and other books.

SHIITAKE (LENTINUS EDODES). These mushrooms boost immune function, have anticancer activity, and increase the body's resistance to infection by bacteria, viruses, and parasites. Studies show that shiitake extracts improve the health of people with chronic hepatitis and AIDS and suggest that this mushroom can also lower cholesterol and triglyceride (blood fat) levels.

Health food stores and many grocery stores often carry fresh shiitake mushrooms. Try sautéing them for tasty and healthful additions to soups, stews, sauces, omelettes, and stir-fried meals. If you're battling a serious illness, Hobbs says you'll need to go with tablets, capsules, or teas made from the powdered extract. Follow the manufacturer's dosage guidelines.

REISHI (GANODERMA LUCIDUM). In laboratory studies, preparations made with reishi mushrooms inhibit tumor growth, reduce blood pressure, slow production of cholesterol and atherosclerotic plaques, lower blood sugar levels, scavenge free radicals, protect the liver, and quell inflammation and allergies. Tests on men and women have found it useful in treating diabetes, insomnia, high-altitude sickness, heart disease, chronic bronchitis, and asthma and other allergic diseases.

Hobbs also uses reishi for chronic stress, anxiety, or insomnia. "I often recommend reishi during menopause to promote better sleep and to support the nervous system and hormonal system. Reishi is safe to use during pregnancy and can be useful with PMS," he says.

Some experts caution that in rare cases, reishi can cause dry mouth or stomach upset when used for more than 3 months. Reishi is available in capsules, tablets, tinctures, and teas. Follow manufacturer's dosage guidelines.

than the recommended dose on the package. Long-term, heavy consumption of the traditional kava beverage can produce a reversible scaly skin rash known as kava dermopathy. If you do develop a rash, stop using it.

Ginkgo (*Ginkgo biloba*)

While perhaps best known for its potential to improve short-term memory in the early stages of Alzheimer's disease, this herb may also have mild antidepressant activity. Ginkgo can also help with the changes in mental clarity, memory, and concentration that some women experience during menopause, Dr. Hudson says.

In one study, ginkgo effectively reversed antidepressant-induced sexual dysfunction in men and women, says Dr. Hudson. So it may boost the flagging sexual desire that rides menopause's wake.

Forms and dosages: For a ginkgo biloba extract standardized to contain 6 percent terpene lactones and 24 percent ginkgo flavone glycosides, take 40 to 80 milligrams three times a day or ½ to 1 teaspoon of standardized tincture three times a day.

Caution: Ginkgo inhibits blood clotting, which is one reason it improves bloodflow to the brain. So don't combine it with aspirin or other nonsteroidal anti-inflammatory medications, or blood-thinning medications such as warfarin (Coumadin). Don't use the herb with antidepressant monoamine oxidase inhibitor drugs such as phenelzine sulfate (Nardil) or tranylcypromine (Parnate). Ginkgo can cause dermatitis, diarrhea, and vomiting in doses higher than 240 milligrams of concentrated extract.

Herbal Hormone Balancers

For centuries, women have been turning to herbal remedies to balance hormones.

Herbalists say that plants seem to have an affinity for the female body, effectively relieving menstrual discomforts and maintaining the health of our reproductive systems.

Here's what can help.

Black cohosh (*Actea racemosa*)

Although best known as a menopause remedy, black cohosh can also ease menstrual cramps, relax muscles, soothe nervous tension, alleviate headaches, reduce the inflammation and pain of arthritis, and regulate menstrual cycles when low estrogen levels cause absent or infrequent periods.

Studies in menopausal women show that this herb alleviates symptoms such as hot flashes, night sweats, vaginal dryness, sleep disturbances, nervousness, irritability, and depression. Research focusing on a standardized black cohosh extract called Remifemin has found it performs on par with estrogen-replacement treatment for such menopausal symptoms.

Scientists have yet to pinpoint how black cohosh works. It seems to suppress the pituitary gland's secretion of luteinizing hormone, a hormone implicated in menopausal symptoms such as hot flashes. At the same time, it appears to mimic estrogen in the body, counteracting the vaginal thinning, dryness, hot flashes, insomnia, and mood swings that result when estrogen levels drop during menopause. (Black cohosh doesn't appear to stimulate cells in the uterus or breast as estrogen does. So, unlike traditional estrogen-replacement therapy, black cohosh carries no increased risk for breast or uterine cancer.)

What isn't known is whether black cohosh can help prevent the two main conditions for which estrogen-replacement therapy is prescribed: osteoporosis and heart disease.

Forms and dosages: To prevent menopausal symptoms, take one or two 40-milligram capsules or tablets of extract standardized to 2.5 percent triterpene glycosides twice a day. The dosage for standardized tincture is ½ to 1 teaspoon (60 to 120 drops) twice a day. If you're trying to ease menstrual cramps, Dr. Hudson recommends ¼ to ½ teaspoon of tincture or one or two capsules of the dried (nonstandardized) root.

Caution: Do not use black cohosh for more than 6 months and do not take it while pregnant or nursing.

Chasteberry (*Vitex agnus-castus*)

This herb is useful for many women, regardless of age or hormonal status, says Shelley Torgove, an herbalist and owner of Apothecary Tinctura, an herb store in Denver.

Also known as vitex or chaste tree berry, this hormonal modulator eases PMS symptoms, including premenstrual acne and headaches, and reduces early menopause symptoms, such as hot flashes. Health practitioners often include it in a treatment plan to increase fertility, reduce uterine fibroids, and regulate irregular bleeding patterns caused by hormonal imbalances.

Chasteberry seems to work by influencing pituitary hormones, Torgove says, increasing secretion of luteinizing hormone, which, in turn, stimulates the ovaries to produce progesterone in the second half of a woman's cycle, after the ovary releases an egg. Progesterone stimulates the glandular growth of the uterus. As progesterone and estrogen drop, in the absence of implantation, a period happens. If you don't ovulate or otherwise don't produce enough progesterone (as happens when periods first occur in adolescence and as menopause nears), then you get irregular or frequent periods, often with heavy bleeding. Low progesterone may also generate PMS symptoms.

In a German study, a chasteberry preparation helped regulate menstrual cycles in women whose chief problem was elevated prolactin, one cause of amenorrhea, or absent menstrual periods. In a German survey involving 1,542 women with PMS, one-third of the women reported complete relief from PMS symptoms while nearly two-thirds reported significant improvement. Physicians surveyed at the same time rated women's responses to chasteberry as very good or good 92 percent of the time.

Forms and dosages: With an extract standardized to 6 percent agnusides, take either 40 drops of tincture or one 175-milligram capsule once a day, recommends Dr. Hudson.

For a nonstandardized tincture, Torgove suggests 90 drops each morning.

This gentle herb acts slowly, often taking 4 to 6 months of continuous use to regulate cycles or tame PMS. To reduce a woman's menopause symptoms, Amanda McQuade Crawford, founder of the National College of Phytotherapy in Albuquerque and author of *Herbal Remedies for Women*, often blends chasteberry with estrogen-like herbs such as black cohosh.

Caution: Chasteberry may counteract the effectiveness of birth control pills, and it is not recommended for pregnant women.

Dang gui (*Angelica sinensis*)

Herbalists use this herb to regulate menstrual periods, ease premenstrual discomfort, and, in combination with other herbs, quell menopausal symptoms.

"It's one of the most useful female tonic herbs," says Rosemary Gladstar, director of Sage Mountain Herbal Retreat Center in Barre, Vermont, and author of *Herbal Healing for Women*. Although this herb has no direct hormonal action, it somehow regulates and normalizes hormone production through its actions on the liver and endocrine system.

Forms and dosages: The standard dosage for a tincture is 3 to 5 dropperfuls, three to five times a day. If you prefer tea, drink two to three cups a day as needed.

Caution: If you already have heavy or frequent menstrual periods, dang gui is probably not the herb for you—it can aggravate these conditions. Gladstar also doesn't recommend it during menstruation or pregnancy.

Licorice root (*Glycyrrhiza glabra*)

Licorice root contains phytoestrogens, plant-based estrogens that sometimes act as weaker versions of our own estrogen hormone in our bodies. It helps balance our hormones, making it useful in reducing PMS and menopausal symptoms such as hot flashes and vaginal dryness.

Forms and dosages: For her menopausal patients, Dr. Hudson often combines licorice with herbs such as motherwort, dang gui, burdock (*Arctium lappa*), chasteberry, and black cohosh in teas, capsules, or tinctures. For licorice taken alone, she recommends ½ to 1 teaspoon of tincture diluted in water one to three times a day.

Caution: Do not use licorice if you have diabetes, high blood pressure, liver or kidney disorders, or low potassium levels. Do not use it daily for more than 4 to 6 weeks because overuse can lead to water retention, high blood pressure caused by potassium loss, or impaired heart and kidney function.

Pregnant or nursing women should not take licorice medicinally without the guidance of a qualified health practitioner.

Red clover (*Trifolium pratense*)

Like licorice root, red clover is also rich in phytoestrogens. Thus, some herbal healers believe that it inhibits the cancerous effects estrogen has on breast, uterine, and ovarian tissues. Herbalist Susun Weed, founder of the Wise Woman Center in Woodstock, New York, and author of *Menopausal Years: The Wise Woman Way*, labels red clover "the most renowned anti-cancer herb."

Herbalists use red clover to increase mothers' milk supplies, boost fertility, relieve menopausal symptoms such as hot flashes and vaginal dryness, prevent osteoporosis, treat eczema and psoriasis, relax spasmodic coughs, and gently calm the nerves.

As this purple-blossomed plant often pops up in gardens uninvited, you may decide to welcome it rather than uproot it, since commercial red

PMS-BE-GONE TEA

This tea supports the liver, diminishes cramps, nourishes the blood, and relaxes and uplifts the spirits, according to herbalist Betzy Bancroft, a professional member of the American Herbalists Guild and manager of Herbalist and Alchemist, an herbal medicine company in Washington, New Jersey. The proportions in this recipe are based on weight, so when you purchase your herbs, have each type of herb weighed and packaged in equal quantities, or use a kitchen scale.

- One part cut and sifted yellow dock root (*Rumex crispus*)
- Two parts chamomile flowers (*Matricaria recutita*)
- Two parts linden flowers (*Tilia europaea*)
- Two parts nettle leaf (*Urtica dioica*)

To make tea, pour boiling water over the herbs (1 heaping or 2 level teaspoons per 4-ounce cup). Cover and steep ½ to 1 hour. Drink three cups a day. Start a few days before you usually notice PMS symptoms and stop after the first days of your period.

Caution: If you have a history of kidney stones, do not take yellow dock root without medical supervision as it contains oxalates and tannins that may adversely affect this condition. This tea is not recommended for use during pregnancy. Very rarely, chamomile can cause an allergic reaction when ingested, and people allergic to closely related plants such as ragweed, asters, and chrysanthemums should drink the tea with caution. If you have allergies, your symptoms may worsen if you take nettle, so take only one dose a day for the first few days.

clover is often of poor quality. Simply pick the flower head, let it dry, make an infusion, and drink up it to three times a day. Before harvesting your own red clover, seek the assistance of a someone well-trained in the identification of plants.

Cramp bark (*Viburnum opulus*) or black haw (*V. prunifolium*)

These related herbs help relax the uterus and other muscles, easing the cramps that accompany menstruation and follow childbirth, Hobbs says. Their high tannin content also helps curb heavy menstrual bleeding. Both also have a traditional use in preventing miscarriage.

Forms and dosages: You can drink two to three cups of tea a day or take 3 to 5 dropperfuls of tincture three to five times a day. Herbalists often blend cramp bark or black haw with other female tonic herbs (such as red raspberry when bleeding is excessive). To ease crampy periods, Gladstar blends equal parts of valerian root, cramp bark, and fresh or dried ginger (*Zingiber officinale*) into a tea. (If you have gallstones, you won't want to use this blend without seeing your doctor. When consumed regularly, dried ginger can increase bile secretions and affect your condition.) She suggests drinking ¼ cup every 15 minutes until cramps diminish.

Caution: While cramp bark is generally considered safe, you shouldn't take black haw without medical supervision if you have a history of kidney stones, as it contains oxalates, which can cause kidney stones.

The Herbal Route to a Healthy Heart

Quick: What's the most common cause of death from disease in women? If you said breast cancer, you're mistaken. It's heart disease. The best prevention is a healthy diet and plenty of exercise. And an herbal remedy can never replace the wonders of pharmaceutical medicines for treating diseased hearts. Yet one particular herb can offer protection, provided you get your doctor's okay.

SLOW-THE-FLOW TEA

If you tend to have heavy periods, herbalist Shelley Torgove, owner of Apothecary Tinctura, an herb store in Denver, offers the following recipe. Drink two to three cups a day beginning 7 to 10 days before your period.

Blend equal parts of the dried leaves of red raspberry, lady's mantle, and nettles—try about a cup each. Store in a tightly sealed jar. To make the tea, steep 1 tablespoon of the herb blend per 8 ounces of hot water for 15 minutes to 1 hour, then strain the tea. Once your menstrual flow begins to wane, decrease the dosage to one to two cups per day until your bleeding is finished.

Hawthorn (*Crataegus,* various species)

This herb boasts a long tradition as a remedy for heart ailments. European and Chinese practitioners still use it to treat early congestive heart failure and to lower blood pressure. Because this gentle tonic herb acts slowly, it may take up to 6 months to see peak benefits.

Crawford uses hawthorn berries in many ways, including in jams or baked into breads.

Forms and dosages: You can drink one to three cups a day of tea or 10 to 30 drops of tincture diluted in water three times a day. The dosage of a standardized extract made from the leaves and flowers is 80 milligrams twice a day.

Caution: If you have a cardiovascular condition, do not take hawthorn regularly for more than a few weeks without medical supervision. You may require lower doses of other medications, such as high blood pressure drugs. And if you have low blood pressure caused by heart valve problems, do not use hawthorn without medical supervision.

The New Nutraceuticals: The Verdict on Specialty Supplements

Supplements used to mean vitamins and minerals. Now anything from melatonin to a basketful of initialized pills like SAM-e, CoQ_{10}, and MSM come in supplement form.

Their manufacturers tout the "new" supplements as natural, yet many begin their lives in the chemist's lab. And although the claims on their boxes might lead you to believe that they are the ultimate cure for everything from heart disease to Alzheimer's, most have barely been tested, and then usually on animals or in very small human trials.

Yet we're buying these "nutraceuticals" in enormous amounts, spending $3.8 billion a year on various dietary supplements, not counting vitamins and minerals.

"The idea that we can attain optimal health by doing something as simple as popping the appropriate pill is incredibly attractive, especially to busy people who can't or don't want to face reorganizing their lives around more exercise and a better diet," says Ruth Kava, R.D., Ph.D., director of nutrition at the American Council on Science and Health in New York City. "I also think that we all want to feel that we're doing something to improve our health, and certainly taking a supplement seems like taking an active role."

At the same time, scientific support for many supplements is growing, as is interest in remedies that not only treat our ailments but also increase our energy and sense of well-being and decrease our pace of aging, says Michael Janson, M.D., past president of the American College for the Advancement of Medicine in Laguna Hills, California. Yet unlike pharmaceutical drugs, there is little, if any, government oversight of nutraceuticals or other dietary supplements to ensure that the pills you take contain what their manufacturers say they do, will do what they claim, supply the appropriate dose, and won't make you sick.

Many nutraceuticals are promising, but need more study.

Heart Helpers

If you're reading this book, you are probably already doing quite a bit to ward of heart disease—eating heart-healthy foods and exercising, for example. But if you have a family history of cardiovascular disease, you're probably wondering what else might help.

Carnitine. A natural proteinlike substance produced by our livers and kidneys from two amino acids, carnitine carries fatty acids to cells—including heart cells—producing energy.

"There is strong evidence that carnitine is just one in a group of natural substances that, when taken together in supplement form, can offer protection against the onset or progression of heart disease," says Stephen L. DeFelice, M.D., author of *The Carnitine Defense*, who coined the term *nutraceutical*. (The other substances include fiber, fish oil, coenzyme Q_{10}, and niacin, among others.)

Dr. DeFelice recommends 1,500 to 3,000 milligrams of L-carnitine a day, divided into two doses 8 to 12 hours apart, for adults over age 35, especially those at high risk for heart disease.

Coenzyme Q_{10} (CoQ_{10}). CoQ_{10}, or ubiquinone as it's sometimes called, is found in the mitochondria, our cells' energy factories. It works as an antioxidant. Several clinical studies have shown the supplement to have a positive effect on heart disease, including improving quality of life for patients who experienced heart failure, reducing arrhythmias in those with angina, and decreasing blood pressure. One study found that on 150 milligrams per day, people with congestive heart failure were 38 percent less apt to need hospitalization than those taking placebos.

In another study, however, Stephen Gottlieb, M.D., of the University of Maryland Medical Center in Baltimore, found that 200 milligrams of coenzyme Q_{10} daily had "absolutely no effect" on heart function. The 6-month study done by Dr. Gottlieb and his colleagues on 46 people with

EVALUATING THE PRODUCTS

If you're considering a nutraceutical supplement, don't just reach for the first bottle you see and start knocking them back with abandon. You could end up doing more harm than good.

- Look for the USP label on the supplement bottle. This label from the U.S. Pharmacopeia indicates that what is claimed to be in the product, including what dose, can actually be found in the product.
- Buy from nationally known food and drug manufacturers who have a good reputation and who are more likely to have created the product under strict controls.
- Always read product labels, follow directions, and heed all warnings.
- Realize that the label NATURAL doesn't guarantee that the product is safe. Even poisonous mushrooms are natural.
- Write to the supplement manufacturer for more information. Ask the company about the conditions under which its products were made.
- Always tell your doctor and pharmacist about any supplements you take; some may interfere or react with prescription drugs or mask signs and symptoms of serious illnesses.

congestive heart failure measured how much blood the heart is pumping out—a way to test the heart's strength—and saw no difference in the subjects before and after.

Until further research is available, it's hard to tell whether individuals with heart problems can benefit from coenzyme Q_{10} or not. And it wouldn't be wise to abandon medical treatment prescribed by your doctor and treat yourself with supplements instead. If you do decide to try coenzyme Q_{10}, don't take more than 120 milligrams for more than 20 days without medical guidance. Though rare, possible side effects include heartburn, nausea, and stomachache, which can be prevented by taking the supplement with a meal. If you are taking the blood thinner warfarin (Coumadin), discuss supplementation with your doctor since coenzyme Q_{10} may reduce its effectiveness.

Memory Boosters

On those days when you call your kid by the dog's name, put your brown-bag lunch in the freezer, and lock your keys in the car with the engine running, a memory-enhancing pill sounds like a godsend.

DHA. A source of omega-3 essential fatty acids, DHA, or docosahexaenoic acid, is the most abundant fatty acid in our brains and retinas. Some research suggests that low levels of DHA may be linked to Alzheimer's disease, and studies in rats show that it can improve their ability to remember and learn new things.

But the bulk of research on DHA focuses on its benefits for depression, with low levels increasing susceptibility to depression. In fact, that may be one reason for postpartum depression—pregnant women are often deficient in DHA.

While little research exists to support the benefits of DHA for memory, it's worth trying for depression, as long as your doctor knows you're taking it. Experts say that it is best consumed as fish oil, not a separate supplement, because it is better absorbed and balanced with other omega-3 fatty acids that way. For depression, the suggested amount is 3 grams of DHA and eicosapentaenoic acid (EPA)—another omega-3 fatty acid precursor, says Ray Sahelian, M.D., a physician with the Longevity Research Center in Marina Del Rey, California, and author of *Mind Boosters*. They're often sold in combination form.

People who are taking prescription blood-thinning medications such as warfarin (Coumadin) shouldn't take fish oil without their doctor's supervision, especially at this level. Fish oil is also a blood thinner, so their dosage for warfarin would need to be adjusted. High intakes may reduce blood-clotting ability, resulting in bleeding or, in extreme instances, hemorrhaging.

Phosphatidylserine (PS). PS occurs naturally in the membranes of nerve cells. "There's evidence that it's quite good for memory," says Dr. Janson. In one study, 149 men and women with age-related memory impairment were treated for 12 weeks with either 300 milligrams of PS or a placebo. Those treated with the drug were better able to learn and recall names, faces, and numbers. The worse their memory had been before the test, the greater their improvement.

The problem is that the type of PS used in most human and animal trials came from cow brains, says Dr. Sahelian. With the possibility of brain-related diseases being passed from cows to humans, it's doubtful that this type would be available. Supplements sold today are made from soy, and few clinical trials have been conducted using them.

"I have a problem with recommending the over-the-counter PS because it has a different chemical structure than the one used in testing," he says. Although it's technically safe, it may not necessarily be effective, and people may want to wait until soy-based PS has undergone adequate testing before taking it as a supplement. If you do want to try it, check with your doctor first and follow his or her recommended dosage.

Choline. Within our cells, choline is translated into the neurotransmitter acetylcholine, the brain chemical involved in memory and learning. Other sources of choline you may see as supplements include lecithin and phosphatidylcholine, or PC.

"Some studies with lecithin show that it slows the rate of decline in early Alzheimer's disease," says Alan R. Gaby, M.D., professor of nutrition at Bastyr University in Seattle. "But in more advanced stages of the disease, it doesn't help. In theory, choline might be beneficial, but that's just theoretical."

In one study, nine volunteers took either a placebo or 20 grams of lecithin 5 hours before a test, but neither group showed any improvement in various learning tasks. When the compound was tested on 24 elderly volunteers with memory problems, however, doses of 300 to 1,000 milligrams a day for 4 weeks significantly improved their performance on word recall tests, leading the researchers to conclude that the compound is suitable for treatment of memory deficits in elderly people.

Don't take more than 3.5 grams of choline or 23 grams of lecithin without medical supervision. Excess choline can cause low blood pressure, and high doses of lecithin may cause sweating, salivation, and loss of appetite. A dose of lecithin close to 5 grams may cause upset stomach, nausea, and diarrhea. Both supplements may cause a fishy body odor in some people.

Huperzine A. This is an extract from the club moss *Huperzia serrata*, used for centuries in Chinese folk medicine to treat fever. It works by inhibiting an enzyme that breaks down acetylcholine. And its action is similar to that of tacrine and donepezil, prescription medications used for people with Alzheimer's disease, possibly with fewer adverse side effects. In China, the purified compound has been used as a prescription drug to treat an estimated 100,000 people with dementia, with low toxicity.

"Preliminary research is encouraging," says Dr. Gaby. So taking huperzine is worth a try under the supervision of a knowledgeable physician.

Energy Expanders

Supplements that promise to recharge your batteries are tempting. Do they work? It depends.

Coenzyme Q$_{10}$. Along with its heart-helping properties, this nutrient is involved in the production of energy in cells. Just as it energizes our cells, it can energize us, says Dr. Janson.

As with the research on heart benefits, studies on the effect of coenzyme Q$_{10}$ on energy are mixed. Of 11 studies of coenzyme Q$_{10}$ conducted in the 1990s, five showed an improvement in physical capacity, five showed no effect, and one actually showed decreased energy.

Don't take more than 120 milligrams of coenzyme Q$_{10}$ for more than 20 days without medical guidance. Though rare, possible side effects include heartburn, nausea, and stomachache, which can be prevented by taking the supplement with a meal. If you are taking the blood thinner warfarin (Coumadin), discuss supplementation with your doctor since coenzyme Q$_{10}$ may reduce its effectiveness.

Octacosanol. This is a naturally occurring, long-chain alcohol commonly marketed as an athletic aid, energy booster, and overall tonic to enhance vigor and vitality. It's also a component of wheat germ oil, which studies from 30 years ago suggested could improve endurance, says Dr. Gaby. But it's not clear whether octacosanol is the active ingredient in wheat germ oil, and Dr. Gaby has seen no studies on the compound specifically for energy.

So for now, you might want to save your money.

Sleep Aids

It typically hits when you're facing major deadlines at work, your checkbook won't balance, and your husband has begun muttering about "life change" and "find myself." Suddenly, you either can't fall asleep or you're snapping awake at 3:00 A.M., ready to scrub down the kitchen. Worried about side effects from prescription sleep aids, you consider trying a natural sleep aid. What's the story on them?

Melatonin. "It's good for jet lag and shift-work insomnia, but I don't recommend it as a general sleeping pill," says Dr. Gaby. That's because melatonin seems to work best if your own levels of the hormone are low—which may not be the case if it's stress that is keeping you up. And a Harvard Medical School study has cast doubt on the common wisdom that our melatonin levels drop as we age. The study compared 34 men and women ranging in age from 65 to 81 and found that their nighttime melatonin levels were basically the same as those of 98 men ranging in age from 18 to 30. Finally, in about 10 percent of people who are followed in studies of melatonin supplements, high doses have actually *caused* insomnia and nightmares.

Dr. Gaby says that melatonin is worth a try for jet lag and shift-work insomnia. The typical dose is anywhere from 0.5 to 3 milligrams. Don't take it more than twice a week, because it may disrupt your natural production of melatonin and other hormones. And if you have sleep apnea—in which you stop breathing for short periods throughout the night—definitely skip it. In a very deep sleep induced by melatonin, you might not wake up.

Take melatonin only under the supervision of a knowledgeable medical doctor, and never before driving. It may cause headaches, nausea, morning dizziness, daytime sleepiness, depression, giddiness, difficulty concentrating, and upset stomach, and may have interactions with prescription medications. Skip it altogether if you have a cardiovascular condition, high blood pressure, any autoimmune disease such as rheumatoid arthritis or lupus, diabetes, epilepsy, migraine, or a personal or family history of a hormone-dependent cancer such as breast, testicular, prostate, or endometrial cancer. Melatonin may cause infertility, reduced sex drive in males, hypothermia, retinal damage, and interference with hormone-replacement therapy. And the long-term effects of melatonin supplements are unknown.

Even when melatonin is advised, choose synthetic melatonin over the animal-derived hormone. It would take 30 million sheep pineal glands, an impossible amount, to provide the melatonin found in one 100-count bottle of tablets, each containing 3 milligrams of the hormone. So even the so-called natural melatonin contains synthetic melatonin. Plus, viruses may contaminate the animal-derived hormone.

Mood Enhancers

The difference between the blues and depression can be life threatening. So this is one arena where you don't want to diagnose and treat yourself. Talk to your doctor, discuss what the appropriate treatment is, and if he or she agrees that natural supplements may help, use the information below to make informed choices.

L-tryptophan. If you're depressed, you may have low levels of serotonin, which your body makes from L-tryptophan. Increasing your level of tryptophan could help with the depression.

But clinical studies are mixed, with only two out of eight showing tryptophan having a better effect than a placebo.

Concern in 1989 that commercial L-tryptophan was contaminated with a substance that was connected with a painful muscular disorder led the FDA to order its removal from the market. It is legally available today only by prescription and should only be used under the supervision of a knowledgeable medical doctor.

5-Hydroxytryptophan (5-HTP). This supplement is marketed as an alternative to L-tryptophan, and, indeed, very small amounts of it are produced in our own bodies from tryptophan. It's also a precursor to serotonin, a brain chemical linked to depression, so the more 5-HTP you have, the more serotonin your brain makes.

There are few significant clinical trials in humans, however, showing 5-HTP's effectiveness in alleviating depression. In one study, researchers reported low levels of impurities in retail samples of dietary supplements containing 5-HTP. One was "peak X," suspected of being the possible cause in one case of eosinophilia-myalgia syndrome (EMS), a serious illness characterized by increased white blood cells and severe muscle pain. Similar impurities were found in L-tryptophan.

The study found that there were, indeed, traces of peak X in all the samples tested. But it did not establish a direct connection between peak X and EMS, says Stephen Naylor, Ph.D., professor of biochemistry at the Mayo Clinic, one of the researchers involved. The FDA has issued an alert on 5-HTP and is continuing to monitor the situation. Pass on this supplement.

SOMETHING NOT RIGHT? HERE'S WHO TO CALL

If you start taking a new supplement and don't feel well, stop taking the product and call your doctor immediately. Then report any adverse reactions to the FDA's MedWatch number at (800) FDA-1088, or on the MedWatch Web site at www.fda.gov/medwatch/. You can also browse the MedWatch Web site and learn about any adverse reactions reported, listed by product.

S-adenosylmethionine (SAM-e). Available by prescription in Europe for nearly 20 years, SAM-e didn't appear in this country until the late 1990s, when it was quickly touted as a natural alternative to prescription drugs like fluoxetine (Prozac) and paroxetine (Paxil).

And studies do show that SAM-e can be just as effective as these medications without side effects like dry mouth, headache, poor concentration, and constipation. Much of the research on SAM-e has been done with the injected form of the supplement, not the oral form, although what little research does exist on the oral form suggests that it also works, says Dr. Gaby.

In one Italian study, 80 postmenopausal women with depression improved more with taking 1,600 milligrams of oral SAM-e a day than with a placebo.

In clinical studies, 400 to 1,600 milligrams of SAM-e were as effective at reducing depression as prescription antidepressants. SAM-e may also help traditional, prescriptive antidepressants work faster. One study comparing a combination of SAM-e and the drug imipramine to a placebo combined with imipramine found that those taking 200 milligrams of SAM-e by injection saw their depressive symptoms decrease faster than those taking the placebo. If you are taking any kind of antidepressant, however, Dr. Gaby says that you must consult a doctor before taking SAM-e. SAM-e is not recommended for bipolar disorder. "In some cases, it has caused depression to switch to mania," Dr. Gaby says.

SAM-e also helps arthritis. "SAM-e gets into the joint and serves as a building block to make more of the substances a joint needs," says Sol Grazi, M.D., assistant professor of family medicine at the University of Colorado School of Medicine. In addition to regenerating cartilage, SAM-e also reduces inflammation, which allows the cartilage cells known as chondrocytes to repair the injured joint. Don't take it if you have any kind of cardiovascular disease, because it may increase blood levels of homocysteine. Anyone taking it should also be taking folic acid and vitamins B_6 and B_{12} to keep their homocysteine levels down.

Alleviating Arthritis Aches

While SAM-e is recognized for effectiveness against arthritis, the big players in this supplement category are chondroitin sulfate and glucosamine, natural substances found in and around cartilage cells, the connective tissue that cushions the ends of bones within the joint.

When glucosamine is taken in pill form, it binds to cartilage tissue and helps rebuild cartilage, says Dr. Sahelian, author of *All About Glucosamine and Chondroitin.* The research on chondroitin is sketchier, he says, because it is still unclear what its role is. Some researchers believe it provides cartilage with strength and resilience.

"I say start with glucosamine, and if it's not effective after 3 or 4 months, then it may be appropriate to add chondroitin," Dr. Sahelian says. So it's worth a try.

The typical dose for glucosamine is 1,500 milligrams a day, taken all at once or throughout the day. The suggested dosage for chondroitin is 500 milligrams three times a day or 750 milligrams twice a day. Glucosamine may cause upset stomach, heartburn, or diarrhea.

In clinical studies, both supplements as well as SAM-e had to be taken for 34 weeks before providing any pain relief. Let your doctor know if you take either of these supplements. Some animal studies suggest increases in blood sugar levels with glucosamine, and chondroitin is molecularly similar to the blood thinner heparin.

Methylsulfonylmethane (MSM). MSM is a sulfur-containing compound found in trace amounts in food. You shouldn't take it if you are allergic or sensitive to sulfur drugs. Theoretically, it decreases inflammation by increasing the effect of cortisol, the body's own natural inflammation fighter.

As with drugs, the best way to study nutraceuticals is by using either the substance or a placebo. Few research studies of this kind have been done with MSM. One, published in the *International Journal of Anti-Aging Medicine,* shows that in 8 out of 10 people with arthritis who took 750 milligrams of MSM three times a day for 6 weeks, pain relief improved 82 percent, compared to an 18 percent improvement for those on a placebo. Other doctors have reported similar success in case studies, especially if combined with glucosamine. Large doses (2,000 to 8,000 milligrams per day) may cause stomach upset or diarrhea, however. So for now, glucosamine with chondroitin appears to be a better choice.

Supplements for the Athlete

Getting in shape—and training for sports—is work. Can popping a pill help?

"Depends on the type of training you're into," says Bruce W. Craig,

Ph.D., professor of exercise physiology at Ball State University in Muncie, Indiana, who has tested and evaluated sports supplements.

Creatine. This is probably the most studied athletic aid, says Dr. Craig. Its benefits seem to support the claims. An amino acid made by the body and stored predominately in skeletal muscle, reserves of creatine replenish ATP (adenosine triphosphate), a substance that gives our muscles their get-up-and-go.

Supplementing with creatine boosts your storage area, so instead of maybe 20 seconds of explosive muscle power, you have 30 seconds. "This might not seem like a lot, but to a football lineman that extra 10 seconds of power in a game can make a difference," Dr. Craig says. But if you're a runner, you'll burn it off just warming up.

It won't build muscle mass, he says, and few studies have looked at creatine's effects on women. There are no long-term studies of its effect on human health. The typical dose is 20 grams a day for 5 days, then a maintenance dose of 2 grams a day indefinitely. Larger doses may lead to stomach cramping, nausea, or kidney disease.

Androstenedione. This is the supplement St. Louis Cardinal slugger Mark McGwire took when he broke baseball's home-run record. But it's doubtful that the supplement, a precursor in our bodies to such hor-

ROYAL JELLY: LEAVE IT TO THE BEES

Supplements of royal jelly, the creamy white substance special nurse bees produce to feed their queen, are touted as a cholesterol reducer, antibiotic, and anti-inflammatory. Anything that makes a queen bee live longer than her worker bees should do the same for you, right?

Wrong.

"That's an old one," says Ruth Kava, R.D., Ph.D., director of nutrition at the American Council on Science and Health in New York City. "You're talking about stuff made from pollen that bugs chew up. I know of no reason to think it's effective."

Worse, it may be harmful. People who've taken royal jelly have experienced asthma attacks, severe allergic reactions, and even death.

It's best left to the bees.

mones as testosterone and estrogen, made much of a difference, says Dr. Craig. In one study in men, the only effect of androstenedione was slightly higher hormone levels with no performance improvement. And there are no good studies on women. Pass on this one.

Other amino acid supplements. These include arginine and glutamine. They're a way to boost protein levels to increase muscle mass. But, says Dr. Craig, "you can do that by eating more meat. You don't need supplements; they'll just give you very expensive urine." That's because you'll excrete any excess amino acids your body can't use. No matter what you've heard, these supplements won't improve your performance, he says. And high doses of arginine may cause nausea and diarrhea. People who have genital herpes should not take it because it may increase herpes outbreaks. Don't take arginine and lysine at the same time, as they compete for absorption in the body. Long-term effects of taking arginine are unknown. If you have problems with your kidneys or liver, check with your physician before taking glutamine.

Hydroxymethylbutyrate (HMB). HMB is a popular dietary supplement that preliminary evidence suggests may inhibit the breakdown of protein, leading to muscle gain. In one study, HMB supplementation during 3 to 8 weeks of training showed significantly greater gains of fat-free body mass and strength in men and women just beginning resistance training. Other studies looking at well-trained athletes, however, showed no effects. Pass on this one.

Weight-Loss Supplements

Just popping a pill to help you lose weight without changing your lifestyle is pure fantasy. "Women are just fooling themselves if they think that they can lose weight without reducing their calories and increasing exercise," agrees Dr. Janson.

Chromium picolinate. Chromium is a trace mineral important in regulating the way our cells absorb glucose, or energy. "Studies show that it can change your body composition," says Dr. Gaby, "but you won't lose weight."

In one study, 123 men and women were randomly assigned to either a diet/exercise/supplement group or a diet/exercise/placebo group. On a regimen of 1,500 calories a day, plus 5 days of walking, those taking the supplement had significantly more muscle and less body fat, but there was no difference in weight loss.

And in one study in which 43 young, overweight women took chromium supplements without increasing the amount they exercised, the women actually *gained* weight. So in 1996, the Federal Trade Commission ordered several chromium manufacturers to stop claiming that their products promote weight loss.

Too much chromium may cause kidney failure. Stick to no more than 200 micrograms unless your doctor advises you otherwise.

Pyruvate. This is a naturally occurring substance that you use in producing energy, and it does show some promising possibilities. Researchers at the University of Pittsburgh put 27 women on very low calorie diets, ranging from 500 to 1,000 calories a day, with half of them getting pyruvate supplements and half of them getting a placebo. The women on the supplements lost considerably more weight than those taking the placebo. The researchers then took 17 women and for 3 weeks had them on 300-calorie diets, during which, as might be expected, they all lost weight. But after the diet, when they were put on a moderately high-calorie, "overeating" diet designed to induce weight gain, those also taking a pyruvate supplement gained back 36 percent less weight and 55 percent less body fat than those receiving placebos.

"It's interesting, but I don't know if it's the pyruvate or a lifestyle change," says Jackie Berning, R.D., Ph.D., assistant professor of nutrition at the University of Colorado at Colorado Springs. Until claims are verified, exercise and improved eating habits are a better bet.

Chitosan. This supplement is derived from chitin, an indigestible type of cellulose from the shells of crabs and other crustaceans. Chitin has been used as an industrial water purifier for years, soaking up oils, grease, and other toxins from polluted waters. Can it do the same in your stomach? Evidently not.

In a British study, 30 overweight people took either 1,000 milligrams of chitosan or a placebo twice daily. After 4 weeks, neither group lost any weight. And in animal studies, chitosan binds with micronutrients, including calcium, iron, and magnesium, while interfering with various fat-soluble vitamins.

Chitosan may also interfere with the absorption of carotenoids (beta-carotene, lutein, zeaxanthin) and cause gas, bloating, and diarrhea. Talk with your doctor before supplementing with chitosan.

Customize Your Supplement Program

Nutrition researchers are well-versed in what vitamins and minerals the typical woman should take every day. In reality, though, we're individuals with very individual needs. No two women eat precisely the same foods or have exactly the same needs.

Some are overly susceptible to colds, others never get a sniffle. Some are overstressed by trying to simultaneously care for aging parents and adolescent children, others are not. Some worry about family histories of heart disease, others, cancer or osteoporosis.

What's more, your health profile is in constant flux (like your life), changing from month to month or year to year as you switch jobs, have children, get divorced, move into menopause, gain or lose weight.

From what she sees in the women she counsels, New York City nutrition scientist Shari Lieberman, Ph.D., is exquisitely aware of these individual needs. Dr. Lieberman, a nutrition professor at the University of Bridgeport in Connecticut and author of *The Real Vitamin and Mineral Book*, believes strongly in the power of nutrition and nutritional supplements to keep us healthy, prevent disease, and work in conjunction with traditional medicine in treating illnesses. In fact, physicians often refer patients to Dr. Lieberman for nutritional counseling.

Dr. Lieberman explains how to customize your supplement program—for today, tomorrow, and into the future.

THE RIGHT WAY TO USE
VITAMIN B-COMPLEX FORMULAS

Unlike vitamin C, there is not one but several B vitamins your body needs: thiamin, riboflavin, niacin, niacinamide, vitamin B_6 (pyridoxine), vitamin B_{12} (cyanocobalamin), folic acid, pantothenic acid, biotin, and choline.

The B vitamins should be taken together, as they interact with each other in a variety of complex ways, and B-complex supplements generally contain all of these. You'll typically find formulas containing 50 milligrams of all B vitamins measured in milligrams (thiamin, riboflavin, niacin, pantothenic acid, choline, and vitamin B_6) and 50 micrograms of all those measured in micrograms (B_{12}, folic acid, and biotin).

Look for a 1-to-1 ratio of the percent Daily Values. In other words, you should get the same percent Daily Values of each vitamin—all 100 percent or all 50 percent. Don't take higher doses of any single B vitamin without increasing the amounts you take of the others. This is important because the B vitamins compete with each other in your intestines for absorption by your body. Too much of one might mean a deficiency of another. Therefore, it's important not to take more than one dose a day of either a B-complex or single B vitamins.

The Basics

Start with a daily multivitamin/mineral similar to the one in "What to Look For in a Multi" on page 198. If you can't find it all in one supplement, add separate supplements to meet these recommended levels. Think of this as the basic black dress of your supplement "wardrobe." Now we want to accessorize.

What's Your Nutritional Type?

Over and above your basic needs, you may need additional nutrients, depending on your health history and lifestyle. Read each of the following 10 profiles, and determine which one describes you best. Then, use the information to customize your supplement program. If you have a health condition or take medication, work with your doctor, pharmacist, registered dietitian, or a licensed nutritionist, to be sure you make the best decision based on your individual needs or to avoid harmful drug interactions.

If more than one profile seems to describe you, do not duplicate supplements. For instance, if you have both a poorly functioning immune system and asthma, you would take at most 800 milligrams of vitamin C per day, not 1,300 milligrams.

Profile 1: The Worried Well

You do everything right. You eat a balanced diet with plenty of fruits and vegetables, exercise regularly, and don't smoke. Your mother lived well into her eighties, and your father is still around to ask you how your car is running. But "what ifs" keep you up at night, and every twinge or minor illness sends you running to the doctor, on the alert for trouble best caught early.

The basic multi described on page 198 coupled with your healthy lifestyle provides solid protection against the vagaries of life in the 21st century.

Profile 2: Blood Sugar Blues

One of your parents had diabetes, or maybe you had gestational diabetes when you were pregnant. Perhaps you're one of those who simply crashes around 3:00 P.M. unless you get something to eat. Maybe you're overweight. All these are risk factors for blood sugar disorders, primarily diabetes and hypoglycemia.

Most likely, your doctor will suggest exercise and dietary changes. Taking the following supplements may offer added protection.

Chromium. For diabetes prevention, take 400 to 600 micrograms daily of chromium of any kind. If you have low blood sugar, 200 micrograms may help. If you already have diabetes and you are chromium deficient, 600 to 1,000 micrograms may be helpful. (If you're taking insulin, it's important that your doctor or pharmacist approves the supplements you're taking, and dosages above 200 micrograms should always be taken under a doctor's supervision.)

Chromium is the major mineral involved in insulin production and the best-studied natural diabetes supplement. Insulin binds to certain sites on cells called receptors. This lets cells take in glucose for energy.

Vitamin E. To reduce diabetes-related damage to your body, take 400 IU a day. If your diabetes is difficult to control, with wildly fluctuating blood sugar levels, it may be helpful to work your way up to 800 to 1,000 IU under the guidance of your physician. If you are considering taking more than 400 IU of vitamin E, talk to your doctor first. One study using low-dose supplements showed increased risk of hemorrhagic stroke.

High levels of vitamin E may be able to reduce some of the harmful effects associated with diabetes, perhaps by regenerating insulin-producing beta cells in the pancreas, thus enabling you to produce more insulin. If you begin taking vitamin E, start with 200 IU and gradually increase.

Profile 3: Creeping Cholesterol

The last time you had a cholesterol test, your LDL (bad cholesterol) was high, your HDL (good cholesterol) was low, and your VLDL (very bad cholesterol) was very high. The fatty globules—LDL and VLDL—stick to your arteries, impeding bloodflow to your heart and putting you at risk for a heart attack.

Most likely, you are trying to cut out saturated fat and eat plenty of fiber. Thanks to heredity, your ratio of total cholesterol to good cholesterol is still high—above 4 to 1.

Here's what to try. (Consult your doctor, especially if you are a candidate for cholesterol-lowering medication.)

Flush-free niacin. Take 250 to 350 milligrams daily. Doses above 35 milligrams should be taken under supervision of your physician. An overwhelming number of studies have shown that niacin reduces total cholesterol and triglyceride levels—another blood fat—even more effectively than a prescription-only cholesterol medication called clofibrate. It also significantly *increases* HDL.

Avoid sustained-release niacin, however, which may cause liver problems. Also avoid regular niacin, which may, in high doses, give you hot flashes. Choose flush-free niacin, which goes by the chemical name inositol hexaniacinate.

Gugulipid. Choose a daily supplement that provides 75 milligrams of gugulsterones. This herb, also known as guggul, has been used in India for thousands of years. In one study, men and women who took guggul lowered their cholesterol levels by 24 percent and their triglyceride levels by 23 percent. Guggul rarely may trigger diarrhea, restlessness, apprehension, or hiccups.

Chromium. Take 600 micrograms a day. Chromium lowers elevated blood sugar and insulin levels and improves insulin resistance, which plays a role in how your body stores fat. Dosages above 200 micrograms should always be taken under a doctor's supervision.

Note: Flush-free niacin, gugulipid, and chromium may be taken together.

Cholestin. Red yeast rice powder, the main ingredient in the over-the-counter supplement Cholestin, contains a natural substance that is chemically identical to lovastatin, the active ingredient in the prescription drug Mevacor. A University of California study found that Cholestin lowered blood cholesterol significantly more than diet changes alone (up to 40 points compared to just 5 points when combined with diet and exercise) with no adverse effects. Follow label directions for the daily dosage, and only take this under the supervision of a medical, naturopathic, or Chinese Medicine doctor. Take this along with your multi.

Profile 4: Blood Pressure Woes

High blood pressure puts you at risk for stroke, heart failure, or kidney failure because your heart has to work harder to move blood through your body. Even if your blood pressure reads normal now, a family history of hypertension puts you at risk for problems later.

Losing weight and getting more exercise can help. So can the following supplements.

Garlic. Take the equivalent of 1 gram of raw garlic per day. Because garlic comes in so many different preparations, check the label carefully to see that you're getting the appropriate dose. Do not use supplements if you're on anticoagulants (blood thinners) or before undergoing surgery, because garlic thins the blood and may increase bleeding. Do not use it if you're taking drugs to lower your blood sugar.

Hawthorn berry. Take 400 to 600 milligrams daily. Garlic and hawthorn berries are thought to act as vasodilators—widening blood vessels so that blood flows more easily through them, thus reducing blood pressure. If you have a cardiovascular condition, do not take hawthorn regularly for more than a few weeks without medical supervision. You may require lower doses of other medications, such as high blood pressure drugs. If you have low blood pressure caused by heart valve problems, do not use hawthorn without medical supervision.

Fish oil. Take a daily dose of around 720 milligrams eicosapentaenoic acid (EPA) and 480 milligrams docosahexaenoic acid (DHA). These are the essential fatty acids found in fish oil. You can get this amount from fish, but if you don't like fish, experts say that it is safe to get up to 1 gram of omega-3's a day from fish-oil capsules. You will need to take several capsules to reach this dose; check the ingredient label on your supplement.

No one knows exactly why fish oil protects against heart disease or lowers blood pressure, but it probably has to do with the way it thins the blood, making clots less likely. It also may reduce inflammation and may help relax arteries. You should not take fish oil, however, if you have a bleeding disorder or uncontrolled high blood pressure, if you take anti-coagulants (blood thinners) or use aspirin regularly, or if you have an al-lergy to any kind of fish. Since it increases bleeding time, fish oil may possibly lead to nosebleeds and easy bruising, and may cause upset stomach in some people.

Coenzyme Q$_{10}$ (CoQ$_{10}$). Take about 100 milligrams per day. Because it's ubiquitous—everywhere in the body—coenzyme Q$_{10}$ is known as ubiquinone. It basically acts as a catalyst for certain cell reactions needed to create ATP, a compound that provides energy to cells. It improves en-ergy supplies to heart muscle cells, helping them pump more efficiently with less effort. That, in turn, helps lower blood pressure. At least one study found a significant increase in survival rate among people with car-diomyopathy, a disease of the heart muscle. Supplementation should be observed by a professional if taken for more than 20 days at levels 120 milligrams a day or higher. Side effects are rare, but tend to be heartburn, nausea, and stomachache, which can be prevented by consuming the sup-plement with a meal. Rarely, a slight decrease in the effectiveness of the blood thinner warfarin (Coumadin) has been observed.

Profile 5: Prone to Bone Loss

You're thin, don't exercise much, crash-diet often, hate milk, and your mother slumps forward with a dowager's hump. Any or all of these put you at risk for osteoporosis. Perhaps a DEXA scan or other bone density screening test has confirmed that you're at risk. Here's what can help re-store bone density.

Calcium. Take 500 to 1,000 milligrams a day. Calcium is just the tip of the iceberg in preventing osteoporosis. Yet women have been told to take massive amounts of calcium while other minerals are ignored.

Magnesium. Take 500 to 600 milligrams a day. Magnesium helps calcium get into the bones and also converts vitamin D to its active form in the body, which in turn convinces organs to release calcium for bone growth. Just over half of our magnesium is found in our bones. Take daily doses above 350 milligrams only under a doctor's supervision.

Boron. Take 3 to 6 milligrams a day. A trace mineral that actually enhances the bones' ability to take in calcium and other minerals, boron works kind of like estrogen—without any side effects.

Ipriflavone. Take 600 milligrams per day. A phytonutrient isolated from soy, ipriflavone has been shown in more than 50 human clinical trials to actually *build* bone, even more than prescription estrogen or the drug alendronate (Fosamax).

Profile 6: Coping with Allergies and Asthma

Whether it's grass, pollen, or dust mites, it seems something always makes you sneeze and sniff. Or wheeze and cough. Allergy and asthma are among the fastest growing maladies in this country. Thankfully, research on safe and effective supplements is keeping pace.

Vitamin C. Take 500 to 800 milligrams daily. Vitamin C acts as a natural antihistamine, blocking the release of histamine, a biochemical that, among other actions, causes constriction of the bronchial tubes, making it difficult to breathe.

Quercetin. Take 250 to 400 milligrams (a 1-to-2 ratio with vitamin C) per day. Quercetin is a flavonoid extracted from certain fruits and vegetables like apples and onions, and behaves similarly to vitamin C. Quercetin dilates blood vessels and causes blood thinning, so women with a history of low blood pressure or problems with blood clotting should avoid using it.

Magnesium. Take 250 milligrams a day. A study conducted at the University of Nottingham City Hospital in the United Kingdom showed that men and women diagnosed with asthma who took 400 milligrams of magnesium supplements daily experienced less airway obstruction than when they did not take these supplements. Magnesium helps muscles relax while calcium helps them contract.

Fish oil. Take a daily dose of around 720 milligrams EPA and 480 milligrams DHA. A natural prostaglandin, fish oil blunts inflammation, halting the actions of compounds that your body produces that cause bronchial constriction and other allergic reactions. You should not take fish oil if you have a bleeding disorder or uncontrolled high blood pressure, if you take anticoagulants (blood thinners) or use aspirin regularly, or if you have an allergy to any kind of fish. Since it increases bleeding time, fish oil may possibly lead to nosebleeds and easy bruising, and may cause upset stomach in some people.

Profile 7: Poorly Functioning Immune System

You catch every cold your kids bring home, can count on spending at least 2 weeks a winter in bed with the flu, and seem to be always just finishing a round of antibiotics when the next infection hits. You need to pump up and strengthen your immune system so that it's better able to fight off hostile invaders.

Vitamin C. Take 500 milligrams a day. One of C's main jobs is to keep your immune system strong. Vitamin C supplementation has helped resistance to infections and cancer, skin graft rejection, and wound repair. It also increases white blood cells' mobility, so that they can eat more bacteria, viruses, and other harmful invaders. What's more, it's a powerful antioxidant.

Vitamin E. Take 400 IU of natural vitamin E daily. Vitamin E increases the levels of interferon and interleukin in your blood, biochemicals the immune system produces to fight infection. Because it's an antioxidant, it can also prevent the kind of cellular damage that may further lower immunity.

Echinacea. Take 900 to 1,000 milligrams in capsule form 4 days on and 4 days off during cold and flu season. Echinacea is an herb well-known for its immune-boosting properties, with many studies showing that it prevents or shortens the duration of viral illnesses. Do not use echinacea if you are allergic to closely related plants such as ragweed, aster, and chrysanthemum. If you have an autoimmune condition, don't use echinacea without the consent of your physician.

Astragalus. Take about 1,000 milligrams of astragalus in capsule form daily for 1 month, then stop for 2 weeks, then take it for another month. For other forms, follow the label directions. Astragalus prevents colds and flu. It may boost interferon production in the body.

Profile 8: Overactive Immune System

An autoimmune disease like lupus, rheumatoid arthritis, or multiple sclerosis brings with it numerous medical challenges. A variety of supplements can help you manage and may even improve your symptoms. (As with any progressive, chronic condition, it's a good idea to let your doctor in on your plans to supplement, and get a medical green light, especially if you're taking medication.)

Vitamin E. Take 800 IU of natural vitamin E a day. Two studies of people with lupus showed that large doses of vitamin E had a beneficial effect, with some seeing their symptoms completely disappear. And in one study of seven rheumatoid arthritis patients given vitamin E and selenium along with their usual treatments (which was no longer effective), joint pain either diminished or disappeared entirely. One reason: E's anti-inflammatory effects.

If you are considering taking more than 400 IU of vitamin E, talk to your doctor first. One study using low-dose supplements showed increased risk of hemorrhagic stroke.

Fish oil or gamma-linolenic acid (GLA). Take a daily dose of four or five fish-oil capsules that contain 180 milligrams of EPA and 120 milligrams of DHA or 240 milligrams of GLA. EPA and GLA seem to work similarly, blocking proinflammatory prostaglandins. In one study, 275 milligrams of GLA a day relieved various immune-related skin disorders, such as eczema and atopic dermatitis. Take both, as GLA and EPA work slightly differently, complementing each other.

GLA may cause headaches, indigestion, nausea, and softening of stools. Take it under the supervision of a knowledgeable medical doctor if you take aspirin or anticoagulants (blood thinners) regularly, have a seizure disorder, or are taking epilepsy medication such as phenothiazines. You should not take fish oil if you have a bleeding disorder or uncontrolled high blood pressure, if you take anticoagulants or use aspirin regularly, or if you have an allergy to any kind of fish. Since it increases bleeding time, fish oil may possibly lead to nosebleeds and easy bruising, and may cause upset stomach in some people.

Coenzyme Q_{10}. Take 100 milligrams per day. Anecdotal and clinical evidence shows that coenzyme Q_{10} benefits autoimmune diseases. While there is no research to back up this belief, some nutritionists report success in alleviating symptoms of lupus, multiple sclerosis, and other immune disorders with the enzyme. Although rare, side effects can include heartburn, nausea, and stomachache (which can be prevented by consuming the supplement with a meal) and a slight decrease in the effectiveness of the blood thinner warfarin (Coumadin).

Profile 9: Approaching (or in) Menopause

Perimenopause—the years just before your menstrual periods disappear for good—manifests itself in a variety of ways. Your periods may be shorter or longer, heavier or lighter, come more frequently or even skip a month. You may start to notice some night sweats and irritability or more intense premenstrual syndrome. Whether you are standing on the diving board of the menopause pool or already swimming in its waters, the same supplements can help.

Black cohosh and chasteberry. Follow package directions for the daily dosage. Both herbs are well-known and widely used for their effects in soothing problems like hot flashes, bloating, and irregular periods. Do not take black cohosh for more than 6 months at a time unless you have been given professional advice to do so.

Vitamin E. For mild hot flashes (ones that don't keep you up at night), vitamin E may help. Some women have found that vitamin E helps reduce the incidence of hot flashes. Research using 800 IU of vitamin E showed that E eased mild hot flashes.

Profile 10: Genetically Cancer-Prone

Although most women who get cancer have no family history of the disease, cancer in a first-degree relative—mother, father, sister, or brother—increases your risk. You can find extra protection in antioxidants that neutralize cancer-causing toxins and destroy cell-damaging free radicals.

Vitamin C. Take 500 milligrams daily.

Vitamin E. Take 800 IU a day of natural vitamin E, in its dry form, not the oil; the dry form is used in vitamin tablets and in breast cancer research. If you are considering taking more than 400 IU of vitamin E, talk to your doctor first. One study using low-dose supplements showed increased risk of hemorrhagic stroke.

Selenium. Take 50 to 100 micrograms a day.

Coenzyme Q_{10}. Take 100 milligrams per day. CoQ_{10} is included here because several breast cancer studies showed that the cancer regressed or even disappeared after treatment with coenzyme Q_{10}, while other studies showed lower levels of the enzyme in women with breast cancer than in those without. A study of women in France with breast cancer showed a worse outcome for those with lower levels of the enzyme than those with more. Although rare, side effects of coenzyme Q_{10} can include heartburn, nausea, and stomachache (which can be prevented by consuming the supplement with a meal) and a slight decrease in the effectiveness of the blood thinner warfarin (Coumadin).

Garlic. Take the equivalent of 1 gram of raw garlic per day. Because garlic comes in so many different preparations, check the label carefully to see that you're getting the appropriate dose. Do not use supplements if you're on anticoagulants (blood thinners) or before undergoing surgery, because garlic thins the blood and may increase bleeding. Do not use it if you're taking drugs to lower your blood sugar.

Most of these supplements are important antioxidants.

In many countries, lower levels of beta-carotene and vitamin A in the diet are associated with an increased incidence of certain cancers, including those of the breast, cervix, bladder, and colon, while higher levels correlate with reduced cancer risk.

Personalize Your Plan

Aside from your personal health status and family history, other factors, including stress, can create various nutritional demands. As with the 10 nutritional types outlined above, don't duplicate supplements recommended for more than one health problem or lifestyle factor.

Your job involves shift work. If your schedule is as haphazard as the stock market, chances are you're not sleeping well. Try 400 to 500 milligrams of valerian each day for the sleep problems. Don't use valerian with sleep-enhancing or mood-regulating medications—it may intensify their effects. It also may cause heart palpitations and nervousness in sensitive individuals. If that happens to you, discontinue use. Wacky eating schedules may throw your blood sugar out of whack; add 200 to 400 micrograms of chromium a day. Dosages above 200 micrograms should always be taken under a doctor's supervision.

You have trouble sleeping. Try kava kava (70 to 210 milligrams of kavalactones per day). Look for kava kava capsules standardized to 30 percent kavalactones. Do not take kava kava with alcohol or barbiturates. Do not take more than the recommended dosage on the package. Use caution when driving or operating equipment as this herb is a muscle relaxant. In addition, the herb is not recommended for use while pregnant. Or try the herb valerian at 400 milligrams. Higher doses of valerian don't seem to have any greater effect. Do not use valerian with sleep-enhancing or mood-regulating medications because it may intensify their effects. It may cause heart palpitations and nervousness in sensitive individuals. If such stimulant action occurs, discontinue use.

You're always tired, even though you get enough sleep. Make sure that you are not eating too much refined sugar and flour and other simple carbohydrates. But if changing your diet doesn't help and you suspect that your dips are due to hypoglycemia, consult your doctor. If she confirms the diagnosis of hypoglycemia, ask her if you might benefit from 200 to 400 micrograms of chromium a day. Dosages above 200 micrograms should always be taken under a doctor's supervision.

You're bothered by PMS. Try fish oil, primrose oil, or GLA supplements. Follow package directions for dosages. You should not take fish oil if you have a bleeding disorder or uncontrolled high blood pressure, if you take anticoagulants (blood thinners) or use aspirin regularly, or if you have an allergy to any kind of fish. Since it increases bleeding time, fish oil may possibly lead to nosebleeds and easy bruising, and may cause upset stomach in some people. GLA may cause headaches, indigestion, nausea, and softening of stools. Take it under the supervision of a knowledgeable medical doctor if you take aspirin or anticoagulants regularly, have a seizure disorder, or are taking epilepsy medication such as phenothiazines.

You're irritable. Snapping at your husband, kids, dog, boss? Try some kava kava (70 to 210 milligrams kavalactones per day) and 50 to 100 milligrams of vitamin B complex per day. Do not take kava kava with alcohol or barbiturates. Do not take more than the recommended dosage on the package. Use caution when driving or operating equipment as this herb is a muscle relaxant. It is not recommended for use while pregnant.

You're depressed. Taking a daily dose of 900 milligrams of the herb St. John's wort may help. Slowly build up to this amount by taking a 300-milligram capsule once or twice a day, then three times a day. In Germany, this herb is prescribed for depression more often than traditional antidepressants. Do not take St. John's wort if you're taking prescription antidepressants—the combined effect can be very harmful. The herb may cause photosensitivity, so avoid overexposure to direct sunlight.

You're under intense stress (over and above the normal daily hassles of life). Try 50 to 100 milligrams of a vitamin B complex a day. Because the B vitamins are essential for maintaining healthy nerves, they're recommended for psychiatric symptoms like depression, anxiety, and irritability. Also take kava kava, known for its calming effect on the nervous system.

Look for kava kava capsules standardized to 30 percent kavalactones and take 70 to 210 milligrams of kavalactones a day. Do not take kava kava with alcohol or barbiturates. Do not take more than the recommended dosage on the package. Use caution when driving or operating equipment as this herb is a muscle relaxant. It is not recommended for use while pregnant.

You smoke or live with someone who smokes. Other than the obvious—quit or try to persuade the person to quit—take 500 milligrams of vitamin C each day. Because smoking depletes your body's vitamin C levels, you need extra to protect your immune function. Also take the equivalent of 1 gram of raw garlic daily because garlic provides antioxidant protection against cancer. Check the label carefully to see that you're getting the appropriate dose. Do not use supplements if you're on anticoagulants (blood thinners) or before undergoing surgery, because garlic thins the blood and may increase bleeding. Do not use it if you're taking drugs to lower your blood sugar.

You work in a city or spend more than 30 minutes commuting by car, bus, or train. You need antioxidants like vitamin C (up to 1,000 milligrams) and vitamin E (400 IU) to detoxify your body.

You bruise easily. Take 500 milligrams of vitamin C a day. Look for supplements that contain bioflavonoids, which are thought by some alternative healers to be important for strengthening veins and capillaries.

You spend a lot of time in the sun. Up your daily vitamin C to 1,000 milligrams and take 400 IU of vitamin E daily, says Dr. Lieberman. You should also consider applying these antioxidants to your skin under sunscreen. Look for skin creams or other products that contain vitamin C or E for topical application. Vitamin C is also important for collagen and elastin—which keep wrinkles and sagging under control.

You're prone to acne or other skin problems. If your face sometimes resembles that of an adolescent, try 200 to 400 micrograms of chromium daily. (Dosages above 200 micrograms should always be taken under a doctor's supervision.) Acne seems to be related in some way to insulin. Also, try fish oil (it works like natural prednisone, decreasing inflammation that can lead to zits), and the herb milk thistle (follow package directions). You might want to talk with your doctor about taking a prescription form of beta-carotene (the precursor of vitamin A) that is called retinoic acid.

You should not take fish oil if you have a bleeding disorder or uncontrolled high blood pressure, if you take anticoagulants (blood thinners) or use aspirin regularly, or if you have an allergy to any kind of fish. Since it increases bleeding time, fish oil may possibly lead to nosebleeds and easy bruising, and may cause upset stomach in some people.

You experience frequent urinary tract infections. Cranberry juice—either in natural or supplement form—and acidophilus are excellent at preventing UTIs. Watch the sugar in your juice, though, since sugar feeds infection-causing bacteria. Make sure that your juice is made from real fruit juice and has little added sugar. You could also try artificially sweetened juice.

You frequently suffer indigestion or other stomach problems. Take acidophilus supplements (follow the directions on the package). If you're susceptible to bloating or gas from a high-fiber diet, don't be afraid to try dietary enzymes like Beano or Lactaid. If you're being treated for serious gastrointestinal problems, check with your doctor before using these digestive aids. If you are taking antibiotics, take them at least 2 hours before supplementing with acidophilus.

You are a vegetarian. The basic multi is going to meet all your needs.

You drink more than two alcoholic drinks a day. Even women who don't have full-blown alcoholism often have blood sugar problems if they drink a lot. Think about cutting back (or quitting if you can't stop at one drink). In the meantime, take 200 to 400 micrograms of chromium a day. (Dosages above 200 micrograms should always be taken under a doctor's supervision.) For a hangover, you might try six to eight capsules of primrose oil, says Dr. Lieberman.

Your hair seems to be getting thin or falling out. Ask your doctor to test you for thyroid problems. To support healthy thyroid function, take 150 to 300 micrograms of iodine every day under your doctor's supervision, and make sure that you're eating enough protein.

You are at risk for macular degeneration or cataracts. Take 400 IU a day of natural vitamin E and make sure that your daily zinc totals 30 milligrams. Also, take at least 500 milligrams of vitamin C daily. Studies show results with these nutrients in preventing or even reversing macular degeneration, the leading cause of blindness as we age.

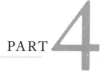

PART 4

PRINCIPLES
OF POWER EATING

Eating Habits of Women around the World

Power Maker #16: To model your eating habits after the healthiest women in the world, center your meal on side-dish foods like beans, rice, pasta, and grains, and make small portions of meat the side dish or condiment.

How's this for a great diet? For the next year, spend 2 months each in China, Japan, France, Italy, and Greece, then spend the final 2 months traveling between Greenland, Polynesia, Hawaii, and Spain. Dine on sushi and soy. Nibble olives and nuts. Wipe your plate with home-made bread and crunch on vegetables so green you can nearly hear the phytonutrients calling. Make lunch your main meal. Eaten with friends, in an open-air cafe or on a wooden table in a flower-bedecked backyard, it might last for 2 hours. Sleep afterward, waking in the cool of the late afternoon for more walking, eating, and conversation.

Back to reality: Most of us don't have the bank accounts of the jet set. But you can adopt some of the eating habits that help Japanese women stay slim, Chinese women stay fit, and women in other countries experience less heart disease and cancers than do women here in the United States.

266

Unfortunately, increasingly more women throughout the world are eating like we do—with the resulting rise in Western diseases like cancers, hypertension, and atherosclerosis.

By following the old ways, you can reverse the trend, notes K. Dun Gifford, president of Oldways Preservation and Exchange Trust, a nonprofit educational organization in Boston. The best habits in the world share certain similarities.

- Diets high in fiber and whole grains, such as rice, beans, and pastas, filled with fruits and vegetables, low in saturated fats, meats, and dairy

- Leisurely meals eaten with others

- Exercise as part of daily life

As a food provider, you can do it. Here's how.

Mediterranean: Many Regions with Much in Common

The man who first publicized the Mediterranean diet in the 1950s is in his nineties, his wife—"just a child," he calls her—is in her late eighties. And yes, Ancel Keys, Ph.D., professor emeritus of public health

THE WORLD'S TWO WORST DIETS

Scotland has one of the worst records in the Western world for coronary heart disease—a problem that is primarily diet-related. Scots are noted for their love of foods high in fat and cholesterol, especially the traditional pub fare—fried fish, meat pies, "chips" (french fries), and beef steaks. Then there's haggis, the national dish—chopped liver, heart, and lungs of a sheep mixed with beef or mutton fat, among other ingredients, and stuffed in sheep's intestine.

Here in the United States, the "mall rat" diet is no better. "Shopping mall denizens—mostly teens—go to food courts in malls and eat terrible food. They don't get any exercise at all except walking from their cars to a seat in the mall and wandering around the mall. Then they go home to watch TV and eat junk food," says K. Dun Gifford, president of Oldways Preservation and Exchange Trust in Boston.

at the University of Minnesota in Minneapolis, and his wife, Margaret, still follow the basic Mediterranean diet: heavy on the vegetables, whole grains, and olive oil, light on meat, dairy, and other fats, with a glass or two of wine during afternoon and evening meals.

Dr. Keys's first studies, showing the remarkably low rates of hospitalization for cardiac problems and the low cholesterol levels enjoyed by men on the Greek island of Crete, eventually grew into the landmark and still ongoing research project called the Seven Countries Study, comparing health conditions and nutritional habits in Greece, Italy, Japan, Finland, the Netherlands, Yugoslavia, and the United States.

Among the findings: The Greeks, a population with few healthy habits outside of eating and exercise, enjoy one of the longest life expectancies in the world, even today. Dr. Keys still remembers the day he watched one farmer leading another by the arm to the fields. Turned out the man needed help because he was blind. It also turned out that the man was 106—yet ready for a day's work under the hot Mediterranean sun.

While the men labored in the fields, the women labored in the kitchens, creating great platters of roasted vegetables, whole grain stews, and loaves of crusty bread.

"The survival of the Mediterranean diet can be attributed almost exclusively to women, who have always been responsible for cooking as well as the household economy," says Dimitrios Trichopoulos, Ph.D., a specialist in cancer prevention and epidemiology at the Harvard University School of Public Health, and a native of Greece.

The Mediterranean region is so diverse, encompassing such countries as France, Italy, Greece, Albania, and Morocco, that to say there is just one Mediterranean lifestyle is like saying there is just one flavor of ice cream. They all have one thing in common, though: olive oil. They believe it is the elixir of youth and health, and they use it generously. As a result, diets there contain nearly 40 percent fat.

They may be right about that elixir thing. Evidence from numerous studies suggests that olive oil may reduce the risk of various cancers, including endometrial and ovarian cancers; provide protection against breast cancer; increase bone density and reduce osteoporosis; and reduce the risk of developing high blood pressure, arthritis, and cataracts.

And when the benefits of the overall diet were tested among 605 men and women recovering from heart attacks, in the Lyon Diet Heart Study, those who ate the way the ancient Greeks did suffered 56 percent fewer deaths and 61 percent fewer cancer diagnoses after 4 years than those eating a typical American diet—a diet heavy in saturated fats, especially dairy fats. They were also less likely to suffer second heart attacks.

But dumping olive oil on your food doesn't make you Greek (or Italian or French or Spanish). Other aspects of the Mediterranean lifestyle may be just as responsible as the diet for residents' extraordinary good health.

Walking. From Italy to Greece, women walk. To the market, to the bus, to the fields. Often across hilly terrain. With cars and gasoline expensive and roads often narrow and winding, walking just makes sense.

Midday siesta. "After lunch, the whole town shuts down," says Gifford of southern Mediterranean regions. The nap itself is refreshing, but men and women often make love at that time, strengthening the bond that research shows is also necessary for a healthy life.

Wine. Whether its *vin ordinaire* in France, or *retsina* in Greece, wine is thought of as a food in the Mediterranean. And, indeed, numerous studies show that wine lowers the risk of coronary heart disease. Other studies suggest that it might inhibit the growth of tumors, reduce your risk of stroke, and improve your memory and age-related eye problems (provided you don't overindulge on a regular basis).

Small dinners, large lunches. Think of the tapas bars in Spain, the bistros in France. The typical Mediterranean meal pattern concentrates the bulk of calories at the midday meal.

So how can you bring the orange-blossom-scented lifestyle of the southern Mediterranean into your life? It's easy—and fun.

Serve fresh fruit for dessert. Mediterraneans eat more fruit than do Americans or people in other parts of Europe.

Dip your bread in olive oil instead of smearing it with butter. But use a good-quality olive oil, and make it a chewy, whole grain bread.

Make pasta the mainstay of your meals. But make it whole wheat pasta, with 5 grams of fiber compared to the 2 grams found in the white stuff.

Start an herb garden, whether indoors or outdoors. The scents of rosemary, lavender, and thyme are indigenous to the Mediterranean region—and these herbs are often used in the cooking. An added benefit is the exercise you'll get from weeding and planting.

Don't eat alone. In the Mediterranean, mealtime is family time. Make it the same for you by inviting friends, neighbors, and family to share a couple of meals a week. (They can share the cooking, too.)

POWER
PIZZA

SPINACH PIZZAS
WITH SUN-DRIED TOMATOES

Easy pizzas like these are a hallmark of the super-healthy Mediterranean diet. They get fiber from vegetables and chewy whole wheat pitas. The tomatoes and spinach contribute beta-carotene, lycopene, and folate. And reduced-fat ricotta and mozzarella furnish a nice helping of calcium without a lot of calories or fat.

4	whole wheat pitas
1	cup water
1	ounce dry-packed sun-dried tomatoes halves, chopped
$\frac{1}{4}$	cup tomato paste with Italian seasonings
1	box (10 ounces) chopped frozen spinach, thawed and squeezed dry
$\frac{1}{2}$	cup reduced-fat ricotta cheese
2	ounces shredded provolone cheese
2	ounces shredded reduced-fat mozzarella cheese

Preheat the oven to 400°F. Arrange the pitas on a baking sheet.

In a small saucepan, stir together the water, tomatoes, and tomato paste. Bring to a boil over medium heat. Reduce the heat to low and simmer for 5 minutes. Spread evenly over the pitas.

In a small bowl, mix the spinach and ricotta. Spoon evenly over the pitas. Sprinkle with the provolone and mozzarella.

Bake for 10 to 12 minutes, or until the cheese is melted and the pitas are slightly crisp. Let stand for 5 minutes before serving.

Makes 4

Per pizza: 279 calories, 18 g protein, 34 g carbohydrates, 8.5 g fat, 28 mg cholesterol, 3 g dietary fiber, 680 mg sodium

Take a nap. No quiet rooms at your workplace? Put your head down on your desk for 15 minutes, or go out to your car and close your eyes for 10 minutes. At the very least, you can catch 40 winks on the weekends when the kids are out playing or in their own rooms napping. Grab your significant other when you head for the bedroom.

China: Stop Before You're Stuffed

The typical Chinese woman is five times less likely to develop heart disease, diabetes, or breast cancer as we are. She also has stronger bones and lower cholesterol. And only 1.5 percent of Chinese women are overweight, compared to more than 35 percent of women in this country. Yet they eat about one-third more calories each day than we do. That said, only about 15 percent of their diet comes from fat, primarily soy oil, not cookies or crackers, says Banoo Parpia, Ph.D., senior research associate in the division of nutritional sciences at Cornell University in Ithaca, New York.

The reason is not just *what* Chinese women eat, but *how* they eat, says Dr. Parpia, who has spent the past decade on the Cornell-China-Oxford project examining the health and nutrition of women in China. From the time they're old enough to swallow a grain of rice, Chinese children are conditioned to stop eating before they feel full.

Meals in China are leisurely, Dr. Parpia says, the food savored. Not like here where we are so pressured that we tend to gobble our food. In China, you take the time to sit down and enjoy a meal, paying attention to what is being eaten, getting involved in the preparation of the meal. "It makes you more aware of what you're putting into your body, which translates to a beneficial effect on diet," she says. And it gives your brain time to signal your body that it's full, since it takes about 20 minutes for the brain to get the message that you've swallowed enough food.

Food is shared, placed on the table in big platters from which everyone takes tiny portions, placing them on mounds of rice in their bowls. So portion control is not an issue—and neither is the voice in your head demanding that you clean your plate.

Compared to women worldwide, Chinese women eat only small amounts of the fattier, richer dishes. In traditional China, rich dishes are reserved for holidays or eaten at special feasts just a few times a year.

To Eat Chinese, Think Balance

Just as there is the *yin* and *yang* of Eastern philosophy, there is the *fan* and *ts'ai* of Chinese cookery: *fan* being the rice and grains, served plain with no adornment; *ts'ai* being the flavor, a bit of meat, and some sauce. Plus lots of ginger, soy, and garlic.

"Eating plain rice three times a day can get boring, so they are wizards at spices," says Gifford.

They also eat lots of vegetables, particularly green, leafy cabbages like bok choy. That's where our Chinese sisters get their calcium because they, like most Asians, are usually lactose intolerant and rarely use dairy products. Those vegetables—coupled with the low amounts of meat in their diets—enable Chinese women to retain calcium. Add in the active lifestyles most of them lead, and you have a country where women rarely get osteoporosis and hip fractures.

Thanks to the rice, the vegetables, and the fruit, Chinese women get about 33 grams of fiber a day on average—three times as much as we do. No wonder, then, that they have so little colon cancer.

Chinese women begin menstruating at 14, compared to our typical age of 12, and enter menopause at about 48, compared to 52 here. That provides an important protection against reproductive cancers like breast and ovarian cancers, Dr. Parpia says, since early menstruation is a risk factor for these cancers.

Chinese women don't eat sweets. So when the 4:00 P.M. doldrums hit, they're reaching not for a candy bar but for a healthy handful of roasted soybeans, says Dr. Parpia.

Here's what you can do to eat more like the Chinese.

Stop eating before you're full. You can always have more later.

Challenge yourself to take the least amount of the dish you like best. Use meat as a condiment, rather than a main dish.

Try your hand at chopsticks. You'll eat more slowly.

Once a week, serve big bowls of rice. Put small plates of vegetables and other condiments in the middle of the table on a lazy Susan.

Japan: The Land of the Rising Soybean

Think about the atmosphere of a Japanese restaurant: quiet, the only sound that of trickling water, the cool air delicately scented with ginger.

Now picture the chaos that is your kitchen at dinnertime.

Japanese women—like women in many other cultures besides ours—savor their food, says Joanne Curran-Celentano, R.D., Ph.D., associate professor of nutritional sciences at the University of New Hampshire in Durham. "If you're eating in a slow, soothing environment, you tend to eat more by your appetite, more in tune to what your needs are. It makes eating part of your existence instead of just episodes."

As for what they eat, Japanese women mimic their Chinese sisters, with rice or noodles forming the basis of their meals. One exception is a higher dependence on saltwater fish and vegetables.

"They don't eat much meat, but they eat a mountain of fish, so their omega-3's are very high," says Gifford. Omega-3's are the essential fatty acids shown to have beneficial effects on heart disease, cancer, depression, and immunological problems like rheumatoid arthritis.

But for Japanese women's nearly invisible rates of breast cancer (three times lower than ours), heart disease (four times lower than ours), and strong bones—look to soy, the Japanese counterpart to olive oil.

For instance, Hiromi Yoshihara, an analyst at the Japanese consulate in New York City, says her typical Tokyo breakfast consisted of rice, soybean soup, and fermented soybeans, with maybe a few dried tuna flakes sprinkled on top. Eating that way, according to numerous studies, probably protected her against breast cancer, osteoporosis, and heart disease.

When researchers gave six women 60 grams of soy protein a day—just under one 3-ounce serving—for 1 month, they found hormonal changes that mimicked those seen with tamoxifen, an anti-estrogen drug used as a breast cancer preventive in high-risk women. In another study, introducing a component of genistein, a form of isoflavone—the plant form of estrogen found in soy—into human breast cancer cells in test tubes slowed the growth of or killed off many of the cells. Still another study suggests that it may have preventive effects on endometrial cancer as well.

When researchers at the University of Illinois at Urbana–Champaign gave women 40 grams of soy a day for 6 months, their "bad" LDL cholesterol dropped, and their "good" HDL cholesterol rose. The higher the level of isoflavones (a beneficial compound in soy), the more bone density and mineral content increased.

As for seaweed, the Japanese eat some 20 different types. Seaweed accounts for about 10 percent of food consumed in the modern Japanese diet, providing an excellent source of trace minerals. It may also provide some cancer preventive effects.

The Japanese also drink copious amounts of green tea, which provides a mother lode of antioxidants. These scavenger chemicals work like a maid-for-a-day in your bloodstream, cleaning up the free radicals that ping around your body and cause damage wherever they alight.

Thus, says Dr. Curran-Celentano, green tea is thought to be an excellent protectant against cancer, heart disease, and age-related eye diseases. When researchers considered the amount of green tea consumed by 472 Japanese breast cancer patients before their diagnoses, they found that those who drank four or more cups a day had fewer lymph node cancers and lower rates of cancer recurrence.

Take a lead from Japan.

Increase the soy in your diet. Introduce it slowly, suggests Dr. Curran-Celentano. If you eat no soy whatsoever, add one serving a day, about equal to the average Asian intake. If you already eat soy in some form, eat more. One serving equals ½ cup of tofu, 1 cup of soy milk, 3 tablespoons of roasted soybeans, or a soy protein shake or bar with 30 to 50 milligrams of isoflavones.

Substitute green tea for coffee or black tea, and add one extra cup a day.

Add seaweed to your diet. Wrap sushi rice (a kind of sticky rice) and pieces of vegetables like cucumber, pickled ginger, and carrots in store-bought nori rolls and top with soy sauce for homemade sushi. Or toss dried or fresh seaweed into salads or soups.

Create a Japanese environment at mealtime. Turn the television and radio off. Eat slowly, putting your fork or chopsticks down between each bite. Consciously try to take more than 20 minutes to finish your meal.

MASKED DISASTER

Chinese Take-Out Dishes

Next time you decide to order Chinese take-out food because you think it's healthier, consider this: According to one analysis, a standard portion of Szechuan Shrimp has 19 grams of fat—more than in two slices of pepperoni pizza. Kung Pao Chicken has a whopping 76 grams of fat per serving—more than an entire day's allotment.

To make Chinese take-out healthy, add a cup of rice and some steamed vegetables to every cup of entrée, and lift the food out of the sauce with a slotted spoon, leaving behind the calorie-laden liquid.

Choose small portions of exquisitely prepared food. The size of the portions in the United States amazes Yoshihara. "Whenever I go out with my friends, we try to share so that we don't leave too much," she says.

Latin America: Not Just Nachos

Forget the taco stand down the street or the cheese-covered burritos at the big chain in the mall. A true Latin American woman would look askance at such food for lunch or dinner. The food we think of as Latino or Mexican—those burritos, tostadas, and tacos—is considered snack food in the countries from which they ostensibly came.

Although the traditional rural Latin American woman's diet differs depending on which country she hails from—more meat in Argentina, for instance, more potatoes higher in the mountains—the basics remain the same: great portions of grains, like corn, maize, and beans, and lots of vegetables and fruits, with maybe a bit of meat or fish for seasoning.

Those patterns mimic healthful eating habits found in other countries. And the simple diets these rural women follow—coupled with the hard physical labor they perform working in the fields, walking where they need to go, and tending to their large families—renders the rates of chronic diseases like heart disease and most cancers low in most Latin American countries.

"They're not total vegans, but they're substantially vegetarians," said Jeffrey Backstrand, Ph.D., assistant professor of nutrition and food studies at New York University in New York City. He studies the diets of rural Mexicans, in particular, and says that some women get nearly 70 percent of their calories from corn. Don't try that at home—he says that's too much.

Until about 1946, those same women (or their grandmothers) spent up to 6 hours a day pounding the corn into flour for tortillas. Now machines do the grinding, freeing the women for other work—like cooking. Many prepare not three, but four meals a day for their families: a small breakfast around 5:30 A.M., maybe just a few tortillas and some beans to break the fast; then a larger, more substantial meal around 10:00 A.M. The main meal of the day is served around 2:00 P.M. and is likely to include some kind of stew made primarily of grains and vegetables with just a bit of chicken or pork for flavor, and then a small meal, really a snack of leftovers, is served around 8:00 P.M.

"I think there are lots of people who would say that this is a healthier pattern of eating than the typical American's three large meals with numerous snacks in between," says Dr. Backstrand. "I would prefer to eat that way."

In the matriarchal Latin American society, where daughters live near their mothers who live near *their* mothers, the traditions are passed down from generation to generation, and the idea of family is a central theme, says Gifford, particularly around mealtimes.

"That's the analogue: the bonding," he says. "We're going to find that more and more, social science is going to tell us that is what makes for good health. Sitting around talking and being together is good for your immune system."

You can adopt south-of-the-border eating habits at your house.

Make lunch your main meal. Just snack on fruit with a bit of cheese and bread for dinner.

Eat small portions of the food you like. Then, if you're still hungry, fill up on bread as the Mexicans fill up on tortillas.

Eschew fat-filled, cheesy "Mexican" dishes. Instead, spread fat-free refried beans on a tortilla, sprinkle with a little low-fat cheese, microwave for 1 minute, then roll it up and eat it. Even better, stuff it with a combination of diced raw tomatoes, broccoli, and cooked corn.

Use beans instead of meat. Add them to stews, mix them into eggs, or stir them into pasta sauce.

Vegetarian Diets:
Strike the Right Balance

Power Maker #17: Eat meatless meals—vegetarian chili, bean dishes, curries—at least three times a week.

Good news! You don't have to become a full-fledged vegetarian to reap the rewards of a vegetarian lifestyle. And those benefits are enormous, says Banoo Parpia, Ph.D., senior research associate in the division of nutritional sciences at Cornell University in Ithaca, New York. Women who follow low-fat, plant-based diets have a lower risk of many chronic diseases from gallstones to high blood pressure.

"Even women who eat substantially less meat but don't go completely vegetarian can get substantial health benefits," says Erica Frank, M.D., associate professor in the department of family and preventive medicine at Emory University School of Medicine in Atlanta.

Equally important, going meatless needn't consume hours of prep time. "Vegetarian cooking can be quick and convenient," says Suzanne Havala, R.D., a nutrition consultant for the Vegetarian Resource Group in Baltimore. "You can certainly eat a healthy diet and put very little time into cooking."

The Benefits of Vegging Out

About 55 percent of vegetarians are over 40, the age many women begin to take steps to protect their future health. Smart move, says Dr. Parpia—a low-fat, nutrient-dense, plant-based diet can help protect women against chronic diseases associated with aging.

A healthier heart. Compared with the average American, vegetarians are half as likely to die of heart disease. No surprise there. As a group, they consume less total fat and saturated fat and more heart-healthy phytonutrients found only in plant foods.

Vegetarian women consume between 50 and 100 percent more fiber than the average woman, much of it the cholesterol-lowering soluble kind found in oats, barley, legumes, and citrus fruits. And because they tank up on fruits, vegetables, and whole grains, vegetarians also consume from 50 to 100 percent more antioxidant nutrients such as vitamins C and E, which help keep "bad" LDL cholesterol from taking up residence in arteries. Vegetarian women also consume more phytonutrients, substances found in plant foods that research suggests stave off heart disease and other chronic diseases.

Reduced cancer risk. Studies from around the world show that vegetarians are less likely to die of cancer than are meat eaters. One British study of more than 6,000 people found an amazing difference—vegetarians were 50 percent less likely to die of cancer than people who eat meat.

Going vegetarian may even reduce your risk of breast cancer. "Women in cultures that consume a plant-based diet, such as China and Japan, have significantly lower rates of breast cancer," says Virginia Messina, R.D., coauthor of the 1998 position paper on vegetarian diets for the American Dietetic Association and author of *The Vegetarian Way*. One possible reason? Vegetarian women have lower amounts of estrogen in their blood, and high blood estrogen levels raise the risk of breast cancer. "Dietary fat tends to raise estrogen levels, while fiber decreases it," says Messina.

Lower incidence of diabetes. There's some evidence that vegetarians have a lower incidence of diabetes compared with the average American. In a study of 25,000 Seventh-Day Adventists, one of the largest groups of active vegetarians in the country, nonvegetarian women were about $1\frac{1}{2}$ times more likely to have diabetes as vegetarian women.

Less intense PMS. Again, a low-fat, high-fiber diet tends to reduce blood estrogen levels, and that can ease some women's PMS symptoms, says Neal Barnard, M.D., president of the Physicians Committee for Responsible Medicine in Washington, D.C. In a study led by Dr. Barnard, 35 women who followed a very low fat vegetarian diet for 2 months reported fewer premenstrual symptoms and less menstrual pain.

Smoother perimenopause. While lower estrogen levels seem to protect against breast cancer, women entering perimenopause may not have enough estrogen. That's where grains and legumes come in. These foods—especially foods made with soybeans, such as tofu and soy milk—contain phytoestrogens, weaker versions of the estrogens women produce naturally. These substances are believed to help balance the hormonal fluctuations

---

MASKED DISASTER

Fast-Food Baked Potatoes

The next time you dine at a fast-food restaurant, think twice about ordering a baked potato with cheese sauce and broccoli. One of these babies contains 403 calories and 21.4 grams of fat—8.5 grams of them artery-plugging saturated fat.

Your best bet is to request a naked spud and drizzle it with some mustard or fat-free salad dressing. You'll consume about 250 calories and less than 1 gram of fat.

DON'T SHORTCHANGE YOURSELF

If you avoid dairy products and eggs as well as meat, you can run low on certain nutrients, says Virginia Messina, R.D., coauthor of the 1998 position paper on vegetarian diets for the American Dietetic Association and author of *The Vegetarian Way.*

VITAMIN B$_{12}$. Our bodies need only a teensy amount of this vitamin—6 micrograms a day. The problem is that Vitamin B$_{12}$, used to make red blood cells and protect nerves, is virtually impossible to get from plant foods. The solution: supplements or fortified foods, such as breakfast cereals and fortified soy milk.

VITAMIN D. You need vitamin D to absorb calcium as well as for overall bone health. You can meet the Daily Value of 400 IU with fortified foods such as soy milk and some breakfast cereals.

CALCIUM. If you eat five to six servings of good sources of calcium a day—such as black beans, chickpeas, canned navy beans, calcium-fortified orange juice or soy milk, and tofu processed with calcium sulfate—you can generally get the recommended 1,000 milligrams a day of calcium, says Messina.

If you have any doubts that your diet is providing you with these nutrients, reach for a daily multivitamin/mineral supplement and maybe calcium supplements.

that occur at perimenopause. It's possible, although not yet scientifically proven, that regular helpings of these foods may also help women experience fewer hot flashes, night sweats, and sleep problems, says Dr. Parpia.

You Won't Miss a Thing

Despite all of this glowing research, you may still wonder if cutting back on meat will allow you to get enough of the nutrients you need, particularly calcium and iron. You bet it can. Here are common misconceptions and the facts that refute them.

Myth #1: "I won't get enough calcium." Every woman should be concerned about osteoporosis—it affects 22.4 million of us in this country alone. But you shouldn't worry that going vegetarian will cause it.

"Studies show that the bones of vegetarian women who eat dairy products and eggs (ovo-lactovegetarians) are at least as strong as those of meat eaters," says Messina.

In fact, there's evidence that their bones may be even thicker. In one study of postmenopausal women, ovo-lactovegetarians lost from 50 to 60 percent less bone mass than nonvegetarian women. One possible reason is that a diet high in animal protein contains more sulfur amino acids, substances that reduce your body's ability to absorb and hold on to calcium.

Many plant foods are good sources of calcium. One cup of turnip greens contains 197 milligrams; 1 cup of fortified soy milk, 200 to 300 milligrams; and ½ cup of tofu processed with calcium, a whopping 861 milligrams.

Myth #2: "I won't get enough iron." Vegetarian women are no more prone to iron-deficiency anemia than those who eat meat. In fact, on average, vegetarians get substantially more iron in their diets than nonvegetarians, says Havala. For example, ½ cup of tofu contains 13 milligrams of iron, a tablespoon of blackstrap molasses contains 3.5 milligrams, and ½ cup of lentils contains 3 milligrams, all of which can make a substantial contribution to the 18 milligrams of iron a day premenopausal women need.

It's true that the iron in plant foods, called nonheme iron, isn't as well absorbed by the body as the heme iron found only in meat, poultry, and fish. To get around this, eat foods rich in vitamin C at every meal, says Havala. They can boost the absorption of iron as much as twentyfold. Broccoli, tomatoes, brussels sprouts, strawberries, cantaloupe, and citrus fruits are high in vitamin C.

If you are past menopause, it may actually be better to get your iron from plant sources, says Messina. Postmenopausal women need less iron than women of childbearing age: 10 milligrams a day. Moreover, some

Waistline

In a study of 2,500 women doctors, 8 percent identified themselves as vegetarians. Their primary reason for going meatless was health.

POWER

CHILI

MEATLESS KIDNEY-BEAN CHILI

It's mostly the spices that give chili its authentic flavor. So no one will even notice the meat's gone from this fiber-filled version. The beans provide lots of filling protein and cholesterol-reducing carbohydrates. And the capsaicin in the chili powder helps prevent cancer—feel free to add as much as you want.

1   large onion, finely chopped

1   green bell pepper, finely chopped

1   small carrot, finely chopped

2   cloves garlic, finely chopped

1   tablespoon olive oil or canola oil

2   teaspoons chili powder

1   teaspoon ground cumin

1   can (15 ounces) red kidney beans, rinsed and drained

1   can (15 ounces) cannellini beans, rinsed and drained

studies have linked high blood levels of iron, particularly the heme iron in animal foods, to increased risk of heart disease, most likely because iron may encourage the production of cell-damaging free radicals.

Myth #3: "I won't get enough protein." All foods contain protein, not just meat. So even strict vegetarians (vegans), who don't eat protein-rich dairy foods and eggs, tend to get enough, says Messina. A 140-pound woman needs 56 grams of protein a day. If you eat a cup of whole grain cereal with a cup of fat-free milk and a banana, that's 17 grams of protein right there.

It's true that the protein in plants is incomplete, meaning that it lacks certain essential amino acids that your body can't produce. If you eat a wide variety of plant foods, however, the amino acids missing in one food will be provided by another.

1   can (14½ ounces) diced tomatoes (in juice)

1   can (8 ounces) tomato sauce

¼   teaspoon salt

¾   cup low-fat plain yogurt or reduced-fat sour cream

2   tablespoons chopped fresh cilantro

In a large saucepan over medium heat, cook the onion, pepper, carrot, and garlic in the oil for 10 minutes, or until the vegetables are softened. Stir in the chili powder and cumin. Cook for 2 minutes, stirring often.

Add the kidney beans, cannellini beans, tomatoes (with juice), tomato sauce, and salt. Simmer over medium-low heat, stirring often, for 45 minutes. If the mixture becomes too thick, add water as necessary.

Serve topped with a dollop of the yogurt and sprinkled with the cilantro.

Makes 6 cups

Per cup: 196 calories, 10 g protein, 33 g carbohydrates, 3.5 g fat, 2 mg cholesterol, 5 g dietary fiber, 581 mg sodium

Don't Make This Mistake

Even a vegetarian diet has pitfalls. By and large, however, shortcomings tend to result from what you do eat, not what you don't.

One potential snare is making cheese and eggs the core of your diet. There's nothing wrong with eating small amounts of these foods every so often, says Havala. But living on quiche or cheese omelettes will send your intake of calories, saturated fat, and cholesterol skyward.

"The health benefits of a vegetarian diet are due primarily to the substances in plant foods," says Messina. "A diet that contains too many dairy foods and eggs doesn't have the same benefits." To avoid this trap, eat no more than one or two eggs a week and use only small amounts of low-fat cheese to flavor foods, advises Messina.

The bottom line? Nutritionists virtually shout it from the rooftops: The key to a healthy vegetarian diet is variety. Eating a wide range of fruits, vegetables, whole grains, legumes, and other low-fat fare protects against nutritional deficiencies while helping to prevent age-related diseases.

Shop-Smart Strategies

Imagine an all-you-can-eat buffet. Now, imagine an all-you-can-eat *vegetarian* buffet. Having trouble? Most people do—and that can mean making less-than-healthy selections at the grocery store or restaurant. These tips can help you get maximum nutrition from your vegetarian menu whether you're eating in or dining out.

Color-code your veggies. Load your shopping cart with deep orange, red, and dark green vegetables, such as sweet potatoes, carrots, tomatoes, red and green bell peppers, broccoli, and kale, recommends Havala. They generally contain the most vitamins A and C, iron, and calcium.

Look for the whole. More often than not, opt for whole grains, such as whole wheat, oats, and barley, over white rice, advises Messina. Unlike white rice, whole grains retain their nutritious bran and germ layers. Further, consuming them regularly may cut your risk of chronic diseases such as cancer and heart disease. To learn more about the health benefits of whole grains as well as tasty ways to get them into your diet, see Grains: Powerhouses of Nutrition on page 62.

Snack vegetarian-style. When you're constantly on the go, as many women are, it's tempting to grab a quick bite at a convenience store or the coffee cart at work. But while chocolate cupcakes may be vegetarian, they're also loaded with calories and fat.

Bring your own snack foods from home and tuck them into your glove compartment or the office fridge. Include low-fat regular or soy yogurt, baby carrots with a container of low-fat dip or salsa, low-fat microwaveable popcorn, and whole grain pretzels. Of course, even healthy snacks aren't calorie-free, so to avoid weight gain, watch your portion sizes.

Splurge on special items. Add interest to meatless meals with exotic fruits, plump portobello mushrooms, spicy jalapeño peppers, or unusual dried beans. Give extra zing to familiar dishes with herb-infused oils and vinegars or ethnic condiments such as the spicy peanut sauce of Thailand.

BURN, BABY, BURN

Getting older has its perks, but a Speedy Gonzalez metabolism isn't one of them. Exercise is one way to raise your metabolism and burn more calories. Another is a vegetarian diet.

In a small study conducted at the University of Maryland in Baltimore, the calorie-burning power of vegetarians at rest was 11 percent higher than that of meat eaters.

The vegetarians also had higher blood levels of a hormone called norepinephrine. It may be that increased norepinephrine accelerates the metabolism, says study coauthor Eric T. Poehlman, Ph.D., now professor of medicine in the department of medicine at the University of Vermont in Burlington. But what caused the vegetarians' greater norepinephrine levels in the first place? Most likely their high-carbohydrate, low-fat diet, he says.

Dine out with confidence. Ethnic restaurants are your best bet, says Havala. The cuisines of China, India, Mexico, and the Middle East tend to be plant-based. But more and more chain restaurants and fast-food drive-thrus also offer meatless or vegetarian items. You might order a veggie burger with a side of steamed vegetables; a bowl of bean soup or meatless chili with a salad and a side of whole wheat toast; or a feta-cheese-and-spinach omelette (made with egg substitute, if you like).

Go Vegetarian Part-Time

It's possible to make quick-and-yummy vegetarian meals in the time it takes to pan-fry pork chops. The tips and tricks below can help make vegetarian cooking such a breeze that even meat eaters will turn to it often.

Devise a "cheat sheet." Make a list of your favorite vegetarian foods and post it on your refrigerator or inside the door of one of your kitchen cabinets, suggests Havala. Your list might include veggie pizza or lasagna, grilled cheese and tomato sandwiches, and bean burritos. Refer to your list when you can't figure out what to cook for lunch or dinner.

Visit your grocer's freezer. Stockpile frozen vegetarian meals for nights when you're too tired or busy to cook, suggests Havala. Somewhere among the frozen dinners you're likely to find a whole section of vegetarian foods, such as meatless hot dogs, veggie burgers, vegetarian burritos, pizzas made with whole wheat crusts, and other microwaveable fare.

Plan a feast from the East. Search out a jar of Indian curry paste (available in large supermarkets and health food stores), says Messina. This thick, pungent mixture of vegetable oil and spices such as turmeric and cumin is the base for a fast, delectable vegetable curry. Simply cook chopped onions in a tablespoon of the paste, then throw in a can of chickpeas and whatever vegetables you have on hand. Fresh or frozen spinach and diced sweet potatoes are especially good. Presto: dinner in under 30 minutes.

Take beans a step beyond. By all means, add beans to soups, stews, and casseroles. And then go beyond that with tips from Nancy Harmon Jenkins, author of *The Mediterranean Diet Cookbook: A Delicious Alternative for Lifelong Health*. Toss cannellini beans with olive oil and fresh herbs for a sumptuous side dish. Make the pasta "fazool" that Dean Martin sang about in "That's Amore": small shells or ziti with cannellini or great Northern beans, a variety of veggies and olive oil. Bake chickpeas in tomato sauce, along with onions, peppers, and olive oil. If you use canned beans, rinse them in a colander to remove the excess sodium.

Make industrial-size batches of grains. When you cook up a pot of brown rice or other whole grain, make double or even triple the amount you need, recommends Havala. Use the leftovers as a base for other meals that week, such as stir-fried vegetables, vegetarian chili, and curries. Grains keep in an airtight container in the refrigerator for up to 4 days.

Stage a weekly cookfest. Set aside a few hours 1 day a week to prepare and freeze entrées for the coming week, suggests Havala. Many women find it most convenient to cook right after grocery shopping or on Sunday afternoons. Eventually, your freezer will be bulging with ready-made meals that you can pop right into the microwave or oven.

While you're cooking, wash, peel, and slice vegetables for the coming week's salads and snacks too. To retain veggies' health-enhancing antioxidants and phytonutrients, store them in tightly sealed plastic bags or airtight containers.

Food/Mood Madness: A New Approach to Emotional Eating

Power Maker #18: For 1 week, write down how you feel every time you eat or drink anything. Then review it for clues as to when and why you seek solace in food.

Karen led a typical time-pressed life: She had two young children at home and a husband who'd sold his business, retired early, and was always underfoot. Even though they could afford it, her husband refused to hire any household help, so Karen's days were a blur of child care, meal preparation, and housekeeping.

In between, she ate. Cake and ice cream at children's birthday parties. Chips and snacks bought for the kids. Leftover dessert and mashed potatoes from dinner. It didn't take long for Karen's weight to creep up, prompting her to seek help from a weight-loss clinic.

"Why do you eat these things?" asked the nutritionist Karen consulted.

"Because I like to eat," she said.

"Why do *you* eat these things?" the nutritionist repeated.

"Because it tastes good."

The nutritionist just looked at her, waiting for the real answer.

"Because it makes me feel good," Karen finally admitted.

A GUILT-FREE GUIDE TO CHOCOLATE

It's the ultimate sin food. No other food is craved the way we crave chocolate, especially for women. Researchers don't know why, but some think it's because chocolate is made up of mainly sugar and fat. The combination seems to send those feel-good brain chemicals known as endorphins into the stratosphere.

Adding to chocolate's appeal is its unique melt-in-your-mouth texture, says Clara E. Gerhardt, Ph.D., associate professor of human development and family studies at Samford University in Birmingham, Alabama, who specializes in food issues. She remembers getting a chocolate craving while on a trip to Japan. The closest thing she could find was red sugared beans, the Japanese version of dessert. "They just didn't do it for me. That's because cultural influences strongly determine our food choices and preferences," she says. "What may be regarded as comfort food in one cultural context may not be appreciated in the same way in another culture." Our childhood experiences also play a role in this learned behavior, she adds.

So give in to chocolate with some guilt-free alternatives suggested by Elizabeth Somer, R.D., author of *Food and Mood: The Complete Guide to Eating Well and Feeling Your Best.*

- Instead of using hard chocolate in baking, try cocoa powder, which has fewer calories.
- Dip pieces of fruit into low-fat chocolate syrup.
- Eat chocolate with meals, not as a snack. You're less likely to overindulge and more likely to choose a small portion.
- Warm reduced-fat fudge in the microwave and spread it thinly on graham crackers for a snack that's low in fat.
- Buy chocolate in small quantities. Avoid the 5-pound box, the oversize candy bar, and the ½ gallon of ice cream. Instead, buy one or two Hershey's Kisses, a Tootsie Roll, or miniature candy bars.

As a child, Karen only had time to herself when she ate. If she was reading or playing, for example, her mother piled on more chores. But mealtime was sacrosanct. So Karen learned that eating equals time for herself, said Judith J. Wurtman, Ph.D., a research scientist in the department of brain and cognitive sciences at MIT in Cambridge, Massachusetts, who worked with Karen.

"If you had one wish, what would you wish for?" Dr. Wurtman asked Karen.

"An hour a day to myself," came the answer.

So Dr. Wurtman convinced Karen's husband to hire a babysitter to watch the kids for at least 2 hours a day so that his wife had time alone. Voilà! With Karen's needs met in ways other than eating, her mindless eating stopped, and she started to drop the extra pounds.

Be Your Own Food Therapist

If you're like most women, you can identify with Karen in some way. The bucket of leftover fried chicken devoured one rainy Saturday while trapped indoors with the kids. The doughnuts consumed after a frustrating meeting at the office. The oversize bag of potato chips that disappeared after the stressful phone call to your mother.

No one disputes the connection between food and mood, says Mindy Kurzer, Ph.D., associate professor of food science and nutrition at the University of Minnesota in St. Paul. "Food cravings are not 'all in your head,' and they're not trivial."

What is less clear is the cause. You eat for lots of reasons, ranging from hunger to boredom to the social settings in which you find yourself. But in recent years, researchers have zeroed in on another reason: the complex network of neurotransmitters and other chemicals in our bodies that turn our appetites on and off. When these various chemicals get out of whack, so can your eating habits.

Which begs the question: Did Karen eat because her stress resulted from out-of-balance brain chemicals, or did she eat because of ingrained feelings about food?

Probably a bit of both. "Eating habits are very complex and probably a combination of many biological, psychological, and behavioral factors," Dr. Kurzer says.

Elizabeth Somer, R.D., calls it the cascade of chemicals. All day long, we're "riding the swells of chemical surges," says Somer, author of *Food and Mood: The Complete Guide to Eating Well and Feeling Your Best*. There are 20 to 30 different hormones, neurotransmitters, enzymes, and amino acids in your body that contribute to your eating habits.

Galanin. Stimulates your desire for fats and carbohydrates.

Neuropeptide Y. Triggers carbohydrate cravings.

Endorphins. These are the same chemicals that give you that super-charged feeling after running 3 miles. Bet you didn't know that eating something sweet like chocolate produces the same feeling.

Serotonin. Of all the chemical messengers that have been studied, serotonin has received the greatest attention, primarily for its ability to improve sleep, diminish pain, and reduce appetite.

Dr. Wurtman and her husband Richard, also at MIT, have a theory about serotonin: Carbohydrates cause the pancreas to release insulin into the bloodstream. That lowers the blood levels of all amino acids except a precursor to serotonin called tryptophan, which is found in proteins like meat, eggs, and cheese. So when carbohydrate levels are low, tryptophan usually has a hard time getting into the brain because the other amino acids arrive first and block its entrance. Think of it as the body's version of rush-hour traffic.

Eating carbohydrates lowers the level of those other amino acids, clearing the freeway and letting the tryptophan zoom into the brain, where it gets to work creating more serotonin. The more serotonin you have, the better you feel. The better you feel, the less you eat.

Dr. Wurtman explores this connection in a special clinic for those with stress-induced weight problems—mainly women. In addition to learning to eat low-fat, healthy diets and incorporate exercise into their routines, they drink a high-carbohydrate liquid in the late morning and midafternoon, in essence "vaccinating" themselves against stress.

In one study, Dr. Wurtman found that compared to those who got a protein or placebo drink, the carb drinkers lost more weight.

You can help "inoculate" yourself against stress and boost your own serotonin levels by eating nearly any fat-free carbohydrate.

- Instead of a doughnut, try an English muffin with a teaspoon of jam. Stay away from cream cheese or butter, because the fat will delay the uptake of tryptophan into the brain.

- Instead of high-fat chips and crackers, choose low-fat popcorn, pretzels, or baked potato chips.

- Instead of chocolate chip cookies, reach for Fig Newtons or graham crackers.

- Try a baked potato spiced with mustard or salsa instead of butter and sour cream.

- Help yourself to a cup of fat-free yogurt, ½ cup of raisins, or a banana.

The Menstrual Mood Cycle

It's like clockwork. It's 10 days before your period, and you're craving things like chocolate, macaroni and cheese, and baked potatoes. Anything sweet, starchy, or creamy—and plentiful.

It's not in your mind. It's in your hormones.

We eat more between the time we ovulate and when our periods start. One theory blames it on increased levels of the female hormone progesterone. You know how this works if you've ever tracked your temperature while trying to get pregnant and seen it rise ½ degree just after ovulation. A higher body temperature burns more calories, impelling us to reach for more food.

Studies show that the dip in estrogen just before our periods reduces serotonin and endorphins, making us hungrier. And lowered endorphins make us reach for the sweet stuff. That's right: c-h-o-c-o-l-a-t-e.

These cravings are not much different from what you typically experience during the month; they just get stronger and more intense before your periods, says Louise Dye, Ph.D., associate professor of psychology at the University of Leeds in England.

What to do? Give in. To bump up the serotonin, eat what Somer calls anti-PMS foods.

- For breakfast, try whole grain cereal sprinkled with wheat germ in fat-free milk, a piece of whole wheat toast spread with all-fruit jam, and grapefruit juice.

- For lunch, fix yourself a chicken breast sandwich with sprouts and honey mustard on whole wheat bread, carrot-raisin-apple salad, melon balls, fat-free milk, and ice water with lemon.

- For dinner, stir-fry tofu and vegetables with safflower oil, and have them with brown rice and 1% milk.

- In the midmorning and midafternoon, snack on either a whole wheat tortilla with 1 tablespoon of low-fat peanut butter or half a whole wheat bagel with fat-free cream cheese and carrot juice.

But if it's the cravings talking and only sweet, creamy foods will do, then have them—in moderation. Start with a small piece of chocolate or a couple of Hershey's Kisses, for example. Then you'll avoid what Dr. Dye calls the what-the-hell effect, as in, "I ate one bite, I may as well eat it all."

The Lady Sings the Blues— And Reaches for Comfort Food

Research studies can feed women specific foods and then measure chemical levels in our blood. The psychological connection between what we eat and how we feel is harder to quantify—but it can't be ignored.

Say you're depressed because you had a fight with your husband. So you eat a bagel—a carbohydrate—and feel somewhat better. (After all, it's raising your serotonin level.) But your husband stormed out in a rage, your best friend's away, and there's nothing on TV. You're bored. So you whip up some fudge and eat half the pan.

Welcome to comfort food land.

It may be Mallomars or mashed potatoes, macaroni and cheese or even something weird like a can of sweetened condensed milk. We all have our food anchors, stemming from associations between what we see, hear, taste, smell, or touch, and from various experiences, says Karen Miller-Kovach, R.D., lead scientist for Weight Watchers International in Woodbury, New York.

"If, when you were a little kid and scraped your knee and it hurt, your mother gave you a chocolate chip cookie to help pacify you, that routine established a connection between the chocolate chip cookie—the anchor—and feeling better," says Miller-Kovach. Then when you're 40 and your teenage son yells that he hates you, you automatically reach for the cookie jar.

This unconscious eating may be one reason that, in scientific studies at least, overweight people tend to underreport what they eat. "They're not lying," Miller-Kovach says. "It's just that so much of the food they consume is not mindful eating."

The key then is to become aware. Even though many women find it a bother, Miller-Kovach stands by the tried-and-true food diary.

- For 1 week, write down everything you put in your mouth. Then record what you're feeling, where you are, and what you're thinking and doing.

- Do it just after you swallow—or you'll forget.

- Read it carefully, noting the patterns. It's important to do this *after* the week is over so that you can detect patterns that are not usually apparent in the heat of the eating moment, Dr. Kurzer explains.

"The key questions to ask are, 'Why was I overeating? What did it get for me?'" Miller-Kovach says. For instance, a new mother who snacks every time her baby takes a nap may be eating because it gives her a sense of indulgence, a rare feeling during the fatigue-numbed postpartum months.

To detour around comfort food land mines:

- Find nonfood things you can do to fill that same need. If it's indulgence you're after, take a bubble bath or a nap, or curl up with a stack of glossy magazines.

NO BAD FOODS

When did eating certain foods become immoral? As in, "I'll be good and order the salad instead of the fries." Or, "I was so bad last night. I ate two brownies."

Food is food. Eating it or not eating it doesn't make you a good or bad person.

Yet at least one study has shown what we all know: Chocolate addicts feel guilty when they eat their favorite food, leading the scientists to conclude that no matter how much pleasure a food provides, if you think you're eating too much, then any pleasure will be short-lived, accompanied by feelings of guilt.

"Why a woman can sit down and eat fat-free frozen yogurt and feel like it's a good food, but if she eats premium Häagen-Dazs, it's a bad food, I'll never understand," says Karen Miller-Kovach, R.D., lead scientist for Weight Watchers International in Woodbury, New York.

But this good food/bad food view of the world is a core belief. The only way to change this thinking, says Miller-Kovach, is to challenge our internal beliefs. Do you *really* believe that Ben and Jerry's will kill you and sorbet will make you live to be 100? Probably not.

Think about it: Three cups of low-fat yogurt has the same amount of fat as ½ cup of premium ice cream. So there's absolutely nothing wrong with eating what you really want. And in fact, if it's more satisfying, it's the "right" thing to do.

- Understand the feeling. Keeping a journal or doing some creative writing can be a wonderful way of understanding the emotion that sends you running for the Häagen-Dazs.
- Have ready a list of at least five alternatives to the food. If you have only one and you can't do it at that time, you'll just give up and eat.
- Wait 20 minutes. Psychologists tell us that an urge, such as a food craving, typically fades in about 20 minutes, whether or not we respond to it.

The idea is to create new anchors. It's kind of like biofeedback, only you don't need a fancy machine.

- Identify how you need to feel in order to reach your goal.
- Think about a time when you had that feeling.
- Choose an anchor—a mental picture, a word, a gesture, or an object—to associate with that feeling.

Say you feel tense every morning when you enter the office, so you make a beeline for the doughnuts. Instead, think about a time when you felt relaxed. For one woman, it was when she rocked her son. She trained herself to connect twirling her wedding ring with that memory and learned to twirl her ring whenever she entered her office.

Sound works, too.

When her husband was overseas during Desert Storm, one woman turned to food to quell her anxiety over his safety. One day, she heard the song "Over the Rainbow." It instantly brought back feelings of safety for her, a sense that everything would work out. She used that song as her anchor to draw upon the inner resources she needed to fight her fear.

Yet another woman found that her personality played havoc with her waistline. When people urged food on her, she was too shy to refuse. She needed to tap into her inner courage. She remembered that she felt especially courageous while delivering a speech when accepting an award. Now she visualizes that award whenever she needs to be more assertive about refusing food.

Most important though, says Miller-Kovach, is deciding that you really want to change. "The bottom line is that if you don't want to change something, you won't; you'll sabotage yourself."

Feed Your Inner Athlete

Power Maker #19: Make sure that you take in an easy-to-digest whole grain carbohydrate 1 to 2 hours before you exercise, a small serving of meat or other good source of protein afterward, and 5 to 12 ounces of water every 15 to 20 minutes while exercising.

Remember Santa Claus? The Easter Bunny? Prince Charming? You left those myths behind when you moved from undershirts to training bras. So what about the myths you haul around when you slip on your sports bra? Whether it's loading up on carbs, avoiding fat like poison, or taking megadoses of protein, misguided notions are common among women who work out to shape up or lose weight, who like to compete, or who exercise just for fun.

Forget supplements and fad diets. Exercise is *natural*. So you don't need to eat like a lab rat on a treadmill. To work at your full potential, reduce your risk of injury, and ensure that you still have enough energy to fulfill your other 15 roles as a woman besides recreational athlete, bust your exercise myths and follow our Power-Eating Tips.

DO YOU NEED A SPORTS DRINK, OR DON'T YOU?

Packed with carbohydrates, vitamins, sodium, and potassium, liquids known as sports drinks are supposedly quicker at restoring energy and replacing electrolytes than plain water. If you've been exercising for more than 1 hour, they can definitely help, say experts at the American Academy of Sports Medicine.

Sports drinks can also provide energy for women who typically exercise without enough fuel, says Jackie Berning, R.D., Ph.D., assistant professor at the University of Colorado in Colorado Springs and a nutrition consultant to the U.S. Olympic swimming team, the Denver Broncos, and other professional teams. A typical 12-ounce sports drink contains 125 calories. Water contains none.

Plus, you're likely to drink more—and avoid dehydration—if you like the taste. In one study, researchers evaluating 50 triathletes and runners found that they drank 25 percent more orange-flavored sports drink than plain water, diluted orange juice, or an orange-flavored, homemade sports drink.

A sports drink may in fact help improve your performance. In one study, men and women exercising in high-intensity spurts, similar to what a basketball or soccer player might encounter, maintained their high-intensity effort longer when they drank a sports drink than when they drank a similar-tasting placebo.

Myth #1

"I need to eat differently if I'm exercising."

Not if you're already eating right. You need what any woman needs—six to nine servings of fruits and vegetables a day, meals heavy on the whole grains and light on the animal protein and saturated fats, and few ooey-gooey desserts or breakfast buns.

But if you're like most women, that's not how you eat. You could probably stand to change your diet even as you're changing your level of physical activity.

"I give all these talks about exercise and nutrition to students who say, 'But you're just talking about general nutrition,'" says Jackie Berning, R.D., Ph.D., assistant professor at the University of Colorado in Colorado Springs and a nutrition consultant to the U.S. Olympic swimming team, the Denver Broncos, and other professional teams. "Guess what? That's it!

If I could just get women who are exercising to make halfway decent food choices, to watch what they eat, to make sure that most of what they eat are the right kinds of carbohydrates, they would have a diet for peak performance *and* a diet that will give them health for the rest of their lives."

Myth #2
"I need to load up on massive portions of pasta and other carbohydrates before exercising."

Eat the spaghetti because you want it, not because you think you need it before hitting the gym. While carbohydrates are important when you exercise, there's no reason that you need copious amounts before a typical workout or 30 minutes to an hour afterward.

When you exercise, your muscles burn glycogen—basically, stored carbohydrates. "It's like the bread inside your muscle cells," says Kristin Reimers, R.D., associate director of the International Center for Sports Nutrition in Omaha, Nebraska. She works with all levels of athletes, from daily walkers to powerhouse triathletes.

But do you need extra carbs? No. "Let's put it this way," says Reimers. "Inside your muscle cells, there are five loaves of bread, and when you go on a ½-hour jog, you burn up four slices. So those who exercise recreationally are fine. It's the marathon runner and triathlete who need to be continually replenishing glycogen (carbohydrate) reserves that they lose—during exercise."

POWER-EATING TIP

Forty percent of your carbohydrate calories should come from complex carbohydrates like potatoes, whole grain breads and pastas, and fruits.

"Balance your carbs," says Kristine L. Clark, R.D., Ph.D., director of sports nutrition at the Center for Sports Medicine at Pennsylvania State University in University Park. The other 60 percent of calories from carbohydrates can come from a variety of sources, like dairy and vegetables. "Athletes fail to realize that carbohydrates also occur in vegetables and dairy products, and thus they consume more starches than they need to," she says.

When to get your carbs depends on how long it's been since you've eaten. A study at Pennsylvania State University found that women who ate high-fiber breakfast cereals 45 minutes before exercising were able to cycle longer than women who just drank water or who ate low-fiber cereals.

POWER-EATING TIP

Eat some sort of whole grain, high-fiber carbohydrate at least 1 hour before you exercise.

Myth #3
"The best fat is no fat."

Wary of weight gain or heart disease, many women shun any kind of fat in their diets. This is a problem for all, including exercisers.

"Too many women are fat-phobic," says Melinda M. Manore, R.D., Ph.D., nutrition professor at Arizona State University in Tempe.

Fat is an essential nutrient for good health, vitamin absorption, brain function, and energy. "Just as many athletes overconsume carbohydrates, they underconsume fats," says Dr. Clark. In fact, the latest research shows that fat may increase your endurance and boost your immune system.

When researchers at the State University of New York (SUNY) at Buffalo had nine female soccer players eat 2.7 ounces of peanuts every day for 1 week—or 450 calories of fat—the women ran nearly 1 mile longer than when they ate their usual fare. When an extra 450 calories of carbs was substituted, there was no change.

Another team of SUNY Buffalo researchers studied trained runners and found that those who limited fat in their diets to about 17 percent compromised their immune systems by depressing the cytokines and immune cells that enhance the way the immune system works. When the level of fat was raised to 32 to 41 percent, performance improved without any jeopardy to the immune system. The results are important even for the recreational athlete, says one of the researchers, Jaya T. Venkatraman, Ph.D., associate professor of exercise and nutrition sciences in the department of physical therapy. "Generally, a low-fat diet is not recommended for when you are working out," she says. Instead, women should maintain a medium-fat diet with 25 to 30 percent of their calories coming from a mix of saturated, monounsaturated, and polyunsaturated fats.

FOOD FIXES FOR EXERCISE DROPOUTS

A lot of women give up on exercise because it leaves them feeling achy, tired, or uncomfortable in some other way, when in fact the problem may be something they're eating. For example, if you feel nauseated after exercise, the real problem could be indigestion, not overexertion. To help you sort through possible causes of problems you may experience, sports nutritionists Chris Rosenbloom, R.D., Ph.D., and Susan Kleiner, R.D., Ph.D., have created this chart. These clues can help you figure out what's really going on.

PROBLEM	POSSIBLE DIETARY CAUSE
Bloating	Beans, cabbage, broccoli, brussels sprouts, sorbitol
Constipation	Low-fiber diet, not enough water, codeine
Dehydration	Insufficient fluids, alcohol, caffeine
Fatigue	Insufficient calories, carbohydrates, iron, or fluids
Gastrointestinal bleeding	Aspirin or other anti-inflammatories
Headache	Monosodium glutamate (MSG), red wine, chocolate
Heartburn	Highly seasoned foods, eating shortly before sleep, fatty foods, alcohol
Muscle cramps	Insufficient sodium, potassium, magnesium, or chloride
Nausea	Eating too soon before exercise, antibiotics
Nervousness	Caffeine or herbal stimulants
Sleeplessness	Caffeine or herbal stimulants
Sluggishness	Consuming too much sugar or high-fat foods
Stomach cramps	Overuse of antacids or anti-inflammatory painkillers

POWER-EATING TIP

If you are eating a typical 2,000-calorie-a-day diet, you should be consuming up to 56 grams of fat—which is about 11 teaspoons—from all food sources, preferably in the form of olive or canola oil, with very little in the form of butter or shortening.

Myth #4

"I need extra protein—from meat, powders, or shakes—to build muscle."

"It's true that protein builds and repairs body tissue, which might be damaged during exercise," says Dr. Berning. You need 0.4 gram of protein per pound of body weight each day if you don't work out. For a 135-pound woman, that's 54 grams of protein—the amount found in 1 cup of yogurt, a veggie burger, ¼ cup of tuna, and 3 ounces of chicken. "Consuming more protein than the body can use will give you the most expensive urine in town."

What's more, too much protein puts strain on your kidneys as they work to get it out of your body, may interfere with calcium absorption, and makes it more difficult to get the recommended 60 percent of your calories from carbohydrates.

If they're burning more calories each day than nonexercisers, athletes do need slightly more protein—but not much more. If she's a recreational athlete, exercising to stay in shape or to have fun, that same 135-pound woman needs about another 41 grams of protein to meet the recommended 0.7 gram of protein per pound of body weight, which can be found in about ¼ pound (4.5 ounces) of chicken or about 2 cups of soybeans. A competitive athlete—training and racing 2 hours a day—needs an extra 68 grams of protein, whether she's a weight lifter or a runner.

POWER-EATING TIP

Eat some protein immediately after exercising. Based on a series of experiments using rats, researchers at the University of Illinois at Urbana–Champaign found that leucine—an essential amino acid found in all protein—helps muscle rebuild itself.

In the tests, the rats were divided into five groups based on activity levels and food (protein, carbohydrates, or both). The exercised rats fed leucine (in the form of the liquid supplement Ensure) plus sugar water right after exercising showed quicker muscle recovery than those fed just sugar water.

"No one has ever studied this recovery process," says lead researcher Donald K. Layman, Ph.D., professor of nutrition. "Usually, they talk about carbohydrates and rehydration after exercise; we think you also need protein to help the muscles recover."

An energy bar or just a few slices of lean turkey or ham equals 12 to 15 grams of protein and will provide enough post-workout power.

Myth #5

"I don't have to worry about getting extra calcium to protect my bones against osteoporosis— working out will do the job."

While weight-bearing exercise is important for strong bones, it's only going to build the bones that you are using the most, says Priscilla Clarkson, Ph.D., professor of exercise science at the University of Massachusetts at Amherst. So if you're a runner, your leg bones will be stronger. But what about your arms and back—which aren't getting such a strong workout? That's where the calcium comes in.

Athletic or not, most women don't get enough calcium. When Connie Georgiou, R.D., Ph.D., of Oregon State University in Corvallis, questioned 104 female exercisers about certain foods, nearly one-third rated macaroni and cheese as unhealthy, and more than 20 percent said that 2% milk was bad for them.

"They're overestimating the amount of fat in dairy products and underestimating their calcium needs," says Dr. Georgiou.

Calcium-poor diets can lead to stress fractures and osteoporosis and may also be a cause of muscle cramps, since calcium plays an essential role in muscle contraction.

POWER-EATING TIP

Drink a glass of low-fat milk or eat another source of dairy with every meal, aiming for about 1,000 milligrams of calcium if you're 50 years old or younger, 1,500 milligrams if you're older.

Myth #6

"I'm active, so I don't need to pay special attention to vitamins and minerals."

On the contrary, you need vitamins and minerals just as much as the next woman. Studies show that female athletes typically consume less than the recommended levels of zinc and B-complex vitamins like thiamin, riboflavin, niacin, folate, and vitamins B_6 and B_{12}, while iron deficiency is one of their most prevalent nutritional deficiencies.

And if you're dieting, chances are slim that you'll get enough vitamins from food.

B vitamins. If you want energy—and who doesn't?—you need your Bs. Even sporadic training increases your need for riboflavin.

Then there's vitamin B_6, involved in metabolizing protein. Studies show that women athletes often get less than two-thirds of the Daily Value of 2 milligrams a day. Blame the deficit on diets high in refined foods, like cookies, cakes, and white bread, or low in calories.

Because exercise stresses the metabolic pathways that use vitamin B_6, athletes and active women need one to two times the Daily Value of this vitamin.

Some of the best sources of B vitamins include chicken breast, acorn squash, watermelon, banana, tomato juice, spinach, broccoli, fortified cold cereals, and rice.

Iron. Exercise should give you more energy. If it doesn't, you may be low on iron. Iron is essential to the production of red blood cells and plays a vital role in transporting and helping the body use oxygen. It's estimated that about 16 percent of all American women are iron depleted—not bad enough to be considered anemic, but still low enough to affect physical performance.

When Cornell University researchers gave 37 iron-depleted women either an iron supplement or a placebo for 8 weeks, they found that the supplemented group increased their energetic efficiency compared with the placebo group.

POWER-EATING TIP

Just a little meat in the diet will help you absorb more of the iron found in the nonmeat portion of the meal, says Jere D. Haas, Ph.D., director of the division of nutritional sciences at Cornell University in Ithaca, New York, and an author of the study. The best sources are beef, chicken, and pork. For vegetarians, Dr. Haas says the vitamin C in orange juice enhances iron absorption from other foods.

WHAT'S SO SPECIAL ABOUT ENERGY BARS?

You notice that your exercise buddies routinely stow energy bars in their workout bags or fanny packs to chow down before, during, or after workouts. But at a dollar or more apiece, aren't energy bars an expensive way to refuel? Wouldn't a bagel or a banana do nearly as well?

Probably. Some energy bars get more than 60 percent of their calories from carbohydrates. Others supply a mix of 40 percent carbohydrate, 30 percent protein, and 30 percent fat, with 250 or more calories and 5 or more grams of fat.

A bagel, on the other hand, has 157 calories and is nearly all carbohydrate, with just 1 gram of fat. And a store-bought bagel costs about 50 cents.

The difference in performance may be negligible. In a small study, David Pearson, Ph.D., of the Ball State University Human Performance Lab in Muncie, Indiana, failed to find any performance difference between cyclists who ate bagels and those who ate energy bars for breakfast before a workout on an exercise bike.

Still, if you're the type who heads to the gym right from work without stopping for a snack, an energy bar might be what you need. Chances are it will survive the day in your gym bag better than a banana or a bagel, too.

Zinc. Think of zinc as the FedEx of the blood system. It's a zinc-containing enzyme in red blood cells—carbonic anhydrase—that helps the cells pick up carbon dioxide in the body and drop it off in the lungs for exhaling. Without it, our muscles couldn't contract and produce energy, and we'd morph into couch potatoes. Even slightly reduced levels of zinc can make you feel sluggish.

That's what Henry C. Lukaski, Ph.D., of the Agricultural Research Service Human Nutrition Research Center in Grand Forks, North Dakota, found when he studied the effects of a low-zinc diet on 12 athletic men in their twenties. For 9 weeks, they ate diets containing 3 milligrams a day of zinc versus their recommended 18 milligrams a day. Then he tested them on stationary bicycles. The result is that they used less oxygen and breathed out less carbon dioxide, reducing their overall performance 6 to 8 percent. "There's no reason these results wouldn't apply to women," he says.

The more fit you are, the more important zinc is to proper functioning, Dr. Lukaski says, because your body uses more carbonic anhydrase when you're working out than when you are resting.

Women typically don't get enough zinc because we often eat less animal-based protein than men do.

POWER-EATING TIP

Snack on some simmered oysters. Just 2 ounces of cooked oysters packs more than the 12 milligrams of zinc a day recommended for women. Other good sources of zinc include lean ground beef, sirloin steak, turkey thighs and drumsticks, and lentil soup.

Antioxidants. Imagine that you are a thigh muscle belonging to a runner. Slam! Slam! Slam! Pretty soon, you begin to feel like a punching bag getting its stuffing knocked out. Now, instead of stuffing, picture that thigh filled with rapidly multiplying free radicals, thanks to the combined effects of the physical stress and the extra oxygen that the body sucks in to power the muscles. In a highly simplified nutshell, that's why exercise increases the level of free radicals in your body, creating oxidative stress. Some free radicals do a good cleanup job, but an excess can contribute to microscopic tears and to enzymes leaking out of muscle tissues.

Animal studies suggest that exercise-induced free-radical increases may be a necessary step toward improving our performance. The increase stimulates the energy generators, or mitochondria, in muscle cells, spurring us to run farther and walk faster. But an excess of free radicals produced by exercise can also damage our muscle tissues.

Antioxidants like beta-carotene and vitamins C and E could rid your body of excess free radicals, counteracting the natural oxidative stress effect of exercise. An impressive array of antioxidant plant substances known as phytonutrients, grouped into families like the carotenoids and the flavonoids, also play a big role.

You can buy phytonutrients as supplements, but they may work better when consumed as food, says Robert Wildman, R.D., Ph.D., assistant professor of nutrition at the University of Louisiana at Lafayette. Smart food choices are the basis of the power-eating plan, supplemented with nutrients if needed on an individual basis.

POWER-EATING TIP

> Eating the "new food group" of phytonutrients—including fruit, greens, tomatoes, and dark yellow vegetables—is especially important for regular exercisers.

Myth #7

"I drink a sports drink before I work out, so I know that I'm well-hydrated."

The chance that you get enough fluid when you exercise is about as high as the chance that when you get home tonight, the house will be sparkling clean and clutter-free, dinner will be on the table, and your kids will have their homework done. It's possible, but not likely.

On average, women drink 4.7 cups of water-based liquids a day. You need a minimum of 9 if you do nothing more strenuous than point the remote control—and at least another 4 if you are doing any kind of exercise. The extra fluid replaces what you sweat out and removes the body heat that you generate during exercise. One danger of becoming dehydrated during exercise is that it takes longer for nutrients to be transported to and from your muscles. Your performance could suffer as a result.

It's really not hard. In fact, women seem to need less fluid than men do in order to stay cool when it's hot. When researchers in Nottingham, England, had 12 male and 6 female runners complete six 1-hour intensive runs, they found that even after making adjustments for body mass, the men lost twice as much fluid as the women.

The difference probably has something to do with the way the menstrual cycle affects electrolytes, electrically charged minerals such as sodium and potassium that power our muscles and hearts, says Mindy Millard-Stafford, Ph.D., associate professor at the Georgia Institute of Technology in Atlanta.

But that doesn't mean that you should leave the water bottle in the car.

POWER

MUFFINS

BLUEBERRY-YOGURT MUFFINS

Have a couple of these whole grain muffins for breakfast or a snack to help fuel your workouts—and boost your body's supply of protein, fiber, vitamin E, and vitamin C. The luscious blueberries make a special contribution: powerful antioxidants that fight the effects of aging.

1½	cups whole wheat flour
2	tablespoons toasted wheat germ
2	teaspoons baking powder
½	teaspoon salt
2	eggs or ½ cup fat-free liquid egg substitute
1	cup low-fat plain yogurt
¼	cup packed brown sugar
2	tablespoons canola oil
1½	cups fresh or frozen blueberries

Preheat the oven to 375°F. Coat a 12-cup muffin pan with cooking spray.

In a large bowl, whisk together the flour, wheat germ, baking powder, and salt.

In a small bowl, whisk together the eggs or egg substitute and yogurt. Whisk in the brown sugar and oil. Add to the flour mixture and stir just until the dry ingredients are moistened. Stir in the blueberries.

Divide the batter among the muffin cups, filling each about two-thirds full. Bake for 20 minutes, or until a toothpick inserted in the center of a muffin comes out clean. Remove to a wire rack and cool slightly.

Makes 12

Per muffin: 128 calories, 4 g protein, 20 g carbohydrates, 4 g fat, 37 mg cholesterol, 2 g dietary fiber, 171 mg sodium

Note: Store the muffins in a covered container for up to 1 day at room temperature or up to 1 month in the freezer.

Dr. Millard-Stafford thinks that one of the major causes of fatigue during prolonged exercise may be due to dehydration, because it affects proper muscle functioning and energy levels.

The simplest way to know whether you're getting enough fluids is to check your urine. If you're urinating about every 2 hours and it's light-colored or clear, you're fine. If it's dark or has a strong smell, you need more liquid.

Another way is through weight loss. Weigh yourself naked before and after exercise. Then for every pound lost, drink at least 2 cups of fluid. In hot weather, you could sweat off as many as 5 to 8 pounds of water weight.

POWER-EATING TIP

Don't wait until you're thirsty to sip, since exercising blunts your thirst receptors. Instead, drink before, during, and after exercise. You need about 1 quart of water for every 1,000 calories you expend during the day—whether it's through exercise or simply sitting on the couch. A good rule of thumb is to take in 5 to 12 ounces of fluid every 15 to 20 minutes while exercising. You'll voluntarily replace only two-thirds of sweat losses. To be safe, keep drinking—even after your thirst is quenched.

Myth #8

"Exercising will make me hungry, and I'll eat more."

"This is one possible excuse why people choose not to exercise," says Neil King, Ph.D., senior research fellow and lecturer in the school of psychology's BioPsychology Group at the University of Leeds in England. "They figure they are going to get hungry and that will counteract the exercise, so why invest the time, getting sweaty and tired five times a week, when it's just going to make them eat more? But in fact, exercise won't automatically make you eat more."

During one of numerous studies he's conducted on this topic, Dr. King brought 12 women into the lab on 4 separate days. Each day, they ate normal breakfasts then either rested or bicycled for 50 minutes. Later, they ate either high-fat or low-fat lunches, and researchers monitored their hunger and how much they ate for the rest of the day.

Regardless of whether they exercised or rested, the women ate about the same amount. But because the high-fat meal was more energy-dense, it more than replaced the number of calories they'd spent exercising, resulting in a net calorie gain.

The moral of the study? "You can't just exercise and then eat high-fat foods and lose weight," Dr. King says. So much for the idea that a quick jog before dinner gives you license to peruse the dessert tray. Yet women persist in thinking that it does, he says. So while we may not actually be hungry, we're so convinced that we burned a large number of calories by exercising and are now entitled to eat more, that we do eat more. Dr. King says that this misconception of exercise relative to food is peculiar to women.

"They think they've burned up lots and lots of calories, but in truth, a single round of exercise doesn't actually burn a lot of energy," he says.

Regardless, it suggests that exercising may contribute more to weight loss than previously thought—not only does it help us burn calories, but it makes good-for-you food taste better, encouraging us to stick to our healthy eating plan.

Pregnancy:
What to Eat, When

From the moment that two pink lines appear on the home pregnancy test, the questions begin. Will it be a boy or a girl? With blue eyes or brown? Your mother's nose and your husband's ears?

You pray nightly for a healthy child. You don't smoke, you walk more often, and you eschew the daily glass of wine.

But what about your diet?

"What you eat during pregnancy may be more important than you ever thought," says Mary Lake Polan, M.D., Ph.D., professor and chairman of the department of gynecology and obstetrics at Stanford University School of Medicine.

Science is discovering that a growing baby retains a memory of life in the womb. The hardwiring of our cells and metabolic, endocrine, and immune systems determines our susceptibility to disease later in life, says David J. Barker, M.D., Ph.D., director of the Medical Research Council (MRC) Environmental Epidemiology Unit at Southampton General Hospital in the United Kingdom.

309

Dr. Barker is the father of a growing body of research linking a fetus's environment and certain birth characteristics, including weight, height, head circumference, and placenta size, to long-term health.

In fetal life, says Dr. Barker, the tissues and organs of the body undergo critical periods of development, which may coincide with rapid cell division. Missing out on key nutrients at these times can set the stage for problems later in life.

Obesity. Trying to avoid weight gain during pregnancy can backfire, prompting your baby to gain too much weight as an adult. Scientists in the Netherlands and United Kingdom studied the daughters of women who conceived during the Dutch famine, a 5-month period at the end of World War II when average calorie consumption often dropped below 1,000 a day. Contrary to what you might expect, 50 years later, the daughters of mothers who had experienced famine early in their pregnancies had higher body weights and body mass indexes (BMI) and larger waists than women whose mothers either hadn't been exposed to the famine at all, or who were affected later in their pregnancies.

It may be that the very young fetus senses metabolic or endocrine changes in the mother's body caused by undernutrition, and adapts accordingly, says lead researcher Jan van der Meulen, M.D., Ph.D., an epidemiologist at the MRC. (It's not certain why male babies in the study didn't react the same way.) So what you eat during pregnancy will affect your offspring as adults, says Dr. van der Meulen.

Diabetes. Skimping on food during pregnancy can also contribute to a baby's risk of diabetes later in life. A comparison of birth weights and later-life diabetes in 69,526 women tracked as part of the ongoing Nurses' Health Study at Harvard found that the smaller the women were as newborns, the greater their risk of developing type 2 diabetes. Other studies also relate development of type 2 diabetes to the thinness of the baby. One theory suggests that malnutrition during certain stages of pregnancy might reduce the ultimate number of insulin-producing pancreatic cells and their effectiveness.

Another reason, suggests Dr. Barker, is that early nutritional deficiencies program the fetus's cells to use energy, or glucose, abnormally, setting the stage for later problems with diabetes.

High blood pressure and heart disease. Low birth weight also seems to predispose women and men to hypertension later in life. In another Harvard study, women who weighed less than 5 pounds at birth are more likely to have high blood pressure as adults than women who weighed between 7 and 8.5 pounds at birth. They also have a greater risk of developing heart disease and of having a stroke.

One theory suggests that stunted kidneys may affect the organs' ability to regulate blood pressure, while a stunted liver, whether too small or simply missing some vital cells, may affect that organ's ability to regulate cholesterol metabolism and blood clotting, which are both factors associated with heart disease. Another possible cause is that changes in fetal bloodflow or hormonal variations in the mother may result in abnormal blood vessels, leading to hypertension as the infant ages.

Breast cancer. At the opposite extreme, a Harvard epidemiological study suggests that baby girls born at the higher end of birth weight—nearly 9 pounds—were twice as likely to develop breast cancer in adulthood as those who weighed less than 5½ pounds. The researchers theorize that the connection may have to do with increased levels of estrogen passing into the fetus before birth.

The message, then, for future moms is simple, says Madeleine Sigman-Grant, R.D., Ph.D., professor of maternal-child health at the University of Nevada Cooperative Extension in Las Vegas. If you're planning a pregnancy, don't crash-diet. To give your baby every health advantage later in life, start eating right before conception.

"You want your uterus to be in as good health as possible," she says. Also, the damage to the women's babies during the Dutch famine apparently occurred as early as 3 weeks after conception—before most women even know that they're pregnant. Animal studies suggest that the fetal growth pattern may be set around day 5 after conception—after which the mechanisms for growth are hardwired into the cells. But when that occurs in humans is as yet unknown, according to Dr. Barker.

What's the Right Pregnancy Weight for You?

Many women, used to lifelong dieting and weight worries, may find it painful to watch the scale inch up like a slow, relentless tide. One survey found that nearly 40 percent of first-time mothers worry that they'll gain too much weight while pregnant, and 72 percent fear that they'll be unable to return to their former weights.

Some are so panicked about weight gain that they make a conscious effort to watch their weight, even admitting to researchers in one study

WHERE DOES ALL THAT WEIGHT COME FROM?

Why do you gain 25 to 35 pounds when you are pregnant, when the baby only weighs 7½ to 8½ pounds, on average? Here's how it breaks down.

Baby	7.5–8.5 lb
Fat and protein stores	7.5 lb
Extra blood in circulation	4 lb
Uterus	2 lb
Amniotic fluid (surrounding the fetus)	1.8 lb
Placenta and umbilical cord	1.5 lb
Breasts	1 lb
Other fluid	2.7 lb
Total	**28–29 lb**

that they chose cigarette smoking and induced vomiting to control their weight.

"That's appalling," says Eileen Behan, R.D., a nutritionist in New Hampshire and author of *The Pregnancy Diet*.

Doctors recommend that you gain anywhere between 25 and 35 pounds during pregnancy. Keep in mind that the weight you gain during pregnancy is temporary: You'll lose most of it at delivery. Most women who gain the recommended amounts during pregnancy retain only 2 to 3 pounds 6 to 12 months after the delivery, she says. If you don't, it probably has more to do with lifestyle than childbirth.

"New moms often don't get enough exercise, and they're apt to eat more if they're staying home with the baby, so they gain weight," Behan says. In fact, women who returned to work 2 weeks after delivery were only 1 pound above their prepregnancy weight by 6 months postpartum, compared to women who didn't return to work and weighed 5 pounds more than their prepregnancy weight.

To figure out how much weight you should gain during pregnancy, start by figuring out your body mass index, or BMI. Calculate your height in inches and multiply the number by itself. Divide your weight by that height figure, then multiply by 705. If you're 5 feet 8 inches tall and weigh

150 pounds, for instance, your BMI before pregnancy should be about 23. You should gain about 30 pounds during your pregnancy. If your BMI is higher before pregnancy—closer to 29, for instance—you probably need to gain 25 pounds.

Most of that weight will come on as the baby and its baggage—placenta, umbilical cord, and amniotic fluid—grow.

Eat for Two—But No More

Overeating during pregnancy is no better than undereating, says Dr. Barker. Women who are overweight also have altered metabolisms, he says, including high circulating levels of glucose, which places the baby in an unbalanced nutritional environment. "So there are reasons for avoiding being overweight that go beyond the health of the mother."

All you need to do is put away another 300 calories. So don't eat as if every day is Thanksgiving. Just add a peanut butter sandwich on whole wheat bread, or yogurt sprinkled with granola, or other nutrient-packed foods each day.

"The fetus requires a balance of nutrients because in order to grow, you can't just give protein to a baby," says Dr. Barker. "To grow, it has to have other nutrients in order to handle the protein."

"Eat 'real food'—that is, food that's not heavily processed," says Behan.

Must-Have Foods

The basic pregnancy diet looks like this, says Behan.

• Two to four servings of whole fruit and one serving of fruit juice every day

• Two to four servings of vegetables daily

• Seven to 11 servings of bread or other starch daily (preferably whole grain)

• Two to three servings of protein-rich foods (preferably fish, lean meats, or poultry)

• Three to four servings of calcium-rich foods, like dairy products or tofu

It's not much different from what you should be eating every day. What may change is how and when you eat.

Small, frequent meals are best, says Dr. Polan. Early in pregnancy they help minimize nausea; later, they are important for maintaining normal blood sugar levels and for getting any food in you at all when the baby is growing and taking up more and more room. It's how you'll be counseled to eat if you develop gestational diabetes during your pregnancy, she says, "But it happens to be a healthy eating practice for all pregnant women."

And don't worry about any kind of strict schedule, Behan says. "Let your appetite guide you."

But if it's guiding you down the road toward cheese-covered fries and Buffalo wings, hang a left. "A double cheeseburger and fries on occasion aren't going to do any harm," says Dr. Polan, although a high-fat diet is going to lead to more weight gain and make it harder to lose the weight after the baby comes. "I urge women not to feel guilty when they have had a french fry or a piece of chocolate."

You need to find healthy foods that taste good, counsels Dr. Sigman-Grant —a challenge during pregnancy when, for some reason, certain foods interest you about as much as donning a string bikini in your ninth month.

For instance, Dr. Sigman-Grant couldn't stomach red meat during the early months of her pregnancy, although she ate so much fish that she swore that her son would be born "with a can of tuna in his hand." Yet another woman we know craved hamburgers morning, noon, and night, while the mere thought of seafood—previously her favorite food—was enough to send her searching for the porcelain throne.

Too bad for her, since seafood, particularly fatty fish, may be about the best thing you can eat for your developing baby.

Fish for the Small Fry

"We encourage at least one serving of fish a week, and two to three are even better," says Dr. Sigman-Grant. "Tuna is fine—it doesn't have to be expensive fresh fish. If you can tolerate them, salmon, mackerel, anchovies, and sardines also fill the bill."

A growing body of evidence suggests that eating fatty fish rich in the omega-3 fatty acid docosahexaenoic acid (DHA) leads to more normal growth of the baby and may even reduce the risk of cerebral palsy, a brain disorder sometimes occurring in premature infants. One theory is that the omega-3 fatty acids may facilitate bloodflow—and thus, nutrients—

to the placenta and may discourage the production of hormones that help initiate labor, so delivery doesn't occur too soon.

The most important time to get your fish—or fish-oil supplements, if you simply can't stomach seafood—is during your third trimester and after the baby is born if you are nursing. That is the time of greatest brain growth, with the DHA in the baby's brain increasing three to five times during the last trimester and tripling during the first 3 months of life.

DHA levels in American women's breast milk, however, are among the lowest in the world, primarily because we don't eat enough fresh fish and are consuming less meat and fewer eggs—all sources of DHA.

Vitamins and Minerals for Your Youngster-in-the-Works

Many women get less than the recommended amounts of several micronutrients critical for a healthy baby, including folate, zinc, iron, and calcium. So if there is even the slightest chance that you might become pregnant, start taking a daily multivitamin, says Matthew Gillman, M.D.,

IS DRINKING COFFEE SAFE?

If you're one of those women who needs her morning cup of coffee to get going, you don't necessarily have to give it up entirely if you become pregnant, says Mary Lake Polan, M.D., Ph.D., professor and chairman of the department of gynecology and obstetrics at Stanford University School of Medicine. The key is moderation.

A study by researchers at the National Institute of Child Health and Human Development in Bethesda, Maryland, found that unusually high levels of caffeine—the equivalent of six cups of coffee per day, primarily in the second trimester—contributes to a higher risk of miscarriage. "But one or two cups of coffee a day shouldn't worry people," says Dr. Polan. That's good news, since three out of four pregnant women consume caffeinated beverages (it's still a good idea to discuss caffeine intake during pregnancy with your doctor).

associate professor of ambulatory care and prevention at Harvard Medical School and Harvard Pilgrim Health Care.

Of these, folate (the naturally occurring form of folic acid) is by far the most critical. Numerous studies show that women who get 400 micrograms a day of this B vitamin before conception and at least throughout their first trimester slash their odds of delivering a baby with neural tube defects like spina bifida by half.

Start early, says Dr. Sigman-Grant. The neural tube—which runs through the center of the spinal cord—is formed in the first 3 weeks after conception, before many women even know they're pregnant.

Other research suggests that women who have a deficiency of the enzyme that metabolizes folate have more than double the normal risk of having a baby born with Down syndrome. More study is needed to determine whether folate supplementation may also help prevent this birth defect.

POWER-EATING TIP

Folate is widely available in green vegetables like asparagus, spinach, and broccoli, as well as in legumes, including pinto beans and lentils. Still, few women get what they need from diet alone, so all refined wheat products are now fortified with folate. To be on the safe side, start with supplements before you start trying to get pregnant. Look for vitamins with the words *folic acid* on the label.

Multivitamin/mineral supplements. The benefits of vitamins don't stop with folate. One study showed that women who used prenatal supplements starting in the first trimester reduced their risk of premature delivery twofold and their risk of very early preterm labor fourfold compared to women who didn't take vitamins at all. Even starting in the second trimester cut the risk of premature delivery in half. The vitamins also sharply reduced the women's risk of having low-birth-weight babies.

And there is growing evidence that multivitamins may prevent other birth defects, including urinary tract and limb defects and, possibly, cleft lip and palate, as well as hydrocephaly (water on the brain) and pyloric stenosis, a narrowing of the outlet from the stomach to the small intestine that requires surgery.

Here are some other nutrients experts recommend that you look for in a prenatal supplement, whether it's one your doctor prescribes or simply a multivitamin you buy over the counter.

Iron. Normally, you need about 18 milligrams of iron a day. You have twice the blood volume when you're pregnant, so it stands to reason that you need almost twice the iron. Some women become anemic during pregnancy because they just can't keep up with their body's demands for this mineral, increasing the chance that they'll deliver smaller, shorter babies.

It's nearly impossible for a pregnant woman to get the 30 milligrams a day she needs from food sources alone. The typical American diet carries 6 to 7 milligrams of iron for every 1,000 calories. So even if you're eating 2,500 calories—about right for a pregnant woman—you'd still only be getting 15 to 18 milligrams.

One study conducted at the University of California, Berkeley, suggests beginning iron supplementation even before conception and continuing through breastfeeding to maintain your body's stores.

The best food sources of iron are red meats, including beef, lamb, and pork; eggs; dark green vegetables (especially green beans and broccoli); and fortified cereals. You can also add iron to your diet by eating cooked clams, potatoes, and tomato juice. Eat a source of vitamin C with every meal to enhance iron absorption.

Zinc. If your doctor has recommended taking more than 30 milligrams of supplemental iron, ask her about zinc supplements. High iron supplementation may interfere with your body's absorption of zinc, necessary for the fundamental process of cell division (which is kind of crucial when you're growing a baby!). Low levels during pregnancy may be associated with preeclampsia (a form of high blood pressure that sometimes occurs in the second half of pregnancy), prolonged labor, excessive bleeding, and impaired growth of the baby.

POWER-EATING TIP

Zinc is highest in protein-rich foods, so turn to meat, fish, poultry, whole grains, and legumes to maintain healthy levels. Whole wheat pita wedges spread with hummus, a zesty chickpea spread, are a good source of zinc.

TACKLE MORNING (OR ALL-DAY) SICKNESS

It's ironic: When you need extra food the most, it appeals to you the least. To call the queasiness that affects many women during the first 3 months morning sickness is misleading: It can occur any time of the day or night.

"We don't know exactly why women get sick at this inopportune time, but it's definitely hormonal," says Madeleine Sigman-Grant, R.D., Ph.D., professor of maternal-child health at the University of Nevada Cooperative Extension in Las Vegas. The main hormones believed to be at fault are estrogen and progesterone, but hormones in the gastrointestinal tract are probably also to blame.

When you're feeling nauseated all day, though, you usually don't care about the mechanisms at work. You just want it to stop. Here are some suggestions.

NEVER LET YOUR STOMACH GET EMPTY. Keep crackers on the bedside table. Eat a few before you even lift your head from the pillow in the morning, says Dr. Sigman-Grant.

ALTERNATE LIQUIDS AND SOLID FOOD. Better to do that than to mix them at meals. "It seems to calm things down a lot," says Dr. Sigman-Grant.

SIP ON GINGER. Whether in flat ginger ale or ginger tea, the tuber may help settle queasy stomachs. In one study, 27 women received 250 milligrams of ginger in capsule form four times a day for 4 days, while others received a placebo. Those getting the ginger found that both their vomiting and nausea were reduced.

MUNCH ON WATERMELON. It's a solid liquid so it will fill your stomach and give you some much-needed fluids, says Miriam Erick, R.D., senior perinatal nutritionist at Brigham and Women's Hospital in Boston and author of *Take Two Crackers and Call Me in the Morning: A Real-Life Guide for Surviving Morning Sickness.*

ASK YOUR DOCTOR ABOUT VITAMIN B_6. Taking 25 milligrams three times a day may relieve symptoms for some women, according to the results of one study. Fifty-nine women received 25 milligrams of B_6 three times a day. Compared to the control group and to women with only mild to moderate nausea, they found significant improvement among those women with severe nausea.

Choline. If you want a smart baby—and who doesn't?—make sure you get enough choline. Researchers at the University of North Carolina–Chapel Hill (UNC) fed pregnant rats diets low in choline, an essential nutrient sometimes treated as a B vitamin. We use choline to make the nerve messenger chemical known as acetylcholine—which helps transfer signals between nerves—and to make cell membranes.

The researchers already knew that pregnant rats offered extra choline during days 12 to 18 of their 21-day pregnancies had babies that performed much better on memory tests for the rest of their lives—even when they lived to be very old.

What, they wondered, would happen if they limited the choline? The result was that the brains of the unborn rat pups showed changes in the hippocampus and septum, the memory centers. Basically, cells didn't divide or migrate the way they should, and many died prematurely.

The research may have implications for human development, says lead researcher Steven H. Zeisel, M.D., Ph.D., professor and chairperson of UNC's department of nutrition. In humans, the memory area of the brain develops from around 30 weeks to just after birth.

Pregnancy and nursing make female rats—and, presumably, women—especially susceptible to choline deficiency, he says.

POWER-EATING TIP

Your body's choline requirements change only slightly during pregnancy. Instead of 425 milligrams, you should try to get 450 milligrams of this nutrient each day. Aside from multivitamin supplements, the best sources of choline are milk, eggs, and peanuts. Keep hard-boiled eggs in a bowl in the refrigerator and reach for one as a daily between-meal snack for a source of choline, iron, protein, and other nutrients.

Vitamin D. During pregnancy and breastfeeding, you should be getting at least 200 IU (5 micrograms) of vitamin D each day. In a Chicago study of five vitamin D–deficient infants, at least two of the deficiencies were caused by low vitamin D levels during pregnancy. Health problems ranged from seizures to rickets to growth failure.

Power-EATING TIP

The best food sources of vitamin D are salmon, sardines, egg yolks, and fortified dairy foods. Also, try a morning and late afternoon walk to increase your exposure to sunlight, one of the primary sources of vitamin D. For most people, exposing the face, arms, and hands to the sun for 10 to 15 minutes a few times a week is sufficient to maintain adequate vitamin D levels.

Magnesium. An estimated 30 percent of pregnant women have problems with leg cramps. And if you've ever seen a 9-months-pregnant woman trying to hobble around on a cramped leg, you know it's not a pretty sight.

But foods and supplements containing magnesium may prevent leg cramps. Researchers from two hospitals in Sweden conducted a double-blind, randomized trial in which 73 women with pregnancy-related leg cramps received magnesium or a placebo daily for 3 weeks. The supplements significantly decreased the severity of the leg cramps with few side effects and no overall increase of blood magnesium levels.

Taking prenatal magnesium may also reduce the risk for cerebral palsy and mental retardation if you are at risk for a low-birth-weight or premature baby. Pregnant women over the age of 19 should consume 350 to 360 milligrams of magnesium. It may also reduce the chance of your having a too-small baby or developing preeclampsia.

Food sources of magnesium include tofu, nuts, seeds, cooked beans, whole grains, seafood, spinach, beet greens, and broccoli. Sprinkle sunflower seeds on top of a seafood stir-fry over brown rice.

Calcium. An Argentinian study showed that children of mothers who took calcium supplements during pregnancy were still reaping the benefits 7 years later with lower blood pressure—especially among overweight children—than those whose mothers didn't take supplements. Other research suggests that taking calcium may decrease your risk of developing preeclampsia. Pregnant women need 1,000 milligrams of calcium every day.

POWER - EATING TIP

Excellent food sources of calcium include all dairy foods, fish with edible bones like canned salmon and sardines, and tofu processed with calcium sulfate. Other sources include broccoli, bok choy, almonds, and molasses. If you are lactose intolerant and usually avoid dairy products, try low-lactose calcium-rich foods such as lactose-free milk and cottage cheese. Yogurt and aged cheeses are often well-tolerated by people with lactose intolerance.

A Diet for New Moms

Once you've given birth, don't be in a rush to get back to your prepregnancy weight, especially if you're breastfeeding.

"It took you 9 months to gain the weight; it's not going to come off in 9 days or even 9 weeks," says Dr. Sigman-Grant.

Losing your weight too quickly if you're breastfeeding could expose the baby to increased environmental toxins that are typically stored in your fat cells, she says. Also, if you're breastfeeding, you need an extra 500 calories a day to keep the milk machine flowing. Even if you're not nursing, you still need a healthy diet to keep up your energy. Dr. Sigman-Grant is surprised by the numbers of women she sees who simply aren't hungry for the first couple of weeks postpartum. "Women will ease into parenthood a lot better if they nourish themselves," she says. "They need that nutrition, even if they have to force themselves to eat. They're repairing their bodies; they may have lost a lot of blood during labor; and to deprive yourself of nutrients while you're also deprived of sleep after a physical strain will really make your life harder."

Dr. Sigman-Grant recommends the following daily plan for new moms.

- Three cups of 1% or fat-free milk (4 cups if nursing)

- Five pieces of fruit or servings of vegetables

- Six servings of whole grain bread, cereal, or pasta

- One or two 3-ounce servings of meat, fish, or poultry

- At least 64 ounces of water—what you'll get in eight 8-ounce glasses; nine is even better

OUT-OF-BOUNDS FOODS

If you're pregnant, handle food with extra care: Pregnancy weakens your immune system, leaving you more susceptible to food-borne illnesses from harmful bacteria like listeria and salmonella.

The bacteria called *Listeria monocytogenes* doesn't always cause symptoms, but some people experience flulike fever and chills or upset stomach. During pregnancy, it can cause meningitis in both the mother and the fetus or cause miscarriage.

Refrigeration isn't enough to kill listeria—you have to cook foods thoroughly or avoid foods associated with listeria altogether. To protect yourself, avoid:

- Soft cheese, such as feta, Brie, and blue-veined varieties (cream cheese and cottage cheese are okay)
- Hot dogs, cold cuts, and other ready-to-eat meats and poultry products directly from the package; cook them until steaming before eating
- Sushi, oysters, and other raw seafood (also because of other seafood-borne illnesses like cholera and hepatitis)
- Undercooked ground beef (like rare burgers) or undercooked eggs (like poached eggs, Caesar salad, or Hollandaise sauce)
- Raw, unpasteurized milk or cheeses and any meals made with them
- Ready-to-eat deli salads, including coleslaw

Power Tips for Breastfeeding Moms

Studies show that breastfeeding your child pays big benefits: It enhances your baby's current and future immune system, reduces the risk of developing allergies, and improves intelligence. One study even showed lower rates of leukemia in children of nursing moms.

Don't view breastfeeding as a weight-loss plan, though. While one study showed greater weight loss for breastfeeding moms 6 months after delivery, by 12 months there was no difference between nursing and bottle-feeding moms. The studies also show, however, that mothers who breastfeed can lose weight without dieting, while those who bottle-feed have to eat less and exercise more to take off those extra pounds.

Shoot for 2,700 quality calories a day. More nutrients are transferred to the infant via the mother's milk in 6 months of breastfeeding than in 9 months of pregnancy, says Mary Frances Picciano, Ph.D., professor of nutrition at Pennsylvania State University in University Park. Yet when she and her colleagues examined the diets of lactating women, the researchers found that, left to their own devices, nursing mothers often failed to meet dietary recommendations.

As with pregnancy, the nutrients most important to breastfeeding moms are calcium, zinc, magnesium, vitamin B_6, and folate.

Continue with your multivitamin. Dr. Picciano also found that the 52 lactating women enrolled in her study were not getting enough zinc, vitamins D or E, calcium, or folate in their diets.

"Breastfeeding is a nutritionally demanding time, which I don't think is appreciated," she said, "and as much effort as women put into diet planning during their pregnancy has to be continued during lactation."

Keep drinking plenty of liquids. Some nursing women are taught that they should increase their intake of beverages and never sit down to nurse without a glass of water at hand. Good advice? Maybe, but studies have yet to prove that women require additional fluid to meet the physiological demands of breastfeeding. Nevertheless, breastfeeding isn't the time to allow yourself to fall short on fluids. Nursing moms should make a special effort to maintain adequate water intake, says Dr. Picciano.

Dine Out
without Filling Out

Power Maker #21: Think of restaurant menus as made-to-order rather than off-the-rack. Then "build" meals that fit your unique calorie and nutrition needs.

Dining out is no longer a special event. If you're like the average woman, you eat out about four times a week, mostly lunch. And even when you eat in, often it's take-out fare that graces the table.

Our fast-paced lifestyles have fueled our demand for both comfort and convenience—and eating out delivers both, says Georgia Chavent, R.D., assistant professor in the dietetics program at the University of New Haven in Connecticut. The problem is, dining out can also mean filling out. Researchers at the University of Memphis found that women who either ate in restaurants or bought take-out food at least six times a week consumed 288 more calories and 19 more grams of fat a day than those who ate out five times a week or less. That easily translates to 25 extra pounds a year! Scary, but hardly surprising.

When you step into a restaurant, you enter the fat zone, a seductive netherworld of jalapeño poppers, baby back ribs, and creamy, cheesy, oily sauces. Further, restaurant portion sizes are

324

mammoth, an obvious fact to those of us who routinely undo the top button of our jeans once we climb back into our car.

But take heart. When it comes to dining out, there are plenty of ways to keep fun on the menu without padding your waistline.

"If you put certain skills and strategies into action, it's possible to eat healthfully—and enjoyably—in 99 percent of restaurants," says Hope Warshaw, R.D., a nutrition consultant in Washington, D.C., and author of *The Restaurant Companion: A Healthier Guide to Eating Out* and *The Guide to Healthy Restaurant Eating*.

Your Eating-Out Action Plan

These skills share one common theme: Master the menu. The power strategies below can help you make healthier choices in any eatery, from fast-food places to five-star restaurants.

Skill #1: Practice portion control. We're suckers for all-you-can-eat buffets, 50-item salad bars, and entrées preceded by words like jumbo, grande, supreme, king-size, and feast. To control portion sizes from the get-go, you need only three magic words: "Wrap it up."

"Even the finest restaurants are happy to wrap leftovers," says Penny Pollack, dining editor of *Chicago* magazine. "There's nothing low-class or embarrassing about it. And if you know you can eat the rest of the meal tomorrow, you'll be more likely to stop eating when you're full tonight."

Waistline

In 1970, we spent 26 percent of our food dollars on dining out. By 1996, the number climbed to 39 percent.

- On an average day in 1998, 21 percent of U.S. households used some form of takeout or delivery.
- Almost 50 billion meals are eaten in restaurants and school and work cafeterias each year.
- The average annual household expenditure for food away from home in 1997 was $1,921, or $768 per person.

Ask if you can order half-, lunch-, or appetizer-size portions, or make a meal of appetizers or side dishes. Mix and match dinner salads, broth-based soups (like vegetable, beef vegetable, or chicken noodle), or appetizer portions of pasta, for instance. If you're a regular at several different restaurants, scrutinize the menus at each and choose three nutritious, low-fat, low-calorie dishes. Order these healthy choices automatically, without even opening the menu. When you get bored, select another few healthy items and rotate among your favorites.

Skill #2: Speak up—nicely. "Making special requests is essential to get foods as you want them," says Warshaw. And chefs are usually glad to oblige. A survey by the National Restaurant Association found that more than 9 out of 10 restaurants would, upon request, serve sauce or salad dressing on the side, prepare foods with vegetable oil instead of butter, and broil or bake an entrée rather than fry it.

Generally, customers make these basic types of requests: asking the chef to omit high-fat, high-calorie ingredients such as cheese, bacon, and sour cream; requesting the substitution of one side dish for another (like steamed veggies or a salad instead of french fries); and asking that a dish be prepared with less fat (cut back on the butter or oil; hold the mayo or cheese). Of course, restaurants that prepare food ahead of time can't always accommodate special requests, which is why it's smart to frequent eateries that prepare food to order.

Skill #3: Learn to say "fat" in five languages. French fries, Buffalo wings, and bacon cheeseburgers are fat bombs. But the word "fat" comes in other guises as well: "chimichanga" at Mexican restaurants, "carbonara" at Italian eateries, "crispy" at Chinese places, and "tempura" at Japanese restaurants. Wherever you dine, remember that items baked, broiled, grilled, poached, roasted, or steamed are typically lower in fat and calories.

Chain Restaurants: Escape from Fat City

Upscale chains like T.G.I. Friday's and Chili's offer so much variety that you have plenty that you can choose other than deep-fried appetizers, huge entrées smothered in cheese, and frozen margaritas at 185 calories a pop. And while nobody goes to these places to pick at cottage-cheese plates, you *can* whittle your intake of fat and calories without feeling deprived. Here are your best bets at the some of the most popular chains.

Top picks:

- Boston Market: Hearth honey ham (210 calories, 9 grams of fat); a quarter of a chicken, white meat, no skin or wing (170 calories, 4 grams of fat); chicken, turkey, or ham sandwich without cheese or sauce (400 to 440 calories, 4.5 to 8 grams of fat). Enjoy a side of homestyle mashed potatoes (190 calories, 9 grams of fat), zucchini marinara (60 calories, 3 grams of fat), or half a piece of down-home cornbread (100 calories, 3 grams of fat).

- Chili's: Go for the Guiltless Grill items, which include veggie pasta or a chicken platter, pita, or sandwich. These items are usually served with black beans or steamed veggies, but again, the portion sizes are overly generous. Eat half the meal—and consume an average of 300 calories and up to 7 grams of fat.

- Denny's: Zero in on the Fit Fare items, such as the Garden Chicken Delite Salad (277 calories, 5 grams of fat), grilled chicken sandwich (434 calories, 9 grams of fat), and the Slim Slam without butter or syrup (495 calories, 12 grams of fat).

SNEAK NUTRITION INTO YOUR ORDER

Here are six pain-free ways to eat healthy away from home.

1. For a calcium boost, order fat-free milk rather than soda. Hate milk? Ask for it mixed with a tablespoon of chocolate syrup—a mere 41-calorie increase.

2. Visit a salad bar for fresh broccoli, carrots, and red peppers—all loaded with disease-fighting antioxidants. Add a tablespoon of low-fat dressing.

3. For more fiber, order sandwiches on whole grain bread. And try to get brown rice rather than white.

4. When having pasta with marinara sauce, request that steamed veggies be mixed in. Especially tasty are carrots, zucchini, and broccoli.

5. Order fruit for dessert—even if it's not on the menu. Orange slices, melons, and strawberries used as garnishes are often available.

6. Look to grilled salmon, rainbow trout, and tuna for a dose of heart-healthy omega-3 fatty acids.

- Olive Garden: Enjoy this chain's Garden Fare menu items, such as capellini pomodoro, capellini primavera, or capellini primavera with chicken. The portion sizes are huge, so ask the waiter to wrap half the entrée before it's even set before you. At that rate, you'll eat hearty for 310 to 365 calories.

- Ruby Tuesday: Enjoy a half-serving of shrimp and veggie pasta (381 calories, 5.5 grams of fat) or a chicken fajita salad—without the cheese or deep-fried tortilla bowl, which has 441 calories and 29 grams of fat.

Oil slicks: Appetizers smothered in cheese and sour cream, such as nachos or potato skins; sandwiches called melts (for instance, tuna melt), which are loaded with cheese and grilled with butter; croissant sandwiches; creamy coleslaw; macaroni and potato salads; salads served in a fried tortilla shell or bread bowl. (Skipping the tortilla shell that comes with a taco salad can save you up to 400 calories and 30 grams of fat.)

Chinese Food: Check Your Oil

Whether you order from the take-out joint down the street or dine at a cozy little place with cloth napkins, Chinese food can be either a healthy eater's nightmare or a dream come true, says Warshaw. It depends on what you order and how much you eat.

The trick is to eat like a woman from the Chinese countryside—lots of steamed rice and steamed fresh vegetables and small amounts of meat, poultry, or seafood.

Perhaps your biggest challenge, though, is to minimize the tremendous amount of fat used in Americanized Chinese cuisine. It's best to avoid deep-fried items, says Warshaw.

If you watch your salt intake, leave the soy sauce on the table. Even the low-sodium kind packs 600 milligrams per tablespoon.

Top picks: Wonton or hot-and-sour soup; steamed dumplings; steamed or stir-fried veggies, seafood, or chicken; dishes prepared with a light wine or lobster sauce.

Oil slicks: The deep-fried, crispy noodles served as an appetizer; egg rolls; fried dumplings; spareribs; Peking duck; dishes prepared with cashews or peanuts; entrées described on the menu as "crispy" or "sweet and sour."

Diners: Healthy Hash-House Fare

There's a reason diners are affectionately nicknamed greasy spoons. They're the home of the deep-fat fryer. Still, many of us love a diner's convenience and casual atmosphere. And if you order carefully and make special requests, healthy choices are plentiful, says Warshaw.

Top picks: Broth-based soups; a small hamburger; a bacon, lettuce, and tomato sandwich (request the mayo on the side); a large Greek or spinach salad, dressing on the side; a turkey, chicken, roast beef, or ham sandwich on whole grain bread (hold the cheese and mayo) with lettuce and tomato. "Use mustard, barbecue sauce, or low-fat dressing to moisten the bread and spice up the sandwich," says Warshaw. For dinner, consider having grilled fish or chicken with a small salad, steamed veggies, and a small baked potato topped with spicy brown mustard or low-fat salad dressing.

If you have room for dessert, opt for a fresh fruit cup (in juice, not syrup) when available or just a few of those after-dinner mints at the cash register.

Oil slicks: Creamy soups; melts; club sandwiches; jumbo burgers; most platters, which are typically served with french fries and creamy coleslaw. Reuben sandwiches "add insult to injury—bread grilled with butter, corned beef, melted cheese, Thousand Island dressing," says Warshaw. "They're a fat and sodium nightmare."

Also steer clear of most "diet" plates, says Warshaw. "They became popular in the 1950s, when protein was in and carbohydrates were out. They're usually a hamburger or cottage cheese, with maybe some canned fruit or crackers."

MASKED DISASTER

Eggplant Parmesan

Eggplant Parmesan (or parmigiana) seems like a smart restaurant choice—it's a vegetable dish, after all. But eggplant soaks up oil like a sponge. And when it's breaded, fried, and buried under mozzarella, the fat content can easily exceed 25 grams a serving. If it is available, order eggplant caponata instead. Or opt for pasta in marinara sauce, or a broth-based soup such as lentil or minestrone with a crusty, whole wheat bun.

HOW A RESTAURANT CRITIC STAYS SLIM

Penny Pollack eats for a living—and fits into size 6 jeans!

For years, the 5-foot-3 dining editor of *Chicago* magazine has eaten out five or six times a week—and we're talking full-course dinners. Here's how she keeps the scales at 108 pounds.

- Pollack starts her day with cornflakes and 2% milk. She lunches at her desk on yogurt, crackers, and fruit.

- On review nights, she takes along three or four friends to share the experience—and the calories. "I only take three or four bites of each dish," she says.

- She lets her companions choose the high-fat courses and opts for low-fat fish, chicken, or vegetarian entrées—and fruit for dessert when available.

- Rain or shine, three times a week Pollack takes a brisk early-morning walk with a friend. Afterward, she hoofs it to work—a 20-minute walk.

Italian Food: More Fettuccine, Less Alfredo

Whether you dine at a candles-in-the-Chianti-bottle trattoria or a four-star hideaway, the rule is this: Follow the path of least mozzarella. While most Italian food is heavily Americanized, there are usually several healthy choices, says Maria Giordano Lupo, chef at Va Tutto restaurant in New York City. Here's what to look for.

Top picks: Grilled meat, poultry, or fish; pasta with red or white clam sauce; pasta pomodoro (sautéed fresh tomatoes, basil, garlic, and a small amount of olive oil); pasta primavera without cream sauce. "I do a three-mushroom fettuccine in a light mushroom stock," says Lupo. "Risotto and polenta are also good picks, as long as they're made with spices and vegetables rather than butter and cheese." Risotto is made with rice, and polenta is a dish made with cooked cornmeal.

If you're ordering pizza, ask for extra marinara sauce and half the cheese. Add some toppings, and you'll barely notice the difference. Request a thin-crust pie rather than Sicilian or deep-dish. And obviously, order your pie piled high with veggies rather than sausage or pepperoni.

Oil slicks: Antipastos with cheeses, olives, and salami; anything carbonara (cream, eggs, cheese, and bacon); anything parmigiana (breaded, fried, and smothered in mozzarella). And watch out for the garlic knots—they're dripping in oil or melted butter. Leave them in the basket or send them away with the waiter.

Indian Food: Savor the Spice, Forgo the Fat

If you like your food spicy, chances are you enjoy Indian cuisine. If you're watching your weight, there's even more to love—like the fact that Indian food is based on healthy complex carbohydrates, particularly legumes like chickpeas and lentils, and veggies such as spinach, eggplant, potatoes, and peas.

The downside is the fat used to prepare many of these dishes. Many appetizers are deep-fried, and vegetables and meats are typically fried or sautéed in the Indian butter called *ghee*.

Still, "most Indian restaurants provide plenty of choices for the low-fat diner," says Priya Kulkarni, an Indian cooking instructor and coauthor of *Secrets of Fat-Free Indian Cooking*. "As a general rule, avoid dishes that have the words 'butter' or 'coconut' in their menu descriptions. And stay away from those that are cooked in a creamy sauce and those that contain large amounts of nuts." Here are her thumbs-up and thumbs-down selections.

Top picks: Mulligatawny soup; naan, roti, and chapati breads, which are baked rather than fried; dals (legume dishes—choose those without cream); chana (chickpea curry); kachumbars (vegetable salads); raitas (salads with a tart yogurt dressing); dishes described on the menu as masala (a combination of spices with sautéed tomatoes and onions) or tandoori (seasoned meat, poultry, or fish roasted in a clay oven).

Oil slicks: Samosas (deep-fried pastry filled with vegetables or meat); puri (a puffy, deep-fried bread); entrées described as biryani, malai, or korma, which are heavy on the oil or cream.

Mexican Food: Sidestep the Guacamole

We *love* Mexican food. Unfortunately, we love it prepared American-style—which means knee-deep in fat, especially at chain restaurants and Mexican fast-food places.

In those establishments, the perfectly healthy staples of Mexican cuisine—corn, beans, and tomatoes—are smothered with cheese and sour cream or heaped into deep-fried shells. "You won't find a salad served in a deep-fried tortilla shell in Mexico," notes Warshaw. And we won't even mention the basket of deep-fried tortilla chips the waitress sets on the table as soon as you take your seat—and keeps refilling.

Yet it is possible to go Mexican and eat healthfully. The goal is to bring this gringo fare back to its healthier, more nutritious roots, says Felipe Gaytan, executive chef at Via Reál, a Mexican restaurant in Irving, Texas.

Top picks: Grilled chicken or fish; items wrapped in a soft flour tortilla, such as fajitas and burritos; *pescado Veracruzana* (fish in Veracruz sauce). "The Veracruz sauce contains green olives and capers, which give it a tangy flavor, along with olive oil and grilled onions," says Gaytan. "It's light but full of flavor." Other options include *mole pollo* (boned chicken breast served in a hot and spicy sauce) and *camarones de hacha* (shrimp sautéed in a red and green tomato sauce). Enjoy them with a side of rice and pinto, kidney, or black beans with no added fat.

Or order à la carte. For example, make a meal of a bowl of black bean soup, a dinner salad dressed with salsa or low-fat dressing on the side, and one bean, seafood, chicken, or beef burrito or fajita, suggests Gaytan.

Oil slicks: Deep-fried tortilla chips; anything topped with cheese, sour cream, or guacamole; refried beans (commonly fried in lard); chimichangas (deep-fried flour tortillas filled with meat and cheese); the Mexican sausage called chorizo; deep-fried taco-shell bowls.

Steak Houses: Easy on the Beef

There's nothing inherently unhealthy about red meat, unless you eat a pound of it at one sitting. Unfortunately, that's the whole idea behind steak houses, most of which serve slabs of meat that would choke Fred Flintstone.

Take Gibsons, a popular steak house in Chicago. The steaks and chops run from 8 to 19 ounces. And some steak houses serve 24- or even 96-ounce steaks (that's 6 pounds of steer).

Stick to one serving of meat—about 3 ounces. Few steak houses offer a cut of meat that weighs less than 8 ounces. So be prepared to split it or ask that half be wrapped before it hits the table, says Audry Triplett, head chef at Gibsons.

Enjoy your 3-ounce portion of, say, filet mignon with a cup of broth-based soup or a salad, a side dish of steamed vegetables, and a plain baked potato. By the way, ask if a small potato is available. Many steak houses present you with a spud that's the size of a football. Many steak houses won't be able to fulfill your request for a smaller potato, but you can share with a friend or wrap part of it to go, says Triplett.

Top picks: Lean cuts of beef such as top sirloin (229 calories, 14.2 grams of fat) or tenderloin (258 calories, 18.6 grams of fat), a well-trimmed lamb chop (172 calories, 8.3 grams of fat), a pork loin chop (178 calories, 8.2 grams of fat). Ask that the extra fat be trimmed away before cooking, or simply request lean meat. Good-for-you appetizers include peel-and-eat shrimp, shrimp cocktail, and dinner salads with low-fat dressing on the side. At the all-you-can-eat salad bar, focus on the fresh veggies and give the bacon bits and croutons a wide berth.

Oil slicks: Deep-fried appetizers, creamy soups such as New England clam chowder, baby back ribs, coleslaw, and macaroni and potato salads.

Drinking for Health:
A Risk/Benefit Report

Power Maker #22: To reap antioxidant and heart-healthy benefits, sip one glass of red wine with dinner (if you can drink alcoholic beverages safely), or help yourself to purple grape juice any time of the day.

To drink or not to drink? It's a conundrum. Drinking alcohol moderately can protect you from heart disease and reduce your risk of stroke. What's more, evidence suggests that in some cases, red wine affords better protection than other forms of alcohol.

Evidence also suggests, however, that moderate drinking—as little as one glass a day or less—might increase your risk of breast cancer and possibly your risk of infertility, too.

Do you auction off the wine collection or invest in a vineyard in Napa? Neither. You just use common sense. All things considered, an occasional glass of wine is more likely to help than hurt you (unless you have problems with alcohol). After all, women in Mediterranean countries have been drinking wine with meals for more than 2,000 years, and they're among the longest-living women. They generally have lower rates of breast cancer than women in the United States.

334

Heal Your Heart with Flavonoids

Researchers and studies agree on one thing: Drinking red wine lowers your risk of coronary heart disease, which is particularly important after menopause, when women's risk of dying from a heart attack tops men's. "No question about it—that's universal," says Andrew L. Waterhouse, Ph.D., assistant professor of viticulture and enology at the University of California, Davis.

It explains the so-called French paradox, where the French, with diets dripping in saturated fats from foods like foie gras, cream, and butter, and cholesterol levels as high as the price of a couture dress, still have 2½ times fewer deaths from heart disease that we do. Could it be the red wine that accompanies their meals?

Quite possibly. And the protective effect most likely comes from substances called flavonoids, says John D. Folts, Ph.D., a flavonoid expert who directs the Coronary Thrombosis Laboratory at the University of Wisconsin Medical School in Madison. Flavonoids are natural compounds that are particularly plentiful in red wine because of the way the wine is produced, using "must," or stems, seeds, and skins of the grape.

White wine has only about one-eighth the amount of flavonoids because the must is removed early in the fermentation process. So stick with the red, says Dr. Folts.

Flavonoids protect the heart four critical ways.

Slowing the activity of platelets, microscopic cells in the blood that stem bleeding. When they collect in coronary arteries, platelets clump together into clots that can block bloodflow and cause heart attacks. Flavonoids act to reduce clot formation before it can become a problem.

Protecting against free radicals—those abnormal oxygen molecules that damage healthy cells. Free radicals are particularly dangerous if they join forces with the "bad" cholesterol, LDL, or low-density lipoproteins, that also hang out in coronary arteries. Put the two together, says Dr. Folts, and you're increasing your risk of heart attack.

Protecting the endothelial cells that line coronary arteries. Think of these cells as a nonstick coating in the arteries that allows blood to swish right between coronary artery walls. When the artery walls are unhealthy, it's as if the coating has been scratched so that things begin to build up and stick. Add flavonoids, and it's like recoating the surface so that cells slide with ease again. Flavonoids also secrete substances that protect against the hardening of the arteries, making clots that may exist less dangerous.

Raising levels of HDL (high-density lipoprotein) cholesterol. This "good" form of cholesterol helps neutralize some of the effects of the bad LDL.

Only the last effect—raising HDL—has been found with other kinds of moderate alcohol intake, not just wine, Dr. Folts says. And while basic alcohol does have some effect on platelets, you'd have to drink enough to nearly kill you before the effects are seen. By then, platelets would be the least of your worries.

Since beer and distilled spirits like vodka and gin barely have any flavonoids, you're better off sticking with red wine.

THE PARTY GIRL'S GUIDE TO STAYING SOBER

It's Saturday night at the neighborhood bar, and the drinks are flowing. You'd love a glass of wine or maybe even one of those cool blue martinis. What you don't want is to get sloshed or to suffer alcohol's wrath tomorrow.

Then go slow, counsels Morris E. Chafetz, M.D., director of the Health Education Foundation in Washington, D.C., and author of *Drink Moderately and Live Longer: Understanding the Good of Alcohol.*

It takes your liver about ½ hour to metabolize the amount of alcohol in a typical drink, so having no more than one drink an hour enables your liver to keep up, says Dr. Chafetz, who was the former director of the National Institute on Alcohol Abuse and Alcoholism.

- Drink water before you start drinking alcoholic beverages.
- Pour nonalcoholic beverages into your wine or martini glass. No one will know the difference.
- Drink nonalcoholic wine or beer, plain tomato juice with a celery stalk in it, or soda water with a lime.
- Only drink when you're with other people, in comfortable, relaxed surroundings.
- Drink alcohol with food, which slows alcohol's absorption into the bloodstream.

If you don't drink now, however, don't start, says Mary C. Dufour, M.D., deputy director of the National Institute on Alcohol Abuse and Alcoholism in Bethesda, Maryland. "There is a lot you can do to improve your cardiovascular risk factors, like exercise and weight loss and maybe taking a baby aspirin every day."

The Breast Connection

Early studies that linked drinking to breast cancer left many women as jittery as a bowl of gelatin. "According to population studies, women who drink are at greater risk for breast cancer than women who abstain. The risk is greatest at high rates of consumption. For light to moderate drinking, the evidence to date is mixed," says Dr. Dufour.

But even those studies are questionable because they don't specifically look at wine, and because everyone defines "drinking" differently, especially if they are relying on women's recall. And in reality, the real risks are relative—and highly individual.

"I think women have to make those decisions based on their own risk profiles," says Sharon C. Wilsnack, Ph.D., a widely recognized expert on women and drinking and the Chester Fritz Distinguished Professor at the University of North Dakota School of Medicine and Health Sciences in Grand Forks. "For instance, I don't have any family history of breast cancer, but I do have a family history of cardiovascular disease. So factoring that in, I think I'm probably in a group where moderate drinking will not be harmful."

Why You Can't Drink like a Man

If you do drink, be aware that alcohol affects us differently than it affects men. Women produce less of an enzyme that begins breaking down alcohol in the stomach. So we absorb about one-third more alcohol than our husbands and boyfriends.

It's also why the USDA defines moderate drinking differently for women than for men: one drink a day for women and two for men. In reality, the amount anyone, male or female, can drink safely is highly individual, depending on genetics, health condition, weight, age, and family history. What's more, few—if any—experts recommend more than three drinks a day.

HOW MUCH *IS* A DRINK, ANYWAY?

Experts define a glass of wine as 5 ounces. But wine goblets come in all shapes and sizes. To find out just how much wine your favorite goblet holds, fill it with wine or water, then transfer it into a measuring cup calibrated in ounces. If it's more than 5 ounces, cut back to the recommended limit. Then do the same for beer (one serving equals 12 ounces) and distilled spirits like gin, rum, or vodka (1.5 ounces of 80-proof spirits).

Smart Tips for Savvy Drinkers

If you have a problem with alcohol, or even a family history of alcohol abuse, you probably shouldn't drink alcohol. But that doesn't mean you have to give up the benefits of those flavonoids.

They can be found in fruits, vegetables, tea, and chocolate as well as in red wine. Dr. Folts has even found the same cardiac protection that is attributed to two glasses of red wine in four glasses of purple grape juice. If you're 21 or older with no religious, medical, or social reasons not to drink, experts offer these guidelines.

- Stick to wine, preferably red wine.

- Drink during meals, slowly. Guzzling alcohol or drinking only to get buzzed undermines the potential benefits.

- Moderate means one 5-ounce glass of wine a day, not filling up the souvenir tumbler from Cancun or the beer stein you picked up during your college semester in Germany.

- Only drink if you don't plan to drive or take part in other activities that require attention or skill. Most women retain some alcohol in the blood up to 3 hours after a single drink.

- Don't drink if you're pregnant, nursing, or even planning to become pregnant.

- Don't drink if you're taking any medications that interact with alcohol.

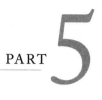

PART 5

DIET POWER

Calories Do Count

No matter what weight-loss plan you choose, the bottom line is still this: "If you take in more calories than you burn, you'll gain weight. End of story," says Louis Martin, M.D., medical director of the Louisiana State University Weight Management Center in New Orleans.

Need further proof that calories count? Ponder these sobering statistics.

• In 1978, the average woman consumed 1,571 calories a day. Today, it's about 1,710. That 139-calorie difference translates to 14 extra pounds of body weight a year.

• We consume less fat than ever before (33 percent of our total calories, down from 40 percent in 1978), yet a record 50 million of us are overweight.

• Less than 40 percent of us get regular exercise, the world's best calorie burner.

The upshot is that you can run from calories, but you can't hide. Because they'll hunt you down, grab onto your hips, and cling for dear life. Fortunately, you can fight back. Your reward will be a slimmer, healthier body and jeans you can breathe in.

Calories Count—But You Don't Have To

Counting calories has all the appeal of preparing for a tax audit. Well, thank goodness the latest word from nutritionists is "don't bother."

"Unless you want to eat with a calculator in hand, there's no need to count calories," says Lisa Tartamella, R.D., an ambulatory nutrition specialist at the Centers of Nutrition, Yale–New Haven Hospital in Connecticut.

The alternative is to eat mindfully. And that boils down to basics like becoming aware of portion sizes, shedding your "super-size it" mindset, cutting back on fat, and monitoring your intake of low-fat snacks and sweets because they can be treacherously high in calories.

And yes, go ahead and splurge on your favorite foods now and again. Because life without ice cream, Buffalo wings, and sausage sandwiches would be bleak indeed. For the most part, though, mindful eating should be nutritious eating. "The goal is to get maximum nutrition with minimum calories," says Franca Alphin, R.D., a licensed dietitian and administrative director of the Duke University Diet and Fitness Center in

WHERE HAVE ALL YOUR CALORIES GONE?

Assuming that you don't take in more calories than you need, here's how your body uses what you give it.

- **Basal metabolism.** From 60 to 65 percent of your calories are spent just keeping you alive and kicking—keeping your heart beating, your kidneys filtering waste, and your temperature hovering near 98 degrees.

- **Physical activity.** Another 25 percent goes to pure movement, from running up and down the field during your kid's soccer game to working up a sweat in step class.

- **Thermic effect of food.** The remaining 10 percent of calories is spent processing food. (Yes, it takes calories to process calories!)

Durham, North Carolina. That means more low-calorie, health-enhancing fruits, vegetables, whole grains, and beans. And less sugary, fatty fare, which is calorie-dense and nutrient-poor. But it's not enough to curtail calories. You need to burn them, too.

If you are ready to achieve a higher state of calorie consciousness, here's an easy guide to calories—how many you need to maintain or lose weight, how to whittle the excess calories from your diet, and how to crank up your calorie-burning power.

The Calorie/Gender Gap

Sure, we love our men. But it can be hard when we see how much more they can eat without gaining weight—or how quickly the pounds melt off when they eat less. It's a gender thing.

Men have a higher resting metabolism, which is the amount of calories burned while doing absolutely nothing. That's because, generally speaking, men have more muscle than women, and muscle burns calories. Every pound of the stuff burns from 40 to 50 calories a day.

By contrast, women average 20 to 30 percent body fat; men average 12 to 20 percent. For good reason, though. We need this extra fat to conceive and bear children. Unfortunately for us, fat is metabolically lazy, burning a miserly 2 calories per pound per day.

"Because of her higher percentage of body fat, a woman's resting metabolism is 5 to 10 percent lower than a man's," says Tartamella. "And that's even if they're the exact same weight."

How many calories you need depends on your resting metabolism, which is influenced by your height, weight, age, gender, activity level, and ratio of muscle to fat, among other variables, says Carmen Conrey, R.D., senior clinical dietitian at the Johns Hopkins Weight Management Center in Baltimore.

Tall, big-boned women typically need more calories than petite women. Active women need more calories than sedentary ones. And, oddly, those of us who are packing a few more pounds than we'd like need more calories than those of us who are at a desirable weight. (It takes more energy to power a larger body.)

Still, without taking muscle-to-fat ratios into account, you can get a quick-and-dirty estimate of your individual calorie needs with a few strokes of the calculator. Simply divide your current weight by 2.2 (to

SQUIRM A LITTLE!

We all know someone who eats whatever she wants and doesn't gain an ounce. Why? It may be because she never sits still—literally.

Researchers at the Mayo Clinic in Rochester, Minnesota, had 16 normal-weight people eat 1,000 extra calories a day and stop exercising for 2 months. Then they tracked what happened to those extra calories—whether they were burned or stored as fat.

During those 2 months, some people gained less than a pound. Others packed on nearly 10. Surprisingly, it wasn't the amount of voluntary exercise that separated the groups; it was the amount of small movements they accrued throughout the day—reaching, strolling around the office, fidgeting, walking up and down the stairs.

The researchers speculate that the people who didn't gain weight unconsciously increased their "nonexercise activity thermogenesis" (NEAT): the calorie-burning power of any activity other than voluntary exercise. "Those people who had the greatest increase in NEAT gained the least fat," says study coauthor Michael D. Jensen, M.D., professor of medicine in the division of endocrinology.

"This study shows that performing lots of small activities throughout the day can increase your calorie-burning potential enormously," he says. In fact, if you can increase your NEAT by 30 percent, it's possible to burn an extra 1,000 calories a week.

"To reap the benefits of NEAT, you have to make a concerted effort to move," says Dr. Jensen. Here's what he suggests.

- At home, get up to change the TV channel.
- At work, use the bathroom on another floor. (Take the stairs.) Ditto at home.
- Every hour, get up from behind your desk at work and take a brief stroll around your floor. At home, go up and down the stairs a few extra times.

Of course, this doesn't mean neglecting regular, planned exercise, such as walking, cycling, or swimming, stresses Dr. Jensen. "It's aerobic exercise that's been shown to protect your heart and keep you healthy."

POWER

MUSHROOMS

BIG BROILED BALSAMIC MUSHROOMS

The neat thing about portobello mushrooms is their meaty taste and texture—but they don't have any of meat's fat and contain just a few paltry
calories. Serve these marinated strips as the centerpiece of a vegetarian
meal or use them to extend a small amount of thinly sliced steak.

2	tablespoons balsamic vinegar
2	tablespoons water
2	teaspoons olive oil
½	teaspoon dried thyme
12	ounces portobello mushrooms, trimmed and thickly sliced

Preheat the broiler. Line a broiler pan with foil.

In a large bowl, whisk together the vinegar, water, oil, and thyme. Add
the mushrooms and toss gently to coat. Arrange in a single layer on the
broiler pan. Broil 3" from the heat for 2 minutes. Turn and broil for 2 minutes longer, or until golden.

Makes 4 servings

Per serving: 49 calories, 2 g protein, 6 g carbohydrates, 3 g fat, 0 mg cholesterol, 1 g dietary
fiber, 5 mg sodium

---

convert pounds to kilograms). Then multiply your weight in kilograms
by 30 (the amount of calories you need per pound of body weight).

So if you're 150 pounds, you weigh a little more than 68 kilograms.
Multiply that number by 30, and you arrive at 2,045 calories, the amount
you need to maintain that weight. If your body mass index (BMI) is 30
or higher, or if you are about 30 pounds overweight, however, this calcu-
lation may overestimate your calorie requirements, because body fat does
not require as many calories as muscle. (For information on calculating
your BMI, see page 312.)

To lose weight, multiply your weight (in kilograms) by 25. To lose about 1½ pounds a week, you'd need to consume 1,700 calories a day—345 fewer calories than the amount needed for weight maintenance.

Once you've done the math, you'll see how shaving a few hundred calories can make a significant difference in your waistline. And it's incredibly simple to do. This three-part calorie-trimming strategy can help.

Strategy #1: Go on Portion Patrol

To trim your calorie budget, you need to trim your portion sizes, says Alphin. But that's not always easy in America, Land of the Free and Home of the Super-Size Portion.

Many restaurants—especially our favorite chains—serve bowls of pasta as deep as a 10-gallon hat, steaks half the size of a Frisbee, and muffins as big as grapefruits. A popular pizza chain actually had to design a new box and cutting board for their latest—and most calorie-dense—pizza.

"It's absolutely unbelievable how restaurant portion sizes have changed over the years," says Alphin. "But restaurants aren't entirely to blame. We're not satisfied unless we're served meals that hang over the edge of the plate."

And boy, do they hang. When nutritionists from the Center for Science in the Public Interest (CSPI) in Washington, D.C., compared restaurant portions of 18 foods with the government's "official" serving sizes, here's what they found.

- The government says that a tuna salad sandwich weighs 4 ounces and contains 340 calories. A typical restaurant tuna sandwich weighs more than 10 ounces and contains 720 calories.

- An official serving of french fries is 3 ounces and has 220 calories. A McDonald's Super-Size Fries is 6 ounces and has 540 calories.

- A standard 3-cup serving of unbuttered popcorn has 160 calories. A small movie-theater tub of unbuttered popcorn has 7 cups and 400 calories; a medium, 16 cups and 900 calories.

"And since then, restaurant portions have gotten larger, if anything," says Jayne Hurley, R.D., the senior nutritionist at CSPI who co-led the study. Fast-food places are no exception. At many chains, the only way to get a reasonable adult-size portion is to order a kids' meal.

We help ourselves to plus-size portions at home, too. Who among us

HOW LONG DOES IT TAKE
TO BURN OFF CHEESECAKE?

You know how much last night's creamy slice of heaven cost you: 273 calories. But how long it will take to burn off those calories isn't so clear-cut. And charts that show how many calories you burn for a given exercise are based on a specific weight—usually not your own. Solve the problem with a few simple calculations.

Divide the calories burned during your exercise of choice by the body weight of the person on the chart. Then multiply that figure by your own body weight.

Say you weigh 138 pounds and want to go walking. The calorie-burn chart says a 150-pound woman burns 264 calories an hour walking. Do the math this way: 264 calories (burned during an hour's walking) divided by 150 pounds (the weight of the person on the chart) equals 1.76, multiplied by 138 pounds (your weight) equals 243 calories you'll burn for that hour. (Okay, it's 30 calories less than the cheesecake—so walk a few extra minutes.)

An hour's walk for a piece of cheesecake? Now *that's* a fair trade.

hasn't eaten half a bag of chips at one sitting or gone back for seconds—maybe thirds—of meat loaf and mashed potatoes?

"In my view, huge portion sizes and inactivity are the reasons that one out of three Americans are overweight," says Tartamella. "When I show women what one serving of pasta or mashed potatoes actually looks like, they're absolutely astonished."

"As obvious as it sounds, we need to start paying attention to the serving size portion of food labels," says Alphin. For example, more often than not, the bottled fruit juice or the bag of chips you have with lunch contains 2 or 2½ servings rather than 1.

Second, practice calorie visualization. "Learn what one serving of a particular food really looks like," says Alphin. For example, one serving of meat is 3 ounces and fits in the palm of your hand; one serving of pasta is ½ cup and the size of a tennis ball. For more ways to eyeball portion sizes, see "Visualize Those Calories" on page 358.

When dining out:

- Limit yourself to one piece of bread. Just one small piece of garlic bread has 186 calories. (Better yet, ask the waiter not to bring it.)

- If the restaurant has a reputation for huge portions, ask the waiter to wrap up half your entrée before he even sets the plate in front of you. Save the rest for tomorrow's lunch.

- When you order a meat sandwich, request only two or three slices of meat. If you're partial to tuna, chicken, or shrimp salad, ask that the chef use a smaller amount. A 3-ounce portion of tuna salad contains 160 calories.

- At all-you-can-eat salad bars, use a tablespoon instead of the large serving spoon to serve yourself macaroni or potato salad and other high-calorie items. The extra spooning time will remind you to exercise portion control.

At home or on the go:

- Keep food on the stove or counter rather than on the table. Those few extra seconds it takes to get off your chair for another plateful will remind you to pass up a second serving.

- If you normally eat 2 to 3 cups of pasta (400 to 600 calories) at one sitting, stretch 1 cup (200 calories) with 1 cup of grilled or sautéed veggies.

- Instead of toting a whole box of cookies or a whole bag of chips to the TV, measure out one serving and put the rest away.

- Dilute fruit juice with water. One serving of cranberry juice is ¾ cup and 108 calories. But bottles of fruit juice routinely contain 16 ounces. Drink that much and you've just swallowed 288 calories. If you dilute it with water by half and drink 8 ounces instead of 16, you'll consume a more sensible 77 calories.

- When you order pizza, eat one or two slices, rather than three or four.

- At fast-food restaurants, order à la carte rather than being lured by the "combo packages" of large burger, large fries, and large drink.

- Avoid "big grab" packages of chips, pretzels, or cheese popcorn. They routinely contain two or more servings.

Strategy #2: Avoid "Low-Fat Syndrome"

It's just another story of love and betrayal. The low-fat or fat-free cookies, pastries, and chips you've grown to love seduce you with their healthy promises—but then blow your calorie budget out of the water.

The truth is, many low-fat products contain as many calories as their full-fat counterparts. Here are a few examples.

• A low-fat apple-cinnamon Pop-Tart contains 191 calories; its full-fat counterpart, 200 calories.

• A fat-free Apple Newton contains about 50 calories. So does a regular Fig Newton.

• An ounce of regular cheese curls has 150 calories, the reduced-fat kind, 130 calories.

Don't blame the cookie makers. They print the appropriate serving size and its calorie content right on the Nutrition Facts label. "But somehow, our brains interpret 'fat-free' or 'low-fat' into 'calorie-free,'" says Alphin. "So we tend to eat huge portions of low-fat foods, which can double or even triple our calorie intake."

The antidote? Once again, portion control. Try these suggestions.

• Look for single-portion low-fat or fat-free snacks, readily available at convenience stores.

• If you buy low-fat snacks by the box or bag, divide them into one-serving portions and store in them plastic bags.

• Store boxes of low-fat pastries, snack cakes, or doughnuts in the back of your highest kitchen cabinet. When you want some, measure out one serving and immediately stash the rest away again.

• Eat a small amount of protein (perhaps a glass of fat-free milk) with your low-fat snacks. "The protein will help you feel a little more satisfied," says Conrey.

Strategy #3: Eat Food with Heft

Try this sometime. Measure out 3 cups of strawberries. Then put it next to 10 large jelly beans.

Both contain about 100 calories. What's dramatically different is the amount of food you get for those calories.

POWER

CHILI

WHITE CHILI WITH CHICKEN AND CORN

Who says that chili has to be red and chock-full of meat? White beans and two kinds of corn make this light-colored version deliciously satisfying (thanks to complex carbohydrates). Chicken breasts keep fat to a minimum. If you like your chili sizzling, add a generous splash of hot-pepper sauce—and reap a little extra protection against heart disease.

1	teaspoon canola oil
1	large onion, finely chopped
1	teaspoon ground cumin
$\frac{1}{2}$	cup fat-free chicken broth
$\frac{1}{2}$	cup finely chopped red bell pepper
$\frac{1}{2}$	pound boneless, skinless chicken breast, cut into bite-size pieces
2	cans ($15\frac{1}{2}$ ounces each) white beans, rinsed and drained
1	box (10 ounces) frozen corn, thawed
1	can (15 ounces) cream-style corn
1	can (4 ounces) chopped green chile peppers
2	tablespoons finely chopped fresh cilantro

Warm the oil in a large saucepan over medium heat. Add the onion and cumin. Cook, stirring, for 1 minute. Stir in the broth and bell pepper. Simmer for 5 minutes.

Stir in the chicken. Simmer for 5 minutes, or until the meat is cooked through and no longer pink.

Add the beans, thawed corn, cream-style corn, and chile peppers. Cook, stirring, for 5 minutes, or until hot. Sprinkle with the cilantro.

Makes 6 servings

Per serving: 277 calories, 20 g protein, 49 g carbohydrates, 3 g fat, 22 mg cholesterol, 5 g dietary fiber, 842 mg sodium

This powerful visual is a perfect demonstration of energy density, or how many calories a food packs for a given weight.

Strawberries—along with other fruits, vegetables, and many grains—have a low energy density, which means you can eat more of them for fewer calories. By contrast, jelly beans—as well as croissants, chips, and doughnuts—have a high energy density and therefore a higher number of calories for their weight.

The lower a food's energy density, the fuller and more satisfied you'll feel, so you'll be less tempted to have seconds or thirds, says Barbara Rolls, Ph.D., professor of nutrition at Pennsylvania State University in University Park and author of *Volumetrics: Feel Full on Fewer Calories.*

Since fruits, vegetables, and grains get their satisfying bulk from lots of water and fiber, they fill you up without filling you out, says Dr. Rolls.

They also tend to be high in complex carbohydrates, which increase blood sugar levels and signal the carbohydrate receptors in your body to tell your brain and belly that you've had enough food, thanks.

Here are a few ways nutritionists say that you can modify recipes so that they include less "dense" ingredients.

• If you make homemade pizza, pile on the veggies and reduce the amount of cheese.

• Add more beans and celery to chili and reduce the amount of ground beef.

• If you crave chips, dry-roasted peanuts, or corn chips, measure out 1 ounce—and eat them with an apple.

Don't Count Calories

Here's a better idea than counting calories: Count *servings* of food, says Alphin. Follow the government's Food Guide Pyramid, which calculates calories based on servings.

"If you follow the Food Guide Pyramid, you'll automatically eat sensible portions," says Alphin. You'll also maximize your intake of fiber, essential vitamins and minerals, and the disease-fighting substances in plant foods.

Here's how Tartamella suggests that you translate healthy, weight-conscious eating guidelines into calories. If you're small and less active,

POWER

GINGERED FLOUNDER

It's no fish story! When researchers identified the 10 foods most adept at quelling hunger pangs, fish came in second, bested only by potatoes. (Hint: serve these savory fillets with a side of spuds for double the satisfaction). You can use this no-fuss cooking method for most any type of mild fish fillets or steaks.

2 tablespoons fat-free chicken broth
1 tablespoon reduced-sodium soy sauce
1 tablespoon finely chopped fresh ginger
1 teaspoon sesame oil
4 flounder fillets (about 5 ounces each)
2 tablespoons thinly sliced scallion

In a large nonstick skillet, whisk together the broth, soy sauce, ginger, and oil. Add the flounder and turn to coat. Sprinkle with the scallion. Let marinate at room temperature for 5 minutes.

Place over medium heat, cover, and cook for 5 minutes, or until the fish flakes easily.

Makes 4 servings

Per serving: 205 calories, 28 g protein, 1 g carbohydrates, 10 g fat, 85 mg cholesterol, 0 g dietary fiber, 226 mg sodium

opt for the lower-calorie allotments; if you're tall, big-boned, or active, pick the higher-calorie options. No matter which calorie amount you choose, limit your intake of fats, oils, and sweets.

To consume about 1,200 calories a day: Eat six servings of grains (at least three should be whole grains); three servings of vegetables; two servings of fruit; two servings of meat, poultry, fish, beans, eggs, or nuts; and two servings of milk, yogurt, or cheese (preferably low-fat).

(continued on page 354)

50 WAYS TO SHAVE 100 CALORIES

If you eat just 100 extra calories a day—that's two chocolate sandwich cookies, ladies—you'll be up 10 pounds in a year. But you can satisfy that cookie craving if you cut 100 calories from someplace else. Here are 50 painless ways to do it.

1. Instead of 1 cup of low-fat granola with raisins, have 1 cup of raisin bran.
2. Have a large caffe latte with fat-free instead of whole milk.
3. Eat half a 4-ounce bagel with an orange rather than the whole bagel.
4. Put 1 tablespoon of mustard on a sandwich, not 1¼ tablespoons of mayo.
5. Instead of 2 slices of cheese pizza, have 2 slices of veggie pizza (no cheese).
6. Order 2 slices of cheese pizza instead of 2 slices of pepperoni pizza.
7. Top your tossed salad with 3 tablespoons of fat-free ranch dressing instead of 2 tablespoons of the real thing.
8. Try a Boca Burger or Gardenburger instead of a regular hamburger.
9. Have a cup of steamed rather than fried rice with Chinese vegetables.
10. Put 1 less tablespoon of butter on your baked potato.
11. Have ½ cup of macaroni and cheese and 1 cup of broccoli.
12. Eat only half that slice of chocolate fudge cake with icing.
13. Instead of 6 cups of theater-style microwave popcorn, have the same amount of low-fat, butter-flavored microwave popcorn.
14. Spread 1 tablespoon of all-fruit jam on your pancakes rather than 1½ tablespoons of butter.
15. Instead of whole milk and eggs for French toast, use fat-free milk and egg whites.
16. Munch 1 ounce of baked mini pretzels instead of 1 ounce of pecans.
17. Snack on an orange and a banana instead of a candy bar.
18. Steam asparagus rather than sauté it in 1 tablespoon of butter or oil.
19. Replace 3 bacon slices with 3 slices of Light and Lean Canadian bacon.
20. Have 1 cup of home-style baked beans, not 1 cup of beans with franks.
21. Use 3 teaspoons of dijonnaise instead of 4 teaspoons of mayonnaise.
22. Eat ½ cup of steamed fresh broccoli, not ½ cup of broccoli in cheese sauce.
23. Replace 1 cup of caramel-coated popcorn with 2½ cups of air-popped.
24. Stuff celery sticks with 2 tablespoons of fat-free cream cheese instead of 3 tablespoons of regular cream cheese.

25. Have two chocolate chip cookies instead of five.

26. Replace a 12-ounce can of cola with a 12-ounce can of diet cola.

27. Thicken cream sauce with 1% milk and cornstarch instead of butter and flour.

28. Have 3 ounces of steak instead of 4½ ounces.

29. Grill a cheese sandwich using cooking spray instead of margarine.

30. Replace 1 cup of chocolate ice cream with ⅔ cup of fat-free frozen yogurt.

31. Snack on 2 ounces of oven-baked potato chips instead of regular.

32. Instead of 1 cup of macaroni salad, eat 3½ cups of spinach salad with 2 tablespoons of low-calorie dressing.

33. Have 1 tablespoon of peanut butter on your sandwich instead of 2.

34. Order a sandwich on cracked wheat bread instead of a croissant.

35. Snack on ½ cup of fruit cocktail in water instead of 1 cup of fruit cocktail in heavy syrup.

36. Dip chips into ½ cup of salsa instead of ¾ cup of jalapeño cheese dip.

37. Use 1 tablespoon of mayonnaise instead of 3 tablespoons in tuna salad.

38. Use 2 tablespoons of light pancake syrup, not 2 tablespoons of regular.

39. Top pasta with 1 cup of marinara sauce instead of ¾ cup of alfredo sauce.

40. Stop tasting as you cook. The following "tastes" have 100 calories: 4 tablespoons of beef stroganoff, 3 tablespoons of homemade chocolate pudding, 2 tablespoons of chocolate chip cookie dough.

41. Eat ¾ cup of pudding made with fat-free milk rather than 1 cup of pudding made with whole milk.

42. Snack on a papaya instead of a bag of chocolate candies.

43. Munch on 1 cup of frozen grapes instead of an ice cream sandwich.

44. Eat two meatballs instead of four.

45. Choose one serving vegetarian lasagna instead of lasagna with meat.

46. Eat two Kellogg's Nutri-Grain bars instead of two Kellogg's Pop-Tarts.

47. Replace one large flour tortilla with one 6-inch corn tortilla.

48. Eat one hot dog, not two, at a baseball game.

49. Order your Quarter Pounder without cheese.

50. Shred 2 ounces of fat-free Cheddar on nachos instead of regular Cheddar.

To consume about 1,600 calories a day: Have eight servings of grain products (at least three should be whole grains); four servings of vegetables; three servings of fruit; two servings of meat, poultry, fish, beans, eggs, or nuts; and two servings of milk, yogurt, or cheese (preferably low-fat).

To consume about 2,000 calories a day: Eat nine servings of grains (at least three of whole grains), five servings of vegetables, four servings of fruit, three servings of low-fat dairy products, and two 3-ounce portions of meat.

For calorie levels between the examples above, adjust the servings of grains, fruits, or vegetables, says Tartamella. Each serving of grains contains about 80 calories; fruit, about 60 calories; vegetables, about 25 calories. A serving of starchy vegetables (such as potatoes or corn) contains between 80 and 100 calories. So to move from 1,600 calories to 1,800 calories a day, you might have an extra piece of fruit at lunch, ½ cup of rice at dinner, and another piece of fruit as an evening snack.

Of course, counting servings trims calories only if you stick to the recommended serving sizes.

- One serving of grains: one slice of bread; half of a bagel or English muffin; 1 ounce of cold cereal; ½ cup of cooked cereal, rice, or pasta; one small roll, biscuit, or muffin; two large crackers

- One serving of fruit: one medium apple, orange, or banana; ½ cup of berries; half of a grapefruit; an eighth of a cantaloupe or other melon; ½ cup of canned, chopped, or cooked fruit; ¾ cup of fruit juice

- One serving of vegetables: 1 cup of raw leafy greens, ½ cup of cooked vegetables, or ¾ cup of vegetable juice

- One serving of dairy: 1 cup of milk or yogurt, 2 ounces of processed cheese, 1½ ounces of cheese

- One serving of protein: 2 to 3 ounces of meat, poultry, or fish (or build your protein serving from these sources: Count ½ cup of cooked beans, one egg, 2 tablespoons of nuts or peanut butter, or 4 ounces of tofu as 1 ounce of meat.)

Burn, Ladies, Burn

Trimming calories is one side of the calorie coin. The other side is burning calories. That's best accomplished by shedding fat and building muscle—in other words, exercise.

POWER

POTATOES

ROSEMARY SKILLET SPUDS

Nothing stops hunger pangs dead in their tracks like potatoes. Just don't sabotage their natural goodness (no fat, modest calories, plenty of potassium, lots of fiber) with careless cooking techniques. Here, we lightly brown spuds in a minimum amount of oil and jazz up their flavor with savory herbs.

1   tablespoon olive oil
1   pound small red new potatoes, quartered
2   tablespoons finely chopped fresh garlic
1   teaspoon dried rosemary, crumbled
1   cup fat-free chicken broth

Warm the oil in a large nonstick skillet over medium heat. Add the potatoes and cook, stirring often, for 5 minutes, or until lightly browned. Add the garlic and rosemary. Cook, stirring, for 1 minute longer.

Add the broth and bring to a boil. Reduce the heat to low, cover, and simmer for 10 minutes, or until the potatoes are just tender. Uncover, raise the heat to medium, and cook, stirring occasionally, for 10 minutes longer, or until most of the broth evaporates.

Makes 4 servings

Per serving: 121 calories, 3 g protein, 20 g carbohydrates, 3.5 g fat, 0 mg cholesterol, 2 g dietary fiber, 127 mg sodium

---

Exercise raises your resting metabolism by replacing do-nothing fat with calorie-burning muscle, says Deborah Ezell, a clinical exercise physiologist at the Johns Hopkins Weight Management Center. The more muscle you build, the more calories you'll burn, even while you sleep. And even as you age.

Once you hit 40, you start replacing muscle with fat. In fact, you can expect to lose ½ pound of muscle every year during perimenopause and

POWER

BEAN NACHOS GRANDE

Don't give up nachos—just be smart when making them. That means baked chips instead of fried, light cheese rather than regular, and fork-mashed pintos instead of lard-laced refried beans. You'll get real taco-stand flavor for a fraction of the calories and fat.

 5   cups baked tortilla chips
 1   cup shredded reduced-fat Cheddar cheese
 1   can (14 ounces) pinto beans, rinsed and drained
 ½   cup prepared salsa
 ½   cup fat-free plain yogurt
 1   tablespoon finely chopped fresh cilantro

Preheat the broiler.

Arrange the chips evenly on a baking sheet. Sprinkle with ½ cup of the cheese. Lightly mash the beans with a fork and evenly scatter over the chips. Top with the remaining ½ cup cheese.

Broil 3" from the heat for 1 minute, or until the cheese is melted. Spoon the salsa and yogurt over the chips. Sprinkle with the cilantro.

Makes 5 servings

Per serving: 267 calories, 13 g protein, 40 g carbohydrates, 7 g fat, 16 mg cholesterol, 4 g dietary fiber, 705 mg sodium

about 1 pound a year during menopause. By the time you're 55, you could be down 15 pounds of muscle and burn about 600 fewer calories per day. Scary thought. But exercise can help you turn back your metabolic clock—even after menopause.

Researchers at the University of Colorado in Boulder studied the metabolic rate of 65 premenopausal and postmenopausal women—27 of them sedentary, the rest long-distance runners and swimmers. They found that, after menopause, the resting metabolism of the sedentary women dropped by about 130 calories a day. But the women who exercised had no drop in metabolic rate.

Muscle Up Your Metabolism

For pure calorie-burning power, you can't beat aerobic exercise, such as jogging, cycling, or cardio kickboxing, says Ezell.

"Aerobic exercise burns a lot of calories," says Ezell. "And when combined with eating fewer calories, it also promotes weight loss."

Further, aerobic exercise boosts your resting metabolism for several hours afterward, as your muscles burn calories to recover and repair themselves.

Say you weigh 150 pounds and you do vigorous aerobics for 1 hour. Besides the 558 calories you burn in that 60 minutes, you'll burn almost 100 more calories for several hours afterward, even if you're sprawled out in front of the tube.

According to the American College of Sports Medicine, you should burn about 1,000 calories a week in physical activity. If you're at 150 pounds, that translates to 1 hour of brisk walking three times a week.

Consider adding resistance training to your exercise program, too, says Ezell. "While resistance training doesn't burn many calories, it does build muscle," she says. "If you stick with it for over a year, you may eventually burn from 150 to 200 more calories a day." Her recommendation is to pump iron at least twice a week.

More Sneaky Metabolism Boosters

Physical activity is the best way to rev up metabolism. But it's not the only way. These tips can help you crank your calorie-burning power to the max.

Don't crash-diet. Those "drop a dress size in a week!" diets can slow metabolism by as much as 15 percent within the first 2 weeks, says Tartamella. So no matter how badly you want to lose weight, don't embark on any diet that offers less than 1,200 calories a day.

"Drastically cutting calories makes your body think it's starving," explains Tartamella. "So it tries to conserve its energy stores by lowering the rate at which it burns calories."

Break your fast. You may plan to eat lunch, but all your body knows is that it's not getting food—and may not for a long, long time. To conserve fuel, it starts burning calories more slowly. Eating breakfast reassures your body that there's no impending famine and that it's okay to "spend" its calories. Eating breakfast also helps keep you from overeating at lunch or dinner, adds Tartamella.

Eat often. Eat five or six mini-meals a day or three squares plus two or three snacks of 100 to 200 calories each, recommends Tartamella. "Grazing" can also act as a binge-proofer—eating every few hours staves off hunger pangs.

Even if you eat the same number of calories, you'll burn them off better if you spread them throughout the day. Researchers at Tufts University in Boston found that older women (average age 72) who ate mini-meals of 250 and 500 calories burned the same amount of calories as 25-year-old women. But when they consumed 1,000-calorie meals, they burned 60 fewer calories each day than the younger women. In a year, that could add up to a weight gain of 6 pounds.

Let your period work for you. Two weeks before menstruation, your

VISUALIZE THOSE CALORIES

To most of us, one portion is whatever our appetite tell us it is. But being unaware of real-world portion sizes is the main cause of climbing calorie intakes—and widening hips. Here's how to eyeball one portion with the precision of a sharpshooter.

- 3 ounces of meat: the size of a cassette tape
- 3 ounces of grilled fish: the size of your checkbook
- ½ cup of pasta: the size of a tennis ball
- 1 cup of mashed potatoes: the size of your fist
- Half of a medium bagel: the size of a hockey puck
- 1 ounce of cheese: the size of four stacked dice
- One medium fruit: the size of a tennis ball
- 1 ounce of pretzels or other snack foods: a large handful
- ½ cup of ice cream: the size of a tennis ball

Waistline

Researchers in Australia have actually identified the foods most likely to quell hunger pangs. The top 10: potatoes, fish, oatmeal, oranges, apples, whole wheat pasta, beefsteak, grapes, air-popped popcorn, and bran cereal.

temperature rises, temporarily elevating your resting metabolism. During this time, you burn an average of 150 extra calories a day—and sometimes as many as 360 extra calories. So if you can withstand premenstrual cravings, you'll actually burn your own stored fat for energy.

Of course, don't compound PMS misery by denying yourself chocolate or chips, says Tartamella. "Better to have a small portion now than to binge later."

Muscle up your walks. Pumping your arms to chin height while you walk burns from 7 to 10 percent more calories than just walking, says John Porcari, Ph.D., professor in the department of exercise and sports science at the University of Wisconsin in La Crosse. "When you get your arms into the act, you're using more calorie-burning muscle."

For even more calorie-busting power, use walking poles (a cross between a ski pole and a baton) or wrist weights. Research by Dr. Porcari has found that walking poles boost the amount of calories burned during a walk by up to 25 percent, while wrist weights increase calorie expenditure by 5 to 15 percent.

Wrist weights are available in sporting goods and department stores and cost $10 to $15. Start with 1-pound weights and, if you like, go to 2 pounds after about 6 weeks. Don't use hand weights. Gripping even a 1-pound weight can cause blood pressure to rise in some women, says Dr. Porcari.

Walking poles, which are available in some sporting goods stores and upscale catalogs, cost about $60. To make your own poles, lop the ends off a pair of old ski poles and cover the ends with rubber tips to provide stability on uneven terrain, suggests Dr. Porcari.

10 Ways to Binge-Proof Your Eating Plan

Like tornadoes, binges seem to strike out of the clear blue sky, leaving in their wake cookie crumbs, empty Fritos bags, and guilt.

But is a binge really the irresistible force it seems to be? "Not at all," says Gerard J. Musante, Ph.D., director of Structure House Center for Weight Control and Lifestyle Change in Durham, North Carolina. "Controlling your impulse to binge— and it can be controlled—comes down to how you choose to act." In other words, your behavior.

But before you can change your behavior, you must confront your feelings, says Dr. Musante. You may find that negative emotions—anger, depression, anxiety—are driving your binges. (To learn more about emotional eating, see Food/Mood Madness: A New Approach to Emotional Eating on page 287.)

Once you've made the feeling/food connection, you can work on changing your response to it. The turning point comes when you realize that you have a choice not to pig out. That's when you learn to think through your impulse to eat, then choose whether or not to give in. Then *you* control a binge, not the other way around.

Each time you manage to resist the urge to eat, you create an "I can" moment. "That's when you're hit with the impulse to eat, and you think 'I can handle this' rather than 'I can't stand it,'" says Lee Kern, a licensed clinical social worker and clinical director at Structure House. "That's a very powerful moment."

To avoid a binge, use the first through fourth commandments, below. To stop one already in progress, use the fifth through seventh commandments. To bounce back from a binge, turn to the eighth through tenth commandments.

The First Commandment: Thou Shalt Not Set Thyself Up

Stop berating yourself: You don't pig out because you lack willpower or self-control. "Women think binges fall out of the sky," says Kern. "The truth is, many women set themselves up."

The biggest unconscious setup is poor time or lifestyle management. Long, seemingly endless days, bereft of friends or meaningful activity, can send you straight to the fridge. "For these women, a binge becomes the pleasure and entertainment of the day," says Kern.

Those who juggle a multitude of obligations—houses, spouses, kids, and career—may use eating everything that isn't nailed down as a way to spend some time alone after a day of being a caretaker. To stop the set-ups, analyze the ways in which you manage your time and your life, recommends Kern. Do you have too little time for yourself—or too much? Do you take time to relax and regenerate? Are some of the obligations in your life self-imposed, and might dropping them make your life less hectic? Once you've answered those questions, you can generate solutions.

HOW MANY DOUGHNUTS MAKE A BINGE?

Three, if you're a woman. Six, if you're a man, according to a survey of 400 college students.

If you have too much time on your hands, take steps to fill it with activities other than eating. Take classes, sign up for volunteer work, or made a standing daily date for a brisk walk with a friend. If your impulse to eat arrives at a certain time—say, 11:00 A.M., 3:00 P.M., or right after work—schedule your chosen activity during this time.

If your family and job leave you overextended, announce to your family that, from now on, you'll be taking a 30-minute breather when you get home or at another specific time. Then head for a bubble bath, the home gym, or a juicy novel.

The Second Commandment: Thou Shalt Not Starve Thyself

Many women, having eaten too much at dinner, feel they have to atone for their extra calories. "So they skip breakfast and lunch the next day," says Shannon Turner, Ph.D., professor of clinical health psychology at the Oklahoma State University College of Osteopathic Medicine in Tulsa.

Big mistake. "All skipping meals does is make you famished—which may push you right into a binge," says Dr. Turner.

Another pitfall is being too busy to eat breakfast or lunch, then arriving home at the end of the day hungry enough to gnaw your kitchen cabinets. If you're a meal skipper, eating three meals a day—including breakfast—will ensure that you never get too hungry.

If your stomach lurches at the very thought of eating in the morning, start small, perhaps with a piece of whole wheat toast and a teaspoon of peanut butter or with a carton of low-fat fruit yogurt. If you dislike traditional breakfast fare, opt for half a sandwich—like thin-sliced deli ham and reduced-fat cheese on a piece of whole grain bread.

If it's hard for you to sit down to three meals, try eating every 3 to 4 hours (roughly five or six mini-meals each day), suggests Dr. Turner. "Some women find that small, frequent meals help them curb their urge to binge." (How many calories each mini-meal should contain depends on your unique calorie needs. To find yours, see page 351.)

As often as possible, make mealtime an event. Eat at the kitchen or dining room table, rather than in front of the TV. Eliminate distractions. "Put the magazine down, put away your work, hang up the phone," says Dr. Turner. At work, if you eat lunch at your desk, put away your paperwork and put your phone on private.

WHEN A CARROT DOESN'T CUT IT

Trying to white-knuckle a craving can put you on the fast track to a binge, says Catherine Christie, Ph.D., president of Nutrition Associates in Jacksonville, Florida, and coauthor of *I'd Kill for a Cookie.*

Her advice? Either feed your craving—in moderation—or choose foods that can stand in for the creamy, crunchy, or greasy sensations your tastebuds demand. Here's a short list of substitutes that satisfy.

When you want chocolate:

- 1 tablespoon of chocolate chips (27 chips: 70 calories, 4 grams of fat)
- Four Hershey's Kisses (105 calories, 3.8 grams of fat)
- 4 ounces of Snack Pack fat-free chocolate pudding (98 calories, zero gram of fat)

When you want salty snack foods:

- 36 Guiltless Gourmet corn tortilla chips (try the chili and lime or Mucho Nacho) and salsa (220 calories, 4 grams of fat)
- Six cheese or nacho cheese mini rice cakes (53 calories, 0.5 gram of fat)
- 33 mini pretzels (52 calories, zero gram of fat)

When you want cookies, cake, or pie:

- A low-fat whole grain cereal bar (136 calories, 2.8 grams of fat)
- 2-ounce slice of angel food cake (73 calories, 0.2 gram of fat) topped with fresh raspberries
- 1-ounce slice of pound cake (131 calories, 7 grams of fat) topped with fresh sliced strawberries
- 7 ounces of light cherry cheesecake yogurt (130 calories, 1.5 grams of fat)

When you want ice cream:

- ½ cup of frozen yogurt topped with 1 tablespoon of fat-free caramel topping (165 calories, 4.3 grams of fat)
- ½ cup of vanilla ice milk topped with 1 tablespoon of fat-free hot fudge topping (142 calories, 3 grams of fat)

When you want fast food:

- A small hamburger (231 calories, 8.6 grams of fat)
- 20 to 25 french fries (235 calories, 12.2 grams of fat)
- One chicken wing or drumstick (140 calories, 10 grams of fat)

The Third Commandment:
Thou Shalt Strip Thy Trigger Foods of Their Power

Every woman knows her trigger food like she knows her Social Security number. It's the one she can't put down until she's demolished the entire package. (Call it the you-can't-eat-just-one syndrome.)

Often, trigger foods are what Dr. Musante calls primary foods—those you've learned to associate with feelings of comfort, security, or happiness, sometimes before you even learned to talk.

Yet you can learn to recreate the positive feelings that trigger foods

DO YOU HAVE BINGE-EATING DISORDER?

Imagine eating a large pizza, three cheese sandwiches, a pint of ice cream, and five pieces of cake—all within 90 minutes.

This isn't the face of gluttony. It's the face of a binge-eating disorder (BED), thought to affect up to two million Americans—60 percent of them women. Experts aren't sure what causes BED, but up to half of all people with the disorder have a history of depression.

Only a specialist can tell you whether your overeating might signal BED. But women diagnosed with this condition:

- Have binged at least twice a week for at least 6 months
- Eat abnormally large amounts of food in a short period of time
- Eat much more quickly than normal
- Eat until they're uncomfortably full
- Eat alone because they're embarrassed by how much they eat
- Find that they can't stop eating, even if they want to
- Feel disgusted, depressed, or guilty about their binges

For more information on BED, including where to find treatment in your area, call Eating Disorders Awareness and Prevention, a Seattle-based nonprofit organization devoted to bringing BED and other eating disorders out of the shadows. The toll-free number is (800) 931-2237. You can also get more information through their Web site at www.edap.org.

evoke—without the food itself, says Dr. Musante. He suggests the visualization below.

Think back to your earliest memory of your trigger food—say, potato chips. Perhaps you first remember enjoying these salty rounds at the age of 5 or 6, at a family picnic by the lake.

Close your eyes and remember the scene. But edit out the chips.

Now you're free to focus on the scene itself. Conjure up its sights, sounds, sensations. The sound of your brother's splashing. The warmth of the sun on your hair. The laughter of your parents from the lake as you lay on the soft grass, watching the clouds. Feel the comfort of that scene, when all your needs were automatically met, when you were carefree.

Hold that image until you're smiling with your eyes closed.

See? You've drawn the comfort you needed from memory alone. You didn't need the chips to take you there.

The Fourth Commandment: Thou Shalt Give Thyself Regular Tune-Ups

Many of us are religious about taking our cars in for their tune-ups, the idea being that it's better to head off problems before they occur.

Use the same principle with yourself, says Kern. If you don't want to drive yourself into the ground, you need to schedule regular "tune-ups" that nourish you in ways that don't involve food.

Take 10 minutes to develop a list of daily, weekly, and monthly tune-ups, advises Kern. "The list of one woman I worked with read something like this: 'Every day, I need to spend at least 15 minutes in inspirational reading. Every week, I need to make an appointment to get my hair done. And every month, I need to spend a weekend in the city alone to go to the symphony and hit the museums.'"

Develop and write your list, adds Kern. Find a quiet 15 to 20 minutes—before bed, perhaps, or in the morning. Hang the list in a prominent place—on the edge of your bedroom mirror maybe. You can even put your tune-ups on your home or work computer's scheduling software. (If you'd rather not advertise your list, laminate it and carry it in your purse. Pull it out when you first feel a binge coming on.)

Feel guilty about your tune-ups? Look at it this way. You already feel guilty about bingeing. Moreover, you're unlikely to stop until you find more positive ways to nurture yourself.

Waistline

In studying the eating patterns of 51 female binge eaters, researchers at the Ohio State University College of Nursing in Columbus found that the women ate an average of 1,809 calories on the days they didn't binge. On the days they let loose, they ate an average of 2,707 calories—a 66 percent increase.

"You have to say, 'These are the things that make me feel good about myself. And if I don't do them, then I'm setting myself up for a binge,'" says Kern.

The Fifth Commandment: Thou Shalt Not Eat around a Craving

We've all done it. Confronted by a Grand Canyon craving for sour-cream-and-onion potato chips, you resist. Then you make do with three pieces of buttered toast, half a box of dry breakfast cereal, and most of the kids' fruit rolls.

Eat the chips, already.

When you resist a craving, you often eat everything else in sight. "That's called eating around a craving," says Catherine Christie, Ph.D., president of Nutrition Associates in Jacksonville, Florida, and coauthor of *I'd Kill for a Cookie*. "I've had clients who craved chocolate but ate 15 graham crackers, a bowl of cereal, and an apple—and then ate the chocolate anyway."

Her advice: Indulge in a reasonable portion of the food you crave, unless it's a trigger food that may lead you into a binge. (In that case, proceed to Commandment #6.)

There's a correct way to feed your craving, too, adds Dr. Turner. Put one serving of the food you crave on a dish or in a bowl, then put the package away. *Then* eat. "Don't read, don't talk on the phone, don't watch TV," she says. "Focus entirely on the food. Concentrate on how good it is. And when you're finished, you're finished."

The Sixth Commandment:
Thou Shalt Use the Five Ds

This is the most difficult of all the Commandments because it asks you to use your brains when you're staring down at the unopened bag of cookies. When your very soul cries out for sugar or grease. But use your gray matter you must.

"When you binge, you stop thinking. Your brain goes AWOL," says Dr. Musante. "The Five Ds give you the chance to turn your brain back on and think through your impulse to eat." When you're about to embark on a binge (or are already started on one), follow these steps.

Determine what's going on. Ask yourself, "Why do I want to eat so badly right now?"

Delay your response by figuring out what's driving your urge to eat. Are you famished because you skipped a meal? Angry? Bored? Lonely? You might feel that, once you've hit this point, there's nothing on God's green Earth that can step between you and your jumbo bag of chocolate candies. And that may be true, says Dr. Musante. "But do you have to eat them at this moment? In the next 60 seconds? You can eat them 5 minutes from now, 10 minutes from now, or an hour from now." The longer you stall, the higher the likelihood that the craving will pass.

THE HIGH PRICE OF BINGEING

Compulsive overeating isn't just unhealthy. Here's the cost of some typical pigout portions.

> One (10.5-ounce) package of corn chips: $2.19
>
> One (8.5-ounce) container of dip: $2.99
>
> One (17-ounce) package of M&Ms: $3.29
>
> One (1-pound, 2-ounce) bag of chocolate chip cookies: $3.19
>
> Two pints of gourmet ice cream: $6.98
>
> One frozen pizza: $5.99

Total: $24.63

The upshot? If you normally binge on foods like these twice a month, learning to resist temptation could save nearly $600 a year!

15 BY-THE-MOUTHFUL MUNCHIES

You want snacks. Lots of snacks. Big, whopping handfuls of snacks. When you reach for the treats below, you get quantity as well as quality. The beautiful part is that each contains no more than 250 calories and less than 10 grams of fat. To avoid too much of a good thing, indulge no more than once a week.

- 80 baked pita puffs
- 68 Sunshine Krispy soup and oyster crackers
- 65 pretzel sticks dipped in 2 tablespoons of fat-free hot-fudge topping
- 43 Ritz Air Crisps (sour cream and onion flavor)
- 40 bite-size baked Tostitos, plus salsa
- 30 Orville Redenbacher's Peanut Caramel Crunch low-fat mini pop-corn cakes
- 30 baby carrots with ½ cup of low-fat dip
- 11 cups of Orville Redenbacher's Natural Light popcorn
- Three cherry Fruit-a-Freeze bars
- Two boxes (3 ounces each) of MicroMagic low-fat french fries
- Two snack-size bags of Baked Lays potato chips
- 2 cups of Quaker Crunchy Corn Bran
- One Veggie Delite sub (6-inch) from Subway
- One box of Nabisco Barnum's Animals crackers
- One baked apple, drizzled with 1 tablespoon of caramel sundae topping and sprinkled with cinnamon

Distract yourself for at least 10 minutes. If you're at home, take a shower or give yourself a manicure. (It's hard to binge when your nails are wet.) If you're at work, take a walk around your building, visit a colleague, or freshen up in the ladies' room.

Distance yourself from temptation. If you're at home, throw your binge food down the garbage disposal or bury it in the trash so you can't fish it out again. Leave the house if you have to. If you're out to dinner, ask the waiter to immediately wrap up half of the lumberjack-size entrée he's just set in front of you. If you go to the movies, arrive just before showtime, so there's no time to hit the concession stand.

Decide how you'll handle the situation. Will you stop—or continue? "Some women decide to keep eating," says Kern. "But they do so consciously. They know what they're doing, understand why, realize the consequences, and choose to proceed. They're exercising the power of choice, which is more advanced behavior."

The Seventh Commandment: Thou Shalt Freeze the Moment

On TV, when a policeman yells "Freeze!", the bad guy usually does. What if you could yell "Freeze!" at the start of a binge—or even midway through?

You can, with a simple technique called freezing the moment, says Dr. Musante. In this technique, you literally stop in your tracks—perhaps with a cookie halfway to your mouth or in the act of cutting yourself a fourth brownie.

Dr. Musante tells his clients to remember a scene from one of those old *Star Trek* episodes in which the characters are frozen in time and space. "When you freeze the moment, you have the opportunity to come to your senses."

Even if you don't stop eating, freezing the moment will at least give you the opportunity to control how much you eat. For example, instead of polishing off the entire pint of gourmet ice cream, measure out ½ cup, put it in a bowl, and put the carton away. Or measure out one serving (1 ounce) of chips into a bowl and seal the bag.

Freezing the moment also reminds you that you're in control, says Kern. "If you've had two cookies and not a third, you restore your sense of control," he says. "And instead of feeling bad that you had two, you can feel good that the lapse didn't become a *collapse*."

The Eighth Commandment: Thou Shalt Make Emergency Stops

When you're on the road and you blow a tire, you're supposed to stay calm and pull over to the side of the road. That's exactly what you need to do, metaphorically speaking, after you overeat.

"After a binge, women inevitably feel incredible anxiety and guilt, which can send them further out of control," says Kern. So in the first minutes after a binge, counter these awful feelings. On paper, reconstruct the entire episode. Pinpoint the circumstances that led to the binge and the strategies you might have tried to halt it at any point along the way.

The very act of thinking and writing may calm you, making you more receptive to what went wrong, says Kern. Which makes it easier to devise strategies that will help you avoid those circumstances next time. "If you learn something, then you've fallen forward rather than backward."

The Ninth Commandment: Thou Shalt Not Beat Thyself Up

To bounce back from a binge, you must forgive yourself, says Dr. Musante. That means you must silence the punishing voice in your head that says you're a glutton with no willpower.

Just as jelly beans are empty calories, shame and guilt are empty emotions. "They teach us nothing," says Dr. Musante. In fact, they may actually trigger another binge. When you beat yourself up, you're likely to turn to snack cakes to soothe yourself, says Dr. Musante. Or to starve yourself the next day, leaving you vulnerable to another pigout.

When that nasty chorus in your head starts to sing, silently shout, "STOP!" says Dr. Musante. (Or shout it out loud, if you're alone.) Then replace the negative message with a positive one, for example: "Yes, I slipped. I don't feel good about it, but I don't have to beat myself up either. I hereby forgive myself. And I'll do better tomorrow."

The Tenth Commandment: Thou Shalt Get Back in the Game

No matter what time of day your binge occurs and no matter how dispirited you feel, eat your next scheduled meal, advises Kern. When you immediately resume your normal eating pattern, you help fight off those "What does it matter? I've blown it so I may as well keep eating" blues.

Say you overate—big time—at lunch. "When dinnertime rolls around, simply eat the meal you'd planned to eat. It's a way to tell yourself that you're back in the game, so to speak, says Kern. And that you've begun to restore control to the person to whom it rightfully belongs—you."

Sticky Situations Solved

T

BY ROBERTA DUYFF, M.S., R.D. hink of your diet as a cross-country road trip. Your goal is to get from New York to Los Angeles without breaking down, getting lost, or colliding with someone or something.

To do that, you need to learn to read the danger signs, avoid the slippery slopes, and navigate the detours with ease and panache. That takes know-how, practice, and skill.

Fortunately, we've already made the trek. And we've not only identified potential roadblocks to success but also figured out ways around them.

Here, then, is your map to reach dietary success.

Navigating the Salad Bar

Don't let the "S" word fool you: The average salad bar plate can pack more calories than a deluxe burger, fries, and a shake, totaling more than 1,000 calories. In fact, in one study researchers found that 60 to 70 percent of the calories in a salad bar salad came from fat.

Here's how to avoid salad bar "potholes."

Take a smaller plate. Fill it rim to rim—but not sky high.

Disqualify fried foods and confections. This is a salad bar. Eat salad. Pass up anything batter-fried, be it chicken or zucchini. Go easy on ice cream or pudding.

Minimize the oil slick. While you may use fat-free mayo at home, salad bar salads do not. So go easy on the macaroni salad, coleslaw, and potato salad—or skip it entirely.

Pile up the veggies, beans, and fruit. They're loaded with vitamins, minerals, and fiber—with little or no fat. For more nutrients, pick dark leafy greens instead of iceberg lettuce. One cup of spinach has five times the calcium, twice the fiber, and several thousand times the vitamin A as the same amount of iceberg lettuce.

Slim down the dressings. Two tablespoons of a traditional dressing adds about 150 calories to an otherwise low-fat plate. Splash on some balsamic vinegar and just a drizzle of olive oil instead. You'll get the flavor plus an added bonus: The olive oil helps you absorb nutrient-rich carotenoids from the vegetables.

Slash the toppings. We're talking Chinese noodles and croutons. An ounce of croutons (½ cup), for instance, packs 65 calories and 2½ grams of fat.

Cruising the Buffet Table

Like a scenic mountaintop vista, buffet tables can be overwhelming. Only you can touch, smell, and taste this scenic wonder. But an expedition through an all-you-can-eat buffet isn't all that different than a trek across the Rockies. Just plan ahead and take it slow.

Map out your route. Survey each part of the buffet table—salads, soups, entrées, side dishes, breads, and desserts—before putting any food on your plate. Decide what you absolutely must have, then take it after thoughtful consideration.

Focus on getting your nutrition's worth, not your money's worth. Opt for steamed or grilled vegetables instead of those swimming in butter or cream sauce; fresh fruit versus pie topped with whipped cream; broiled poultry or fish rather than fried, and lean roast meats. Flavor them with just a drizzle of olive oil, if anything, for veggies and even bread. Use a splash of soy sauce for roasted meats, if needed, instead of gravy.

Take a one-way trip. Sit at a table on the other side of the room from the buffet so you won't be tempted by its aromas. Otherwise, it's just too easy to make a return trip.

Slow down. It takes about 20 minutes for your stomach to tell your brain that you're full. So put your fork down each time you try a different food.

Take it natural. Choose foods that are prepared simply: steamed shrimp, carved turkey breast, cherry tomatoes. If it's sitting in sauce or hidden under breading, go easy or skip it.

Chocolate Speed Bumps

Chocolate is a major treat for many women, and it's not hard to understand why. Nothing quite equals chocolate for flavor, creaminess, and pure indulgence. In fact, researchers now admit that a psychological chocolate craving does exist. So although we wouldn't recommend anything called the chocolate diet, we still think the luscious flavor can have a place in a woman's life. Go easy, though, because chocolate candy is loaded with calories and fat.

Consider cocoa. One ounce of cocoa powder has about 100 calories and 0.5 gram of fat, compared with 146 calories and 0.5 gram of fat in a 1-ounce chunk of unsweetened chocolate. Try substituting cocoa powder in baking recipes and puddings. You can even puree it with fat-free milk and ice for a low-fat smoothie.

Keep it small. Satisfy your craving with a small handful of chocolate chips, a miniature chocolate bar, or just two or three chocolate kisses. Always put them on a plate or a napkin and put the rest away.

Go for the best. Buy the very best chocolate you can, then freeze it. When the craving hits, pop one piece and see how much longer the lusciousness lingers. For fewer calories, choose chocolate-dipped fruit instead of chocolate fudge, chocolate angel food cake instead of devil's food cake with icing, and low-fat chocolate milk instead of a chocolate milkshake.

Cocktail Party Patrol

You're all dressed up, feeling beautiful, and networking your brains out when you realize that every other time you open your mouth it's not words going out but hors d'oeuvres going in. To eat (and drink) smarter on the cocktail party–reception–company shindig circuit, try these tips.

POWER

B R O W N I E S

NUTTY BROWNIES

These fudgy squares are the perfect antidote to a chocolate craving. We lowered the fat by using cocoa powder instead of baking chocolate and replacing some of the butter with applesauce. As a result, this recipe has about half the fat and twice the fiber as traditional walnut brownies. And because these brownies are dense, just one may be enough to get that yen for chocolate under control.

2	tablespoons melted butter
⅓	cup unsweetened applesauce
¾	cup sugar
½	cup unsweetened cocoa powder
1	egg or ¼ cup fat-free liquid egg substitute
1	teaspoon vanilla extract
½	cup whole wheat flour
⅓	cup finely chopped walnuts
	Confectioners' sugar (optional)

Preheat the oven to 350°F. Coat an 8" × 8" glass baking dish with cooking spray.

In a large bowl, stir together the butter and applesauce. One at a time, stir in the sugar, cocoa powder, egg or egg substitute, vanilla, flour, and walnuts until well-mixed. Spread the batter in the prepared pan.

Bake for 25 minutes or until the sides begin to pull away from the pan. Cool in the pan on a wire rack. Cut into squares and sprinkle with the confectioners' sugar, if using.

Makes 16

Per brownie: 88 calories, 2 g protein, 14 g carbohydrates, 4 g fat, 17 mg cholesterol, 1 g dietary fiber, 21 mg sodium

Water down the drinks. Just two glasses of wine or spiked punch, two mixed drinks, or two beers, and you've already downed more calories than a ½-hour walk later can use up. Not to mention that the more you drink, the less willpower you may have for avoiding the buffet table. But holding a drink isn't all bad. After all, it keeps one hand away from the chicken croquettes and baked Brie.

- Drink a glass of water in between each alcoholic beverage; you can even fill your empty beer bottle with water.
- Cut your wine with seltzer water and your mixed drinks with extra mixer.
- Load up your glass with ice before pouring anything into it.
- Make your own drinks in order to control the alcohol.
- Volunteer to drive. Then drink club soda or diet cola with no apologies.

Eat something beforehand. Have a bowl of soup or a piece of fruit before you arrive, so you're not facing temptation on an empty stomach. When the hors d'oeuvres make the rounds, graze selectively. Take one bite of whatever you want. Then discreetly discard your plate, pick up a clean one, and fill it with raw vegetables, steamed potstickers (small Chinese dumplings), and shrimp. (Be aware, though, that if the dumplings seem browned, they were probably pan-fried in small amounts of peanut oil.)

Pick the right hors d'oeuvres. This means making a wide turn around the Buffalo wings (200 calories and 15 grams of fat per one fried wing) and heading over to the vegetable lane. Watch out! You nearly got side-swiped by the onion dip (50 calories and 4 grams of fat per 2 table-spoons). Park over by the steamed shrimp (10 calories and no fat per shrimp) and sushi (71 calories with 1 gram of fat per piece), and you can even pop a bacon-wrapped scallop in your mouth if the bacon just wraps around once (39 calories with 2 grams of fat).

Stay active. Dance, take photos, admire the artwork and the view, or help your hostess serve. There's plenty to do besides eat and drink.

The Holiday Slide

So you're driving along doing just fine on your new eating plan—note, that it's a plan, not a diet—when suddenly the weather cools and the leaves turn color. In stores everywhere, Halloween candy has replaced summer lawn chairs. In back, they're unpacking Christmas ornaments.

POWER

C O O K I E S

TOASTED-ALMOND KISSES

Keep a batch of these little "snowballs" on hand for when your sweet tooth demands attention. Since they're made with egg whites—and little else—they're very low in fat. And what fat they do contain comes from the almonds and is the cholesterol-lowering monounsaturated kind.

4	large egg whites, at room temperature
$\frac{1}{8}$	teaspoon salt
$\frac{3}{4}$	cup confectioners' sugar
$\frac{1}{2}$	cup granulated sugar
$\frac{3}{4}$	teaspoon vanilla extract
$\frac{1}{4}$	teaspoon almond extract
$\frac{1}{2}$	cup toasted and very finely chopped blanched almonds

Preheat the oven to 250°F. Line two baking sheets with parchment paper.

Caution: detour ahead. For the next few months, you may find yourself trying to swerve to avoid rich holiday cookies, trying not to get hit with fat-laden appetizers, and pushing through a blinding storm of baking, parties, and other temptations.

"I Brake for Cookies." We know. What's Christmas without Christmas cookies? All 12 varieties, 36 dozen of them. The problem is that when you go to pack them into gift tins, you may only have half that amount left. The rest may be providing some winter warmth around your hips. So try this.

• Use applesauce, mashed bananas, or pureed fruit for half the fat in cookie recipes.

• Toast nuts to bring out the full flavor, then use only half the amount called for.

Place the egg whites and salt in a large bowl. Beat with an electric mixer on low speed until foamy.

In a small bowl, combine the confectioners' sugar and granulated sugar. Gradually add 1 tablespoon at a time to the egg whites, beating well after each addition, until the whites are stiff and shiny. Beat in the vanilla and almond extract. Gently fold in the almonds.

Drop heaping teaspoonfuls of the batter, 1" apart, onto the baking sheets.

Bake for 35 minutes, switching the position of the sheets halfway through. Turn off the oven and let the cookies stay in the oven for 30 minutes longer.

Let cool on a wire rack. Peel the cookies from the paper and store in an airtight container.

Makes 72

Per cookie: 16 calories, 0 g protein, 3 g carbohydrates, 0.5 g fat, 0 mg cholesterol, 0 g dietary fiber, 4 mg sodium

Note: It's best to bake meringue cookies on a cool, dry day, or they will be too sticky.

- Cut calories per cookie by making cookies smaller.

- Try gingersnaps instead of chocolate chip cookies or oatmeal cookies instead of peanut butter cookies.

- Schedule your holiday baking right after dinner, when you're full. Then package the cookies into tins the minute they're cool, seal them with brightly colored plastic wrap, and store them upstairs in a cool, dry, out-of-the-way place until it's time to serve or deliver them.

- Buy, don't bake. A great idea if you really don't enjoy baking but need the cookies as gifts or for school parties. Just wait until the day you need them to buy the cookies, so you're less likely to raid them.

Survive the holiday dinner calorie pileup. Why do all of our celebrations revolve around at least one really big, no-holds-barred dinner?

There's turkey at Thanksgiving, fried potato pancakes at Hanukkah, stuffed goose at Christmas, baked ham at Easter. . . . It takes a day or more to prepare the meal and all of 10 minutes to demolish it—and the rest of the month to work it off.

True, Christmas (and Thanksgiving, Easter, the Fourth of July, your birthday, and your husband's birthday) only comes once a year. Add your niece's wedding, your nephew's graduation, ad infinitum, and celebrating soon becomes a way of life. To avoid too many just-this-once pounds:

- Take a tablespoon-size serving of each dish. By the time you eat it all, chances are you'll be satisfied.
- Discard the turkey skin. You'll save 140 calories per drumstick.
- Skip the butter for the rolls, or use one pat, not two, and say so long to 35 calories that you'll never miss.
- Choose cranberry sauce (¼ cup has 110 calories and almost no fat) instead of gravy.
- Have cookies or dessert, but not both.
- Eat just a sliver of pie, not a whole slice.
- Stick to your regular schedule. Just because dinner is being served at 3:00 P.M. doesn't mean you should skip lunch. So have a light lunch at noon; then you won't be starving when dinner is served.
- Make an after-meal walk part of the holiday tradition.

Weekend Blowouts

Your weight-control strategies may stay on track during the routine of the workday, but let the weekend hit and all bets are off. It's like hitting the road in your father's car just after getting your driver's license for the first time. Here's how to avoid a crash.

Get out of the house. Get away from the refrigerator. Try hiking, biking, walking, or gardening. In bad weather, walk at the mall (just leave your wallet home so that you're not tempted by the cinnamon buns).

Watch out for festival food. By all means, take in craft fairs, art walks, antique shows, or jazzfests. But watch those food stands: If sausage and sandwiches, cheese fries, and fried crabcakes leave your hands greasy, think of what eating too many can do to your waistline and arteries. Still, sampling food is part of the experience. Here are the alternatives.

• Stroll ahead and scout out all of your options. Opt for healthier fare (yes, it does exist) like a grilled turkey leg or fruit smoothie.

• Carry a couple of dollars and a credit card with you. Many food vendors won't take plastic, so you're limiting the temptation.

> ### MASKED DISASTER
> #### Caesar Salad
> A Caesar side salad may have only 210 calories, but it has 17 grams of fat—mainly from the anchovies, egg, oil, and cheese in the dressing. Your best bet is to get the salad without the dressing or try the romaine lettuce with oil and vinegar instead.

Skip the Sunday brunch. It is very tempting to grab the newspaper and head out for a "real" (that is, diner) breakfast when you don't have to report to the office. But figure that two slices of bacon, two fried eggs, and two pieces of buttered toast mean nearly 500 calories and 33 grams of fat. Instead, treat yourself to a special breakfast and the Sunday paper but keep it healthy with a cup of egg substitute, one slice of toast spread with 1 tablespoon of jam instead of butter, and one slice of Canadian bacon. This totals 295 calories, with about 6 grams of fat.

Movie Minefields

A few years ago, a consumer watchdog group reported that movie-theater popcorn is swimming in saturated fat. A large popcorn cooked in coconut oil with butter topping has about 80 grams of fat, more than 50 of them saturated. That's almost 3 days' worth of the recommended limit for this artery-clogging saturated fat, or what you'd get from six McDonald's Big Macs.

Sitting in a movie without a box of popcorn or a candy bar is like hitting the beach without shaving your legs first. You just can't do it. So instead:

Bring your own. Three-and-a-half cups of air-popped popcorn has about 110 calories; the same amount of theater popcorn has as much as 301 calories—and you know you aren't going to stop at $3\frac{1}{2}$ cups. Even a kid-size order in the theater has twice that much.

POWER

BAKED POTATOES
WITH MUSHROOM STROGANOFF

Stroganoff? We're not kidding. This notorious Russian fat trap gets a slimming makeover thanks to lower-fat yogurt and sour cream. The shiitake mushrooms lend more than just meaty taste and texture to this tater topper—studies show that they contain a variety of cancer-preventing compounds.

4	medium baking potatoes
1	small onion, finely chopped
1	tablespoon canola oil
8	ounces shiitake mushrooms, thinly sliced
¼	teaspoon dried thyme
¼	teaspoon salt
¼	teaspoon ground black pepper
2	tablespoons balsamic vinegar
1	cup low-fat plain yogurt
½	cup reduced-fat sour cream

Pick Jujubes. They'll take you so long to chew, the closing credits will be rolling before you finish the box. And at 120 calories for 54 pieces (and no fat), you won't be blowing your entire diet.

Mr. Potato Head at the Wheel

You say tomato, he says french fries. You say veggie burger, he says New York strip steak. Even if you're married to a meat-and-potatoes guy who eschews "diet" food, you can plan meals that make everyone happy.

Go for the grill. He can have his meat, and you can have grilled vegetables or fish or chicken, without dirtying another dish.

Preheat the oven to 400°F. Place the potatoes on a baking sheet and bake for 1 hour, or pierce them several times with a fork and cook in a microwave oven on high for 15 minutes. When done, they will be easily pierced with a knife.

In a large nonstick skillet over medium heat, cook the onion in the oil for 3 minutes. Add the mushrooms, thyme, salt, and pepper. Cook for 5 minutes. Stir in the vinegar and cook for 1 minute, or until the liquid evaporates.

In a small saucepan, whisk together the yogurt and sour cream. Stir over low heat for 5 minutes, or until warm. (Do not allow the mixture to get too hot or it will separate.)

Split the baked potatoes. Top with the yogurt mixture and the mushrooms.

Makes 4 servings

Per serving: 250 calories, 9 g protein, 38 g carbohydrates, 8 g fat, 4 mg cholesterol, 4 g dietary fiber, 209 mg sodium

Build a better burger. Add nutrients by jazzing up burgers. Start with lean meat. Try ground turkey or chicken breast, or even vegetable or salmon patties. Flavor them with great herbs like fresh dill, basil, or oregano. Use chutneys, horseradish, or gourmet mustards instead of high-fat mayo. Layer the burgers with tomato and onion slices, grilled peppers and mushrooms, or spinach leaves and pineapple slices. Also, exchange plain white-bread buns with whole wheat bread for more fiber.

Challenge him to a duel. A nutritional duel, that is. If you're trying to lose weight, chances are he could lose a few pounds, too. See who can lose 4 to 5 pounds within a month. Or see who can actually get those six to nine servings of fruits and vegetables and 30 grams of fiber a day. The loser has to do the laundry—and put it away—for the next month.

Picky Kids in Tow

How many times have you felt so proud of yourself for cooking a healthful, nutritious meal, only to have your children react as if you'd just handed them a summer reading list? It's enough to make you buy stock in frozen chicken nuggets.

But the munchkins need a healthful diet as much as you do. Here are some ways to get your kids to eat the nutritious meals you cook without bringing child protective services to your door.

Let picky kids pick. Give them choices: Chicken or fish? Broccoli or carrots? Brown rice or polenta? But always keep the choices to two and keep both equally healthful. You're giving your child a sense of control—without giving up smart eating yourself.

Let 'em help. Yeah, this might be asking for trouble, but it's amazing how much more delectable that swordfish looks to your 7-year-old when he's the one who got to sprinkle on the soy sauce and chopped ginger.

Sneak in the healthful food. If macaroni and cheese is all she'll eat, mix in some peas or carrots, some tuna or chicken. Instead of fried chicken nuggets, make your own and bake them. Use prepared pizza shells and load the pie with vegetables instead of pepperoni and cheese. If your child is a peanut butter lover, try stuffing celery with peanut butter, or make a peanut butter sauce to go with a stir-fry.

Build your own. With these dinners, kids will be so busy creating, they won't have time to notice all the—*gasp!*—healthful ingredients.

- Build-your-own-pita-pockets night. Put out whole wheat pita bread sliced in half; small pieces of sliced turkey breast or low-fat cheese; and veggies including lettuce, sliced tomatoes, sliced onions, cucumbers, sprouts, or whatever else you like.

- Build-your-own-burrito night. Put out cooked ground turkey, cooked kidney or black beans, hot sauce, black olives, rice, torn lettuce, diced tomatoes, and warmed flour tortillas.

- Build-your-own-baked-potato night. Put out grated Parmesan cheese, fat-free plain yogurt flavored with curry or dill, ratatouille, canned or frozen peas, salsa, steamed broccoli, and grated low-fat Cheddar cheese.

POWER

MACARONI AND CHEESE

QUICK PASTA AND CHEESE

No baking needed for this fast stovetop recipe. But what really makes this dish special is the flavor boost it gets from horseradish and tomato paste. Better yet, these two ingredients contain potent cancer-fighting compounds.

12	ounces elbow macaroni or medium shells
1	tablespoon butter or margarine
2	tablespoons unbleached or all-purpose flour
2	cups 1% milk
2	tablespoons tomato paste
2	teaspoons Dijon mustard
2	teaspoons prepared horseradish
3/4	teaspoon salt
1½	cups shredded sharp Cheddar cheese

In a large pot of boiling water, cook the pasta according to the package directions. Drain and return to the pan.

In a medium saucepan, melt the butter or margarine over medium heat. Whisk in the flour and cook, stirring, for 2 minutes. Slowly whisk in the milk and cook, stirring, for 5 minutes, or until the sauce begins to thicken. Whisk in the tomato paste, mustard, horseradish, and salt. Add the cheese and stir for 1 minute, or just until melted.

Pour the cheese mixture over the pasta. Stir over medium heat for 1 minute, or until the pasta is hot.

Makes 6 cups

Per cup: 406 calories, 20 g protein, 51 g carbohydrates, 12.5 g fat, 38 mg cholesterol, 2 g dietary fiber, 691 mg sodium

Stick to your guns. Missing a meal won't hurt them. If they continually refuse to eat what you've fixed, then just set the rule: This is dinner. Eat it or don't, but the kitchen is now closed. You'll be amazed at how quickly they begin eating what you serve.

Office Oil Slicks

"Cake in the break room" flashes the e-mail. Before you know it, two pieces have disappeared down that dark hole otherwise known as your mouth. Then there's the jar of chocolate candies on your boss's desk. Ever wonder why she has to refill it after every meeting with you?

And let's not even go to the snack machine. Did you know that a daily bag of 1 ounce of chips (calorie content: 150) adds up to an extra 750 calories a week? That could explain the extra pound a month you've been mysteriously accumulating.

Saunter, don't stuff. Stressed by work? Take a walk—and we don't mean to the cafeteria. If the weather won't allow walking outside, walk the halls or up and down the stairs. Walk on a different floor where no one knows you. And don't feel guilty: Everyone is entitled to a break once in a while.

Join in—on your terms. Fit your coworkers' treats, such as a muffin or cookies, into your day's meal plan. Take one to enjoy later with lunch, rather than adding that muffin as a second dessert. If it's a midafternoon pick-me-up, take the treat home for an after-dinner dessert. When it's your turn to supply the munchies, set the standard with exotic fruits, whole grain bagels, or baby vegetables.

Stick with water. While everyone is standing around the break room nibbling cake, keep your hands and mouth busy with a bottle of water. After all, you need at least 9 cups of fluid daily. As an added bonus, water won't leave a sticky mess on your computer keyboard.

Road Trip

It feels like you've been on this interstate for days. Everything looks the same—billboards, road signs, monster trucks. Then you see it: a rest stop ahead, complete with kiosks selling cinnamon buns. Watch it. If you're not careful, you could actually end this car trip weighing more than when you began, since 1 hour of driving uses only about 110 calories and a Cinnabon contains 670 calories and 34 grams of fat (including 14 of them saturated).

There are alternatives.

Get off the main road. Instead of the ubiquitous burger and pizza chains lining interstate highways, pull onto a secondary road and look for family-style restaurants that offer more variety and other options, including grilled foods, fish that's not battered and fried, vegetables, and local specialties (unless it's chicken-fried steak).

Have a picnic. Stop at a grocery store or roadside stand and buy an instant picnic: lean deli meat, cheese, crusty whole grain bread, fresh fruit, cartons of yogurt, raw veggies, juice, and bottled water. Keep paper plates, napkins, and a few utensils in the car and find a picturesque (or at least quiet) spot to enjoy. Even that rest stop usually has picnic benches. Take a quick walk before getting back in the car.

Shop for the car. If you're like most women, you probably spend more time in your car than you do in your kitchen. So keep it stocked with long-lasting, healthful snacks like crackers, cereal bars, juice boxes, dried fruit, nuts, pretzels, rice cakes, whole wheat crackers, and bottled water. You may not necessarily save a huge number of calories. But your meal or snack will consist of nutritious, lower-fat foods.

> **MASKED DISASTER**
> ### Fried Fish
> Baked, broiled, steamed, or grilled, fish is a great choice. But fast-food restaurants typically offer fried-fish sandwiches—with plenty of tartar sauce—at 430 calories apiece. You're better off ordering a grilled chicken breast sandwich at 310 calories or even a small burger at 275 calories.

Excess Vacation Baggage

Just because you're leaving behind the computer, e-mail, cell phone, and deadlines doesn't mean that you should leave behind your healthy eating plan. After all, an extra 5 pounds wasn't exactly the souvenir you had in mind.

Pack appropriately. We're talking exercise clothes and athletic shoes. And use them at least once a day.

Make lunch your main meal. We figure you're going to be eating all your meals out, so save your main meal for lunch. Lunch portions are typically smaller than dinner and usually cost less. Take the afternoon to work off calories on a walking tour.

Eat like the natives. Especially if you're traveling overseas, you'll find that most countries have a great many more fruits and vegetables and whole grains served with meals. Take advantage of it.

Choose the right vacation. A spa, for instance, typically features meals and snacks consisting of fruits, vegetables, whole grain foods, low-fat dairy foods, and lean meat, poultry, and fish. Or try an adventure vacation like skiing, visiting a dude ranch, hiking, or taking a bike tour. You'll be burning up so many calories that how much you eat probably won't be an issue.

Missing the Exit for Breakfast

When *Prevention* magazine asked women about their fantasy foods, high-fat breakfast foods like doughnuts and cinnamon buns made the top 10. Yet women are notorious breakfast skippers. We're either too busy, not hungry, or think we'll save the calories for later.

Big mistake. Studies show that thin people tend to eat breakfast, while overweight people tend to skip it. They just make up for it later by overeating or making poor food choices. Here's how to eat a better breakfast, quickly and painlessly.

Drink your breakfast. Fruit smoothies are nutritious, quick, and portable. Slug yours down in the car on the way to work. Just puree fruit (peaches, bananas, kiwifruit, melon, berries, or even applesauce), fat-free yogurt, and ice into a thick, refreshing drink. Sprinkle some wheat germ, wheat bran, or instant oatmeal on top for a nutritional boost. All together, this first-thing-in-the-morning powerhouse breakfast provides nutrients, including calcium, not to mention that it's low in fat.

Skip it now; eat it later. When mornings are too hectic or you just can't stomach food first thing, plan ahead. Tuck some fruit, a bagel, cheese and crackers, or a muffin in a bag. Stock your office refrigerator with cartons of yogurt and fat-free milk and an empty file drawer with single-serving sizes of high-fiber cereal.

Jump-start your morning the night before. Fill your cereal bowl, slice fruit, hard-cook an egg, reconstitute juice, set the timer so your bread machine bakes while you sleep, or assemble a breakfast sandwich (perhaps raisin bread, lean ham, and cheese)—wrap it up and have it waiting in the fridge.

Forget dessert for breakfast. It's tempting, what with sweet muffins, pastries, and doughnuts all considered breakfast foods. But if you grab a large almond croissant, you'll get more fat and calories than in two Dove Bars.

Watch out for the fast-food breakfast. McDonald's bagel sandwiches have at least double the fat and the calories of the 290-calorie Egg McMuffin.

Try these great grab-and-go breakfasts:

- Spread 2 tablespoons of hummus (chickpea spread) on half a pumpernickel bagel.

> **MASKED** DISASTER
>
> **Jumbo Bagel with a Smear**
>
> Doughnut or bagel? If you're slathering a super-size bagel with cream cheese, you might as well have the doughnut. Two tablespoons of regular cream cheese adds 100 calories and 10 grams of fat to that 195-calorie, practically fat-free bagel for a total of 295 calories. The doughnut isn't much different, supplying about 245 calories and 15 grams of fat.
>
> Try half a bagel with fat-free cream cheese, which has just 32 calories and 1 gram of fat in 2 tablespoons.

- Stuff half a whole wheat pita with ½ cup of 1% cottage cheese and sliced peaches, pears, or banana.

- Roll up a tortilla with scrambled egg substitute and salsa.

Lunch on the Lam

In between running errands to the dry cleaner, bank, and drugstore, you realize you're starving. Small wonder. It is, after all, your *lunch* hour. So you see a burger haven and hit the blinker.

Go beyond burgers and fries. Search for the unique. A box of sushi from the ready-to-eat grocery section. A turkey sub from Subway. A bagel sandwich with low-fat fillings.

If you can't get out of your car and fast food is the only thing for miles, then order smart. A deluxe bacon cheeseburger, large fries, and a 12-ounce soft drink can weigh in at a whopping 1,185 calories and 52 grams of fat. A plain hamburger and a small salad with fat-free dressing has only 345 calories with 9 grams of fat. A grilled chicken sandwich with no sauce has about 300 calories with 5 grams of fat. Add a carton of low-fat milk; you need the calcium.

Eating at Your Desk

If you're not out running errands during lunch, you're probably wolfing it down at your desk between phone calls and e-mails. We call this mindless eating. Taste anything? Feel anything? A better strategy is to eat deliberately. Here's how.

Order smart to eat in. Keep a file of interesting take-out menus—with their nutrition facts, if possible—so your choices stretch beyond burgers and fries or a pale vending machine sandwich of cold cuts and white bread.

Prepare once, eat twice. You're cooking healthy for dinner these days, so double the recipe, then pack a portion in a container for lunch the next day.

Grocery shop for the office. Chances are there's a refrigerator somewhere in your building and a few inches of space in a desk drawer. Stock up on low-fat soups and bean stews, single-serving cans of tuna packed in spring water, low-fat crackers and whole wheat breads, canned fruits and unsweetened applesauce, yogurt, bananas, apples, and oranges. Keep plastic forks, spoons, and knives in the drawer and a stack of paper plates for impromptu lunches.

DON'T EAT AND DRIVE

Half of all auto accidents occur because the driver isn't paying attention, according to the National Highway Traffic Safety Administration. If you have to run those errands at lunch, don't try to eat on the run. Instead, pack a sandwich and fruit and find 5 minutes at a picnic table somewhere, or even sit in your car at a park.

Waistline

A typical restaurant meal without an appetizer or dessert contains 1,000 calories.

The Business Lunch Binge

If you're like the average woman, you eat out about four times a week, usually lunch. And if you're on an expense account, you're likely to overdo it. Unless you:

Order simply good foods. Go for something broiled or grilled, without gravies and rich sauces. See how many servings of fruits and vegetables you can get at this meal—even without the ubiquitous chicken Caesar salad.

Make it your main meal. Promise yourself that supper will be some cut-up fruit, raw veggies, yogurt, and two crackers.

Be first. Order before anyone else to avoid letting others' choices influence you.

Order extra veggies. They'll fill you up without the calories of french fries.

Maintain balance. Have one splurge per restaurant trip and then round out the meal with healthful favorites. If you have to have the fettuccine Alfredo, have a big tossed salad as an appetizer and fruit for dessert.

Take charge. Pick the restaurant yourself, preferably one that offers healthful choices and is good about special menu requests, like no butter sauce on the fish and salad dressing served on the side.

Blinded by Night Eating

You gave the counter a final wipe, hung up the kitchen towel and turned out the lights at 7:15 P.M. So why are you back in the kitchen 2 hours later rooting around in the fridge like a wild boar in a patch of truffles?

Here are some ways to avoid the late-night nibbles.

Waistline

On any given day, 7 percent of Americans eat at McDonald's. The corporate goal is to have no American more than 4 minutes away from one of its restaurants. And that's only one fast-food chain.

Get enough during the day. Make a concerted effort to eat breakfast, midmorning snack, a healthful lunch (not an iceberg lettuce salad), midafternoon snack, and a complete dinner (not a bowl of air-popped popcorn).

Save your dinner dessert. Is it a sweet craving? Then have dessert later. Try low-fat, low-calorie choices like fresh peaches over frozen yogurt, berries on angel food cake, apple cobbler with oatmeal crumb topping, or fresh fruit–topped custard.

Reach for fruit. This is your last chance to get the recommended minimum quota of six servings a day of fruits and vegetables for the day. Because they're high in carbohydrates, fruits leave your stomach faster than gooey, rich desserts, so you may feel more comfortable at bedtime. Another filling, healthful evening snack is a bowl of high-fiber cereal with fat-free milk.

Just do something. Walk the dog, call a friend, put a load of clothes in the wash, or light an aromatic candle and take a bubble bath. And if TV is your version of Pavlov's bell, turn it off. Break the habits that make you eat at night, and you'll break the night-eating habit.

What to Do When the Scale Gets Stuck

Power Maker #25: Before you get worked up about those last 5 to 10 pounds, ask yourself whether you may already be at your ideal weight. You may not achieve your goal *weight*. But if you look and feel great, you certainly have achieved your *goal*.

Nutritionists define a plateau as the cessation of weight loss at any point in a diet and exercise program. Many of us would describe it as the special circle of hell reserved for dieters.

For what better words describe the frustration of stepping on the scale and finding that, although you're watching what you eat and exercising faithfully, you weigh the same amount you did last week . . . and the week before that . . . and even the week before that?

No one knows what triggers a plateau or why some women are especially vulnerable to them, says Franca Alphin, R.D., a licensed dietitian and administrative director of the Duke University Diet and Fitness Center in Durham, North Carolina. "Some women may never hit a plateau, while others may hit one 3 weeks into their program and stay there for 4 weeks," she says.

So why does the scale get stuck in the first place? There are a few possible explanations. One theory is that a plateau may be your body's way of saying, "Hey! I need time to adjust to those lost pounds."

"When you eat less and exercise more, your body's hundreds of thousands of physiological processes change somewhat," says Alphin. "A plateau may be a catch-up mechanism that allows your body to adjust to these changes." Another possible cause is water retention. "The theory is that, over time, your body accumulates water, which is the end result of fat metabolism."

Or—and this is tough to admit—perhaps you've simply let your good intentions slide a bit.

"You're either consuming more calories than you did at the start of your weight-loss program or you're not exercising as much. Or possibly both," says Geralyn Coopersmith, an exercise physiologist, certified strength and conditioning specialist, and certified personal trainer at Trainer's Place in New York City. But regardless of what caused your plateau, one thing is certain: It's at this point that the tough keep going.

"Plateaus are a normal part of losing weight," says Susan Bartlett, Ph.D., assistant professor of medicine and a psychologist specializing in

STRIKE A BALANCE

The trimmer you get, the less effective your current diet and exercise program becomes—and the more likely you are to hit a plateau.

Why? Because the regimen that whittled you down from 175 to 150 pounds is unlikely to burn enough calories to get you to your goal weight of 140 pounds.

If you were 175 pounds when you started, your body burned 1,829 calories a day without exercise to maintain that weight. During exercise—for example, a daily 60-minute walk—you burned an extra 366 calories. In short, you burned 366 calories a day more than your body needed to maintain your "before" weight. Voilà!—the pounds peeled right off.

But at 150 pounds, your body requires only 1,568 calories. Further, at your new, lighter weight, your same hour-long walk burns only 312 calories. If you're still consuming 1,829 calories a day, you're not expending the amount of calories necessary to drop to your goal weight of 140 pounds (1,464 calories).

weight management at Johns Hopkins University School of Medicine in Baltimore. "The best thing to do is carefully evaluate whether or not you really are following your program. In most cases, there's been a slow but gradual return to old habits, and that is what is causing the plateau. If you really are doing what you need to do, the plateau is a temporary blip. Stay the course, and soon your weight loss will resume."

There are, however, a few tips and tricks you can employ to help bust a plateau, says Alphin, "assuming that your goal weight is realistic and achievable." The following two-part plan may just unstick the needle on your scale—quickly and safely.

Get Calories under Control

Whether your plateau is a normal, natural part of weight loss or the result of a few too many run-ins with your favorite treats, the answer is to burn more calories than you're taking in. Here's how to get started.

Monitor "portion drift." Many women who get tantalizingly close to their goal weights unconsciously start eating larger and larger portions, says Michelle Munyon, R.D., outpatient nutrition specialist for the Kennedy Health System, a community-based hospital system in Voorhees, New Jersey. To get back on track, arm yourself with a measuring cup and a food scale and measure out portions every day for 1 week, she suggests. Once you've reacquainted yourself with what one serving of pasta or chicken salad actually looks like, measure or weigh your food choices 1 day a week to keep yourself honest.

Simplify portion control. Stock your freezer with frozen "light" meals. You'll know exactly how many calories you are consuming—and save yourself the hassle of measuring portions.

Eat some skinny minis. Eating mini-meals every 3 to 4 hours can help keep your blood sugar steady, which can quell hunger pangs and thereby make it easier for you to stick to your diet, says Lorna Pascal, R.D., a nutrition consultant for the Dave Winfield Nutrition Center at the Hackensack University Medical Center in New Jersey.

For example, instead of "spending" all your calories on three meals, you might eat five or six mini-meals a day—three squares plus a midmorning, midafternoon, and prime-time snack, says Pascal. Limit each mini-meal to 250 to 350 calories. For best results, include some protein. Here's an example of a day's meals.

Breakfast: ¾ cup of whole grain cereal with half a banana, sliced, and ½ cup of fat-free milk (192 calories)

Midmorning: 1 cup of seedless grapes and a container of low-fat yogurt (257 calories)

Lunch: One small whole wheat roll, ½ cup of sliced fresh fruit (339 calories)

Midafternoon: 1 ounce of Cheddar cheese, five whole wheat crackers, one small apple (266 calories)

Dinner: 3 ounces broiled lean meat, one small baked potato, 1 cup of steamed asparagus, one small melon wedge (345 calories)

Prime-time snack: 3 cups of air-popped popcorn flavored with Butter Buds (97 calories)

Total calories: 1,496

One caveat: "Women who are binge eaters or compulsive eaters are usually not good candidates for the mini-meal approach because they may not be able to limit how much they eat at one sitting," says Alphin.

Redistribute your calories. Do you tend to skimp on breakfast and lunch and eat a huge dinner? Bad idea, says Alphin. You tend to burn calories consumed at night more slowly, because you are not as physically active then. Instead, consume the bulk of your calories at breakfast and lunch and eat a lighter dinner. "You're more physically active during the day, so you have higher calorie needs. You'll also burn off the bulk of those calories during the day."

Eat more. If you've been following a diet of less than 1,200 calories a day (think of those "Lose 5 pounds in 5 days!" diets in the women's magazines), your metabolism assumes that your body is starving, says Pascal. So it starts burning calories more slowly—just what you *don't* need. Her advice is to consume an extra 100 to 200 calories a day for 1 week. It may be enough to flip off your metabolism's starvation switch.

Make like a sponge. Drink a minimum of nine 8-ounce glasses of water a day. "When you're dehydrated, your body conserves fluid," says Alphin. "Drinking more water may allow you to shed some of it."

Revamp Your Workout

Shaking up your workout may also help propel you out of a plateau. The following strategies can help you burn more calories during your workouts—and may nudge the needle on the scale southward once again.

IS IT A PLATEAU,
OR IS IT YOUR IDEAL WEIGHT?

Sometimes, what seems like a plateau isn't. Should you even bother trying to lose that extra 10 pounds? Before you decide, consider the following questions.

ARE YOU STRENGTH TRAINING? Muscle gained during strength training is heavier than fat. But it's also healthier—and it looks better, too.

WHERE'S THE WEIGHT? If your extra pounds are around your middle, they could be increasing your risk of heart disease, diabetes, and some types of cancer.

WHAT DO THE NUMBERS SAY? Developing high cholesterol, high blood pressure, or high blood sugar may be the first indications that your weight is affecting your health.

ARE YOU LIVING ON PLANET EARTH? Is it realistic to eat any less or exercise any more than you already are?

Become a workout klutz. You've heard the expression "Work smarter, not harder." That's exactly what your muscles do when they have been performing the same workout over and over. And the more efficient your body becomes, the fewer calories you burn.

The solution? Switch to a different workout, says Coopersmith. Let's say walking is your exercise of choice. "If you start swimming, your body will be very inefficient because it will be using different muscles and movements," she says. "The good news is that inefficiency burns more calories." While the increased calorie burn amounts to only a few calories per minute, "those calories really add up during the course of a workout."

Stretch out your workout. "Another way to burn more calories is to exercise longer," says Coopersmith. She suggests extending the length of your workouts by 10 percent every 2 weeks. For example, if you normally walk 30 minutes, start walking another 3 minutes. After 2 weeks, shoot for just over 36 minutes. In 3 months, you should be able to walk a whole hour.

Too busy for an hour-long workout? Break it into two 30-minute sessions. You might walk for 30 minutes at lunch and then get on the treadmill for the length of your favorite prime-time sitcom.

Waistline

In a *Prevention/NBC Today* survey, 70 percent of women reported hitting weight-loss plateaus, despite following their diet and exercise programs to the letter.

Lift pounds to drop pounds. When you lose extra pounds, you typically lose muscle right along with them. This loss of your body's calorie-burning machinery depresses your metabolism, so you burn fewer calories.

To lose fat without losing calorie-burning muscle, add resistance training to your workout program, recommends Melyssa St. Michael, a certified personal trainer and owner of UltraFit Human Performance, a personal training and nutrition facility in Lutherville, Maryland. For every pound of muscle you build, you burn an extra 40 to 50 calories per day.

What's more, strength training for 45 minutes at a moderate intensity also increases your resting metabolism from 25 to 30 percent for 4 hours afterward, says St. Michael, and that further increases your calorie burn.

Pump up the intensity of your workouts. Incorporating interval training (alternating short, intense bouts of exercise with slower "recovery" phases) is another primo calorie burner, says Coopersmith.

Let's say you walk at a pace of 4 miles per hour. "To pump up the intensity, walk for 1 minute at a 4.5- to 4.8-mile-per-hour pace, and repeat this every 3 minutes," she says. "During that higher-intensity minute, you burn slightly more calories than normal." Alternate between these speeds for the entire length of your workout. If you use a treadmill or stationary bike, "try their built-in, preset interval programs," says Coopersmith.

How intense your intervals are depends on your level of fitness, she adds. If you're reasonably fit, you might want to do intervals at the highest intensity for 30 to 45 seconds. If you're working toward getting in shape, try doing intervals of moderate intensity for 1 to 3 minutes.

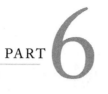

PART 6

FOOD POWER TO FIGHT DISEASE AND AGING

Food-as-Medicine Breakthroughs for Women

DIETARY CHANGES COULD PREVENT AT LEAST 30 PERCENT OF CANCERS WORLDWIDE!

DIET REDUCES BLOOD PRESSURE AS WELL AS DRUGS—IN AS LITTLE AS 14 DAYS!

"REVERSAL DIET" STOPS EVEN SEVERE HEART DISEASE IN ITS TRACKS!

The headlines are simulated. But the message is real: Food—our fuel and our bliss, our prime source of physical, and perhaps emotional, sustenance—is also medicine.

And when it comes to the science of nutrition, it's a brave new world. Research into the potential healing power of food and diet is ever more sophisticated, and the breakthroughs more rapid—and compelling.

"Nutrition is truly a dynamic area of research," says Barbara Schneeman, Ph.D., assistant administrator for human nutrition at the USDA Agricultural Research Service in Washington, D.C. "We're still at the tip of the iceberg in terms of understanding the role that various food components play in promoting health and preventing disease. And we're discovering new functions for nutrients we've known about for over a half-century. Our emerging research is providing new insights into the health benefits of diets rich in plant foods."

Phytonutrients, compounds found only in plant foods, protect against a Pandora's box of maladies, from cancer and heart disease to yeast infections.

Calcium, long known to protect against the bone-thinning disease osteoporosis, also helps reduce blood pressure. The B vitamin folate (the naturally occurring form of folic acid), which helps prevent birth defects, may also reduce the risk of heart disease, the number one killer of American women. Avoiding certain foods can help relieve women-only conditions such as premenstrual syndrome and fibroids.

In short, the diet/disease connection is evident—and the discoveries just keep coming. Here's a roundup of common health conditions and the foods that research suggests may help prevent or treat them.

Anemia

The Power Foods: Iron-rich foods such as meat, oysters and mussels, beans

Anemia is definitely a woman thing. From 3 to 5 percent of us have this blood condition, characterized by a reduction in the size or number of our red blood cells. As a result, our bodies can't make enough hemoglobin, the protein in red blood cells that ferries oxygen from our lungs to the rest of our bodies. Basically, our tissues are starving for oxygen, leaving us weak, pale, breathless, cold, and depressed.

In men or women, anemia can result from a number of conditions, such as severe blood loss or chronic internal bleeding. Menstruation makes women vulnerable: We can lose from 1 to 2 milligrams of iron each day of our periods. (Those of us who don't menstruate don't usually lose much iron.) But another cause of anemia is not eating enough iron-rich foods. Fully 75 percent of us don't get the recommended 18 milligrams of iron a day, the Daily Value (DV) for premenopausal women.

The antidote is to fill our plates with high-iron foods. Three ounces of oysters contains 6.6 milligrams of iron. The same amount of steamed blue mussels has 5.7 milligrams. Some other good sources of iron include 3 ounces of top round or top sirloin, a baked potato, or ½ cup of navy beans or black beans.

POWER-EATING TIP

Eat enough iron-rich foods such as meat, oysters and mussels, and beans to meet the Daily Value of 18 milligrams of iron.

Arthritis

The Power Foods: Cold-water fish (or fish oil), a vegetarian diet low in total and saturated fats

Experts predict that by the year 2020, almost 20 percent of Americans will have arthritis, a disease that affects the areas in or around our joints. Arthritis comes in many varieties. In rheumatoid arthritis (RA), which affects 2.1 million Americans, the immune system attacks the synovium, the membrane lining the joints. The resulting inflammation can damage bone and cartilage, the shock-absorbing material that cushions the ends of our bones. RA affects two to three times more women than men.

Osteoarthritis (OA), which affects more than 20 million Americans, is the result of years of wear and tear on cartilage. While the odds of developing OA rise with age, other factors have a significant impact on risk. For example, being overweight can lead to osteoarthritis of the knees.

Claims abound that certain foods, diets, or supplements can ease the pain and swelling of arthritis. While some of these claims are pure quackery, there's reason to believe that diet does affect arthritis, especially RA.

There's strong evidence that fish—especially fish high in omega-3 fatty acids such as salmon, mackerel, brook trout, bluefish, and herring—helps decrease the risk of RA. Eskimos and other ethnic groups who eat lots of fish are less likely to develop the condition than those who don't. One American study of 1,569 women found that those who ate two or more servings of fish a week were half as likely to develop RA as those who ate less than one serving. Researchers speculate that fish's high content of omega-3 fatty acids may affect the immune response that causes RA.

A low-fat vegetarian diet also seems to ease arthritis symptoms. When researchers in Norway put men and women with rheumatoid arthritis on such a diet for a year, their symptoms improved significantly. Moreover, a follow-up study on this same group found that those who continued on the plan continued to experience less pain, morning stiffness, and joint tenderness and swelling than those who returned to their regular diets.

POWER-EATING TIP

Eat two servings of cold-water fish a week, and focus on a vegetarian diet filled with fresh fruits and vegetables, whole grains, and low-fat or fat-free dairy products.

Asthma

The Power Foods: Foods high in vitamins C and E and magnesium, cold-water fish, fruits and vegetables, green tea

More than 17 million Americans experience the shortness of breath, chest tightness, coughing, and wheezing of asthma. In this chronic lung condition, the muscular bands that regulate the size of the bronchial tubes in the lungs tighten, making it difficult to breathe. The lungs of people with asthma are "twitchy," meaning that they overreact to substances that are harmless to others. These include allergens such as dust mites, pet dander, and pollen, irritants such as cigarette smoke or cold air, exercise, and emotional stress.

There's some evidence that vitamin C and vitamin E, as antioxidants, may help protect the lungs against the damaging effects of free radicals. In a study of 77,866 women, researchers found that women who got the most vitamin E from diet—not from supplements—were 47 percent less likely to have asthma than those getting the least.

Some research has linked magnesium—found in spinach and beans—with an improvement in asthma symptoms, presumably because this mineral helps relax the smooth muscles that line the airways, allowing more air to get through. In one study, researchers exposed 2,633 people with asthma to an airway-constricting chemical. They found that those whose diets were lowest in magnesium were twice as likely to have their airways close up as people who consumed the most.

The omega-3 fatty acids in cold-water fish such as mackerel, herring, and salmon, known to reduce the body's inflammatory response, may also help reduce asthma-caused inflammation in the lungs. In one large survey, researchers found that in families that ate very little oily fish, less than 16 percent of the children had asthma. But in families who didn't eat fish, the rate of asthma in children was 23 percent.

One group of phytonutrients called bioflavonoids has been shown to block the release of histamines, leukotrienes, and prostaglandins—chemicals that trigger contractions of the smooth muscle of the airways—and to slow inflammatory reactions. One particular bioflavonoid, quercetin—found in fruits, vegetables, tea, and red wine—is chemically similar to cromolyn, a drug that slows the release of histamines.

POWER - EATING TIP

Research suggests that 200 milligrams of vitamin C a day—the amount in about 2 cups of sliced strawberries—will help keep lungs strong. Other excellent sources of vitamin C include papaya, cantaloupe, broccoli, and tomatoes. Shoot for 30 IU of vitamin E per day from food and a multivitamin supplement. Good sources are nuts and seeds and wheat germ. Be sure to get 400 milligrams of magnesium, which is the Daily Value and the amount used in research. Include one to two servings of cold-water fish a week—anchovies, tuna, herring, or salmon. Try to eat nine servings of fruits and vegetables a day. One serving equals one medium fruit, ½ cup of chopped fruit, ½ cup of cooked or raw veggies, 1 cup of raw greens, or ¾ cup of fruit or vegetable juice.

Breast Cancer

The Power Foods: Soy; all vegetables, especially onions and garlic and carrots; olive oil

Breast cancer ranks behind only heart disease and lung cancer as the leading annual cause of death among women. While some risk factors can't be changed (such as genetics, aging, and family history of breast cancer), others are well within our control. For example, research suggests that women who are overweight and get little or no regular exercise increase their risk for the disease.

Diet also influences risk. A diet high in fiber and "good" monounsaturated fats (as opposed to saturated fats, found in animal foods such as sausage, cheese, and butter) may reduce risk. Similarly, a meat-heavy diet has been linked to increased risk, possibly because meat raises a woman's estrogen levels, and high estrogen levels are thought to fuel the development of breast cancer. Having three to four alcoholic beverages a week also increases risk.

Other studies have linked certain foods or groups of foods to reduced risk. Here's the dynamic quintet of breast cancer battlers.

Soybeans, soy milk, and soy foods. Soybeans and the foods made from them, such as soy milk and tofu, are rich in phytoestrogens. These plant-based compounds, such as isoflavones, weakly mimic a woman's natural estrogen. Isoflavones are thought to reduce the effects of estrogen in pre-menopausal women and—strangely—to enhance its effects in post-

ESCAPE OF THE WOMAN-SAVING NUTRIENTS

When it comes to getting the recommended daily amounts of calcium, folate, and iron, women are missing the boat. That's serious, because these vitamins and minerals can reduce our odds of developing a trio of woman-targeting conditions: osteoporosis, heart disease, and iron-deficiency anemia. Here are the government's recommendations—and our average intake through diet.

VITAMIN/ MINERAL	WE NEED	WE GET	CONDITION ASSOCIATED WITH DEFICIENCY	TOP SOURCES
Calcium	1,000 mg per day (women under 50); 1,500 mg per day (women 50 and over)	About 750 mg a day	Osteoporosis	Low-fat milk and milk products, sardines with bones, tofu, greens (spinach, kale), broccoli
Folate	400 mcg a day	About 235 mcg a day	Heart disease	Beans, leafy green vegetables (spinach, turnip greens), broccoli, green beans, asparagus, legumes
Iron	18 mg a day	About 12 mg a day	Iron-deficiency anemia	Canned clams, tofu, red meat, fish, poultry, shellfish, eggs, legumes

menopausal women. So including soy foods as part of an overall healthy diet may lower breast cancer risk in premenopausal women by counteracting the tumor-promoting influence of estrogen. In one study of 620 women with and without breast cancer, premenopausal women who ate soy products regularly reduced their risk by 60 percent. Eating soy did not decrease risk significantly in postmenopausal women.

Nutrient-dense vegetables. They're teeming with antioxidants such as vitamin C and beta-carotene, along with untold numbers of phytonutrients. Among a group of women with family histories of breast cancer, those who began eating more vegetables (five servings a day plus 16 ounces of fresh vegetable juice), three servings of fruit, and less beef and pork sustained less damage to their DNA, the genetic material that controls the workings of every cell. That's important, because there is strong evidence that damaged DNA can promote cancer. In this study, the strongest protection came from cooked veggies—possibly because the vegetables that we cook tend to be the most nutrient-dense, such as sweet potatoes, brussels sprouts, and broccoli.

Onions and garlic. Their organosulfur compounds block the access of cancer-causing substances to cells, suppress cancerous changes once they're underway, and stimulate the production of phase-2 enzymes, natural cancer blockers that help give cancer-causing toxins the boot. In a French study comparing 345 women with breast cancer to 345 healthy women, women who ate onions and garlic 7 to 10 times weekly had about half the risk of developing breast cancer as women who ate them less than 6 times a week. Women who ate them more than 16 times weekly had 70 percent less risk.

Carrots. They are a *numero uno* source of beta-carotene, a potent antioxidant that research has linked to a lower risk of breast cancer. In one study, researchers compared the eating habits of 3,543 women with breast cancer and 9,406 women without. Those who ate cooked carrots once a week or more had a 29 percent lower risk of developing breast cancer than those who never ate them.

Olive oil. Like Asian women, Greek women have significantly lower rates of breast cancer deaths than their American sisters. Some experts believe it's because most of the fat in their diets comes from olive oil and fish. Olive oil is a monounsaturated fat research links to a reduced risk of cancer in general, including breast cancer. It contains phytonutrients thought to protect against oxidation, one of the mechanisms thought to kick off the cancer process, and it's a good source of the supreme antioxidant vitamin E. In one study, researchers found that women who used olive oil more than once a day had a 25 percent lower breast cancer risk than women who used it only once a day.

POWER-EATING TIP

Include 1 or 2 servings of soy a day; if you have breast cancer, 1 serving a day. One serving equals ½ cup of tofu, 1 cup of soy milk, 3 tablespoons of roasted soybeans, or a soy protein shake or bar with 30 to 50 milligrams of isoflavones. Eat no fewer than 5 servings of vegetables a day; 10 is even better. Shoot for ⅛ cup of chopped onion a day and one clove of garlic a day. Count one carrot toward your daily high–beta-carotene food. Rely on olive oil for part of your daily 5 to 10 servings of healthy fats.

Cancer

The Power Foods: Tomatoes, cruciferous vegetables, whole grains, garlic and onions, soy

Only heart disease kills more Americans—male and female—than cancer, which occurs when cells become abnormal and keep dividing, forming new cells in a wild way. But cancer is the leading cause of death in women between the ages of 45 and 64. Lung cancer is the leading cancer in women, followed by cancers of the breast, colon and rectum, uterus, and ovary.

While sobering, the facts aren't as grim as they seem. Although genetics are a factor in who develops cancer, there's overwhelming evidence that what you eat—or don't eat—can dramatically reduce your risk. In fact, experts estimate that dietary changes could prevent at least 30 percent of cancers worldwide.

The stacks of research on the link between diet and cancer boil down to a few golden rules.

The first: Eat a plant-based diet. One of the most exciting discoveries in cancer research is the cancer-battling potential of phytonutrients, substances in fruits, veggies, and other plant foods that have been found, among other things, to stop the growth of cancer cells and activate certain enzymes that kill cancer-causing toxins. Plant foods are also rich in fiber—long associated with reduced cancer risk—and antioxidants.

The second rule: Slash dietary fat to 30 percent of total calories, or even less. Evidence points to a link between dietary fat—especially the saturated fat found in animal products such as meat, milk, and cheese—and specific kinds of cancer, particularly of the colon, uterus, and breast. Dietary fat is linked to the promotion of cancer. A high-fat diet also accelerates the production of free radicals, which damage DNA, the genetic material inside cells that tells them what to do. DNA damage can lead to cancerous changes in cells. Finally, a high-fat diet increases the body's production of estrogen, which in large amounts can fuel the growth of breast tumors.

Research suggests, however, that specific foods are cancer-fighting warriors. Include the following in your anti-cancer shopping list.

Tomatoes. Eating a diet rich in tomatoes and tomato-based foods can lower your overall cancer risk 40 percent compared with people who eat the least amount of these foods. That's according to a review of 72 studies. Researchers hypothesize that lycopene, the phytonutrient that gives tomatoes their red hue, may be the source of its cancer-thwarting powers. Lycopene is a potent antioxidant and appears to be even better at stemming free-radical damage than its better-known relative, beta-carotene.

Here are just two examples of tomatoes' cancer-fighting power. An Italian study comparing the eating habits of men and women with and without cancer found that those who ate the most tomatoes cut their risk of stomach and colon cancers by 57 and 61 percent, respectively, compared to those who ate the least. They were also 35 percent less likely to develop cancer of the mouth and esophagus. In another study, conducted in the Netherlands, women who consumed tomatoes three or more times a week reduced their risk of cervical dysplasia—characterized by precancerous changes to the cervix—by 40 percent.

Cruciferous vegetables. These include cabbage, cauliflower, brussels sprouts, broccoli, and collard, mustard, and turnip greens. All contain an arsenal of phytonutrients, such as indoles and isothiocyanates, which seem to stimulate cancer-fighting enzymes in the body. In one study, researchers at Rockefeller University Hospital and the Institute for Hormone Research, both in New York City, extracted a compound called indole-3 carbinol from cabbage and gave it to women for 2 months. The compound reduced the women's levels of estrogen, which can fuel the development of breast cancer. In another study conducted in the Netherlands, people who ate 10.5 ounces of brussels sprouts a day (about 14 sprouts) for 1 week had higher levels of protective cancer-fighting enzymes in their colons than people who didn't eat them.

Whole grains. Whole grains are those that retain their nutritious outer layer (bran) and inner kernel (germ). And they're richer in cancer-battling nutrients—including fiber, antioxidants, and phytonutrients such as indoles, isothiocyanates, and phytoestrogens—than refined grains, such as white flour. In Italy, people who ate the most whole grains had half as much colon cancer over 13 years of follow-up as those who ate the least. And in yet another study that analyzed the relationship between whole grain intake and various kinds of cancers, whole grains were found to exert protective effects against 17 types of cancer, including those of the breast, endometrium (the lining of the uterus), ovary, and colon and rectum.

Garlic and onions. Smelly, yes. But, oh, what healing power. Large population studies in China, Italy, and the United States have found lower rates of cancer in people who frequently eat raw or cooked garlic. Both contain a slew of organosulfur compounds such as diallyl sulfide

POWER

S P U M O N I

RICOTTA CREAM WITH FRUIT

This is like the thickest, richest cannoli filling you've ever had, with one important difference: It's paired with luscious ripe fruit (lots of antioxidants, fiber, and potassium) instead of an empty-calorie fried pastry shell.

1	container (15 ounces) reduced-fat ricotta cheese
⅓	cup sugar
1	teaspoon vanilla extract
½	teaspoon grated orange rind
1	ounce semisweet chocolate, finely grated
2	cups sliced strawberries
1	cup blueberries
1	large banana, halved lengthwise and thinly sliced

In a food processor, combine the ricotta cheese, sugar, vanilla, and orange rind. Process for 2 minutes, or until very smooth, scraping down the sides of the container as necessary. Add the chocolate and pulse just to incorporate. Divide among individual dessert bowls.

In a medium bowl, mix the strawberries, blueberries, and bananas. Spoon over the ricotta mixture.

Makes 6 servings

Per serving: 190 calories, 9 g protein, 29 g carbohydrates, 5 g fat, 23 mg cholesterol, 2 g dietary fiber, 177 mg sodium

and allicin, which stimulate the production of cancer-battling phase-2 enzymes, protect cells from marauding cancer-causing substances, and slow the growth of certain cancers, particularly those of the stomach and colon. These compounds are also potent antioxidants and may protect against cellular damage from free radicals, thereby helping to thwart cancer.

Onions contain quercetin, a powerful antioxidant in the flavonoid family of phytonutrients found to halt the progression of tumors in the colons of animals. Apparently, onions' healing power extends to humans, too. In one large study in the Netherlands, researchers who examined the diets of nearly 121,000 men and women found that the more of these eye-watering bulbs folks ate, the lower their risk of stomach cancer.

Soy. Tofu, soy milk, soy nuts, and other soy foods contain rich stores of isoflavones, plant compounds hundreds of studies suggest may prevent cancer. Lab research has shown that genistein, one isoflavone in soy, stunts the growth of cancer cells and keeps them from multiplying. It's also been shown to thwart the growth of new blood vessels, which help tumors grow.

In a study at Michigan State University in East Lansing, researchers added 39 grams a day of either soy protein or a soyless protein to the diets of 29 men and 10 women who had either previous colon cancer or polyps, which tend to develop into cancer. One year later, changes in the cells lining the colons of the men and women eating soy protein indicated that their risk of colon cancer had been cut in half.

As for breast cancer, studies are inconclusive, but promising. Studies in women suggest that soy foods may reduce the risk of breast cancer in premenopausal (but not postmenopausal) women. The theory is that in premenopausal women, high blood-estrogen levels fuel hormone-related cancers such as breast cancer. Isoflavones, which act as a weaker form of a woman's own estrogen, steal real estrogen's "parking places" on cells, called estrogen-receptor sites. With no place to park, real estrogen can't attach to cells—and its potentially harmful effects are reduced.

MASKED DISASTER

Ready-to-Eat Cereals

Many ready-to-eat cereals may be low in fat, but many healthy-sounding breakfast cereals contain more sugar than Scarlett O'Hara encircled by her ardent male suitors. One brand of oat flakes "touched" with brown sugar lists sugar in various forms no less than five times and contains nearly 2 teaspoons of sugar per ¾-cup serving. The coup de grâce: It contains only 1 gram of fiber. And one brand of "healthy" low-fat granola contains 4 grams of fiber but 16 grams of sugar per ⅔-cup serving. Your best bet is to stick to high-fiber, whole grain, low-sugar cereals such as shredded wheat or bran flakes.

POWER - EATING TIP

Include one tomato, 1 cup of sliced tomatoes or cherry tomatoes, or ½ cup of tomato sauce as one of your daily deep yellow or orange vegetables. Eat ½ cup of cooked or 1 cup of raw cruciferous vegetables a day. Eat at least three servings of whole grain foods a day, in place of foods made with white flour. One serving equals one slice of whole grain bread, 1 cup of cold cereal or ½ cup hot, or ½ cup of whole grain pasta. Aim for ⅛ cup of chopped onion a day and one clove of garlic a day. Help yourself to one to two servings of soy a day. One serving equals ½ cup of tofu, 1 cup of soy milk, 3 tablespoons of roasted soybeans, or a soy protein shake or bar with 30 to 50 milligrams of isoflavones.

Cataracts and Macular Degeneration

The Power Foods: Vitamin C–rich foods; spinach, kale, and collard greens; wine

The vision of people with cataracts, a clouding of the lens of the eye, has been compared to trying to see through oil-smeared glasses. And trying to see when you have macular degeneration, in which you lose central vision but maintain peripheral vision, is like wearing glasses with a penny taped to the center of each lens.

Aging is the main cause of cataracts, but eye disorders or injuries and years of sun exposure without wearing protective sunglasses can also increase risk. Women with diabetes are at significantly increased risk. In macular degeneration, aging, heredity, high cholesterol, and smoking are prime suspects.

Oxidation—specifically, the oxidation of proteins inside the lenses of the eyes—appears to play a major role in cataract formation. (Think of oxidation—a harmful chemical process that occurs when a substance meets up with oxygen—as the body's equivalent of rusting.) So researchers have focused on the potential of antioxidants, which reduce oxidation's damaging effects, to prevent or treat cataracts. Especially vitamin C. Researchers in Boston compared the vitamin C intake of 247 women ages 56 to 71. They found that those who had taken vitamin C supplements for 10 or more years reduced their risk of cataracts by 77

POWER

VEGGIES

MUSTARD-CRUSTED BRUSSELS SPROUTS

You'll love what happens to brussels sprouts when you toss them with spicy condiments and caraway-flavored bread crumbs. It makes these supercharged cancer-preventing crucifers so tasty that you'll want to serve them often.

1	slice rye bread with caraway seeds
2	boxes (10 ounces each) frozen brussels sprouts
2–3	tablespoons Dijon mustard
1	tablespoon prepared horseradish
2	teaspoons olive oil

Preheat the broiler.

Tear the bread into pieces and place in a food processor. Pulse until finely ground.

In a large saucepan, cook the brussels sprouts according to the package directions. Drain and return to the pan. Stir in the mustard and horseradish. Spoon into an 8" × 8" glass baking dish. Sprinkle with the bread crumbs and drizzle with the oil.

Broil 3" from the heat for 3 minutes, or until the crumbs are crisp and golden.

Makes 4 servings

Per serving: 112 calories, 7 g protein, 16 g carbohydrates, 4 g fat, 0 mg cholesterol, 5 g dietary fiber, 400 mg sodium

percent. Researchers defined high intake as more than 359 milligrams of vitamin C a day, the amount in almost six 6-ounce glasses of orange juice or 3 cups of cooked broccoli.

Making like Popeye and eating your spinach may also deter cataracts. In a 12-year study of almost 78,000 nurses, researchers found that those who ate the most foods containing lutein and zeaxanthin, members of the carotenoid family of phytonutrients, were 22 percent less likely to develop cataracts than those who ate the least. Spinach and kale appeared to be the most protective.

Similarly, spinach, along with other greens such as collards and kale, may stave off macular degeneration. In a study of 876 people with and without the disease, those who ate the most carotenoid-rich foods—carrots and other fruits and veggies—reduced their risk of macular degeneration by 43 percent. What's more, those who ate lutein- and zeaxanthin-rich spinach or collard greens two to four times a week were almost half as likely to develop the disease as those who ate them less than once a month. Lutein and zeaxanthin concentrate in the retina, the part of the eye that—much like the film in a camera—processes visual images. It's thought that they filter out certain ultraviolet rays, leaving the macula (part of the retina) and retina less vulnerable to damage.

Because alcohol has been linked to several forms of eye disease, some experts have thought that it also promotes macular degeneration. But one study of 3,072 people found that drinking wine in moderation appears to protect the light-sensing cells normally damaged by the disease.

POWER-EATING TIP

Eat plenty of vitamin C–rich foods, with the goal of getting 250 to 500 milligrams a day. Eat spinach, kale, and collard greens two to four times a week. If you drink, allow yourself one 5-ounce alcoholic beverage a day.

Common Colds

The Power Foods: Citrus fruit, strawberries, broccoli, kiwifruit, sweet red peppers, carrots, sweet potatoes, cantaloupe, tomatoes, yogurt, garlic, chicken soup, hot peppers

Each year, we collectively suffer nearly 61 million colds, which we catch when one of several hundred cold viruses enters our noses or throats. Alas, scientists have yet to find a cure. But eating foods proven to boost immunity may help bar cold viruses from taking up residence in your body in the first place. Other foods can make you feel better.

IMMUNITY-BUILDING EATS

On any given day, all manner of viruses and bacteria vie for the opportunity to give you your kid's cold. Or your coworker's flu. Or a sinus infection. If you tend to get cold after cold or infection after infection, you're not likely to receive this news with much enthusiasm.

Don't despair; smart eating can help pump up a run-down immune system, boosting your body's ability to fight illness. Start filling your plate with these immunity-boosting eats.

BROCCOLI, ESCAROLE, KALE, SWEET POTATOES, SQUASH, AND CARROTS. These foods are good sources of beta-carotene, which fights infection well and protects the mucous membranes of the nose, mouth, throat, and sinuses. In one study, just 15 milligrams of beta-carotene a day—the amount found in two small carrots—heightened immune cell activity.

GARLIC. This pungent bulb has antiviral and antibacterial power. In studies, garlic has been shown to kill *Candida albicans*, the fungus that causes yeast infections, on contact. Plus, garlic appears to stimulate the activity of neutrophils and macrophages, immune cells that fight infection.

Fruits and vegetables. To renew your cold "insurance" year-round, eat plenty of fruits and vegetables, especially those high in the antioxidants vitamin C and beta-carotene.

Sweet red peppers, kiwifruit, citrus fruit, broccoli, and strawberries are excellent sources of vitamin C. While the jury is still out on its effectiveness as a cold remedy, studies consistently show that, taken at the onset of a cold, vitamin C does help reduce a cold's severity and duration. Carrots, sweet potatoes, cantaloupe, and other orange and yellow fruits and vegetables are brimming with beta-carotene. One British study found that as little as 15 milligrams of a day—the equivalent of 1½ medium or 2 small carrots—increased the activity of immune cells.

Get your tomatoes, too. In one small study, 10 people ate a tomato-rich diet for 3 weeks. Then, for another 3 weeks, they ate no tomatoes. While these folks were eating tomatoes, their infection-fighting white blood cells sustained 38 percent less free-radical damage than when they

MAITAKE AND SHIITAKE MUSHROOMS. These Asian mushrooms contain polysaccharides, large chains of sugar molecules with immune-stimulating properties. Polysaccharides are similar to the cell membranes of bacteria, which may fool the immune system into mounting an immune response against them.

OYSTERS, BEEF, AND WHEAT GERM. All are excellent sources of zinc, an immunity booster that is essential to the production of white blood cells.

POTATOES AND BANANAS. They're rich in vitamin B$_6$, long known to influence immunity.

SWEET PEPPERS, STRAWBERRIES, PAPAYA, CANTALOUPE, BROCCOLI, AND TOMATOES. They're rich in vitamin C, another powerful antioxidant that revs up the body's production of gamma interferon, a protein that helps stimulate white blood cells to fight disease.

YOGURT. It contains *Lactobacillus acidophilus,* benevolent bacteria known to shore up the immune system. In one study, people who ate 2 cups of yogurt a day for 4 months had about four times more gamma interferon than people who didn't eat yogurt.

were on the tomato-free plan. It's thought that lycopene, an antioxidant abundant in tomatoes, helps white blood cells resist free-radical damage. Bonus: Tomatoes are also high in cold-clobbering vitamin C.

Yogurt. Like a shoe sale perks up our spirits, yogurt boosts the immune system. Researchers at the University of California, Davis, had 60 people eat either 1 cup of yogurt with live cultures a day, 1 cup of pasteurized yogurt a day, or no yogurt at all. Over the course of a year, those who ate either type of yogurt had a lower incidence of colds, coughing, and wheezing.

Garlic. Dubbed the "poor man's antibiotic," garlic contains a treasure chest of therapeutic compounds that stimulate immune function. Test-tube studies have found that garlic increases disease resistance by stimulating the activity of lymphocytes, one type of infection-fighting white blood cell, and increasing the production of phagocytes, cells that engulf and devour foreign microorganisms. In people, studies show that garlic stimulates immunity by increasing the number of natural killer cells, a particular kind of lymphocyte.

Chicken soup. Don't forget the ultimate grandma remedy. In a classic study, researchers had 15 people slurp hot chicken soup, hot water, or cold water. After each liquid, the researchers measured how well their subjects could breathe through their noses. The winner: chicken soup. Researchers speculated that the soup may help relieve colds by increasing "nasal mucous velocity" (meaning, it makes your nose run like a faucet). And the more your nose flows, the less time cold germs may spend there.

Hot peppers. Consider adding a small amount of minced hot peppers or hot-pepper sauce to the broth. The little fireballs contain capsaicin, a chemical that closely resembles guaifenesin, an expectorant used in many over-the-counter and prescription cold remedies such as Robitussin.

A low-fat diet. If you tend to catch a lot of colds, consider adopting a low-fat diet. Current government guidelines call for getting no more than 30 percent of your calories from fat. But research shows that trimming the fat just a smidgen more—to 25 percent of calories—can increase the effectiveness of immune cells.

POWER-EATING TIP

Eat nine servings of fruits and vegetables a day, focusing on antioxidant-rich varieties. The Daily Value for vitamin C is 60 milligrams. But it's safe, and possible, to consume 500 milligrams a day. Eat one or more daily servings of beta-carotene–rich fruits or veggies. Count one tomato, 1 cup of sliced tomatoes or cherry tomatoes, or ½ cup of tomato sauce toward one of your daily deep yellow or orange vegetables. Eat 1 cup of yogurt a day. Opt for low-fat or fat-free varieties. Eat two raw cloves of garlic a day. To make the raw bulb more palatable, mince it and blend it into foods. Drink chicken soup as needed. (The nose-clearing effect wears off in 30 minutes.) Add hot peppers or hot-pepper sauce to food—as much as your tastebuds can tolerate.

Constipation

The Power Foods: Fiber, plus water and other fluids

The medical definition of constipation is the passage of small amounts of hard, dry stools, usually fewer than three times a week. At last count, about 4½ million Americans, many of them women, said they were constipated most or all of the time. To get relief from the resulting bloating, discomfort, and sluggishness, Americans spend $725 million on laxatives each year.

The simplest remedy is a diet high in fiber—the tough, indigestible part of plant foods such as fruits, vegetables, and whole grains—and getting more fluids. Fiber absorbs water; makes stools heavier, softer, and easier to pass; and speeds up the time it takes for the colon to move stools to the rectum for elimination.

The average woman, however, eats about 11 grams of fiber daily, far short of the recommended 20 to 35 grams. To minimize potential gas and cramping, increase your intake of fiber slowly, over several months.

Consume at least 20 to 35 grams a day from high-fiber cereals, fruits and veggies, whole grains, and beans. Choose cereals that contain 3 or more grams of fiber per serving. Buy whole grain bread. Check the label to make sure the first ingredient is whole grain. Eat at least five servings of fruits and vegetables a day, raw or cooked. (Cooking doesn't significantly reduce their fiber content.) Eat legumes frequently. Choose fiber-full snacks such as popcorn, whole grain crackers, fresh fruits, raw vegetables, and nuts and seeds. Add 2 to 3 tablespoons of 100 percent bran cereals or unprocessed wheat bran to meat loaf, casseroles, and home-baked breads and muffins.

While you're eating all that fiber, remember to drink enough water and other fluids. Fiber sucks up fluid like a sponge, so you'll need it. Drink nine 8-ounce glasses a day, primarily healthy beverages such as

MASKED DISASTER

Jumbo Juice

In itself, fruit juice isn't so bad. (Although you do miss out on the fiber in the fruit itself.) But the portion sizes can do us in. The bigger bottles of juice routinely contain two or more servings, and each serving packs a considerable amount of calories and sugar. For example, drink a 17.5-ounce bottle of one popular orange-mango juice cocktail, and you're ingesting 260 calories and 58 grams of sugar!

If you love juice, here's the smart way to enjoy it. Measure out one serving. Then, dilute it by half with water or club soda. You'll consume just 65 calories and 15 grams of sugar.

water, juice, and fat-free milk. Juice can be extremely high in calories. Try diluting it with water, which will quench your thirst and slash calories. Limit caffeine, found in coffee, tea, and many soft drinks, or avoid them entirely. All are diuretics, which pull water from your body.

Depression

The Power Foods: Vitamin B_6–rich foods; foods rich in the minerals calcium, iron, magnesium, and zinc

We all get the blues at one time or another. But there are different "shades" of blue—and they all have different causes. For example, fluctuating hormones just before a woman's menstrual period can cause the blues, better known as PMS. By contrast, grief or a traumatic event such as the loss of a job or a divorce can lead to major depression.

Whatever the reason, depression doesn't just affect your mood. In women, it's linked to an increased risk of death from heart disease and other illnesses. In one study, researchers from the University of California, San Francisco, tracked the physical and mental health of more than 7,500 older women for 7 years. Those with no symptoms of depression had a 7 percent death rate. But the death rate of women with six or more symptoms was more than three times higher—24 percent.

No one is saying that you can eat your way out of a major depression. But there is at least some evidence that what you eat may help brighten your mood.

While evidence is scant, some research suggests that eating foods rich in vitamin B_6, such as poultry and red meats, could make a difference in your mood. Fish and spinach are good sources of B_6, and even shellfish has a bit. Apparently, when your diet is low in vitamin B_6, brain cells can't produce enough serotonin, a brain chemical that plays a vital role in the regulation of sleep, appetite, and mood. (Interestingly, in one study out of Harvard, more than one out of four people with depression was B_6 deficient.) Be especially vigilant about getting the recommended 2 milligrams of vitamin B_6 a day if you're on the Pill. Oral contraceptives may make your body less able to use vitamin B_6, perhaps causing a deficiency that may lead to depression.

Include plenty of foods high in calcium, iron, and magnesium in your diet, too. Low intakes of these minerals have been linked to depression and mood swings. Calcium and magnesium help regulate nerve impulses and make brain chemicals that affect mood. Not eating enough iron-rich foods can lead to iron-deficiency anemia, a blood condition that can cause depression and irritability.

POWER-EATING TIP

Include several daily servings of leafy green vegetables, legumes, fruits, and whole grains. Eat two to three 2- to 3-ounce servings of fish, poultry, or meat a day. Be sure to consume 1,000 milligrams of calcium a day if you are under 50 and 1,500 milligrams if you are 50 or over. Choose low-fat and fat-free milk, yogurt, and cheese or calcium-fortified orange juice. If you're lactose intolerant or dislike dairy products, opt for calcium-rich vegetables such as broccoli (72 milligrams per cooked cup) and dark greens such as kale (93 milligrams per cup). Aim for 400 milligrams of magnesium from spinach and beans. Eat enough high-iron foods to meet the Daily Value of 18 milligrams of iron.

Diabetes

The Power Foods: Beans; whole grains; vitamin C− and E−rich fruits and veggies; a low-fat, meat- and dairy-free diet

Diabetes is a disorder of metabolism, the way our bodies use digested food for growth and energy. Most of the food you eat is broken down by your digestive juices into glucose, a simple sugar that is the main source of fuel for your body. After digestion, the glucose passes into your bloodstream where it is available for body cells to use for energy. For the glucose to get into your cells, insulin, a hormone produced by the pancreas, must be present. With type 2 diabetes—which usually shows up in adulthood—your body can't use the insulin effectively. The end result is that glucose builds up in your blood and spills out into the urine. Cells go hungry. And all that backed-up sugar becomes toxic.

Men and women with diabetes are vulnerable to a host of other chronic diseases, including high blood pressure, heart disease, stroke, circulatory diseases of the legs and feet, and disorders of the nerves, kidneys, and eyes. The scariest part is that out of the estimated 14.9 million Americans with type 2 diabetes, about a third don't know they have it.

Now for the bright spot. Along with getting regular exercise and maintaining a healthy weight, what you choose to eat can help treat type 2 diabetes—or perhaps even prevent it completely. The guidelines are easy: Follow a low-fat diet brimming with fruits, vegetables, and complex carbohydrates such as whole grains. And fill up on the foods listed below. There's evidence that they can put the kibosh on diabetes.

MASKED DISASTER

Bagels

Sure, bagels are low in fat. But most bagels are made with white flour, the nutritional equivalent of cardboard. They're also low in fiber: only 2 grams in a 3-ounce bagel. Better to opt for a toasted whole wheat English muffin. While smaller than a bagel, the muffin contains twice the fiber. Plus, you'll reap all that whole grain goodness—namely, the vitamins, minerals, and plant chemicals that are stripped from white flour.

Beans. All varieties are excellent sources of fiber, shown to have a beneficial effect on diabetes. They're also low in fat, which helps protect against obesity, a major risk factor for the condition. Beans have also been shown to steady levels of blood sugar and help the body respond better to insulin, crucial for women with diabetes. In one English study, researchers fed people either 1¾ ounces of a variety of beans or other high-carb foods like bread and pasta. After ½ hour, the bean-eaters' blood sugar levels were almost half that of those who ate other high-carbohydrate foods.

Whole grains. Whole oats, brown rice, and whole wheat are good sources of protective fiber, along with phenolic acids, phytic acid, and antioxidants such as vitamin E. In a study of 65,173 nurses, those who ate the least whole grain cereal fiber and the most white bread and other refined carbohydrates had 2½ times greater risk of developing type 2 diabetes over 6 years of follow-up.

Vitamin C– and E–rich fruits and veggies. Strawberries, tomatoes, broccoli, and other fruits and vegetables, along with wheat germ, are excellent sources of powerful antioxidants. They may help prevent the legacy of uncontrolled diabetes: blindness, kidney disease, and nerve damage.

Both vitamins prevent glycosylation, a detrimental chemical reaction between sugar and protein thought to contribute to many diabetic complications. But C and E also work alone. Vitamin C prevents sugar inside cells from being converted to sorbitol, a substance implicated in diabetes-related nerve damage, and some evidence suggests that vitamin E may help insulin do its job more effectively.

A low-fat and meat- and dairy-free diet. While you may not want to go this far, a preliminary study suggests that a low-fat diet free of meat and dairy products (called a vegan diet) can dramatically reduce blood sugar. Researchers had 11 people with type 2 diabetes follow either a low-fat, vegan diet or a standard low-fat diet. After 12 weeks, those following the standard low-fat diet reduced their blood sugar levels by an average of 12 percent and lost about 8 pounds. None reduced or eliminated their medication. But those in the vegan group reduced their blood sugar levels an average of 28 percent and lost an average of 16 pounds. Virtually all of them reduced or eliminated their medications.

POWER - EATING TIP

Try to eat five or more ½-cup servings of beans a week. Research has shown that as little as 3.4 ounces a day helped people with diabetes manage their blood sugar levels. Eat at least three servings of whole grains a day in place of foods made with white flour. One serving equals one slice of whole grain bread, 1 cup of cold cereal or ½ cup hot, or ½ cup of whole grain pasta. Get 500 milligrams of vitamin C a day and 800 IU of vitamin E a day, from food and supplements. Research has shown that the blood sugar levels of people with diabetes fell significantly when they consumed this amount.

Diverticular Disease

The Power Foods: Fiber-rich foods, specifically fruits, vegetables, beans, and whole grains

Diverticular disease comes in two types. In diverticulosis, tiny pockets, called diverticula, form in your colon (large intestine). The problem seems to start when two or more of the muscles that encircle the colon begin to contract at the same time, hindering the colon's ability to move stools and other waste to the rectum. This trapped waste presses against your colon wall, creating diverticula. If one of these pockets becomes inflamed, you have diverticulitis, an extremely painful and serious condition accounting for 440,000 hospital stays a year.

The risk for diverticular disease increases with age: Nearly half of Americans ages 60 to 80 and almost everyone over age 80 has diverticulosis. Only 10 to 25 percent develop diverticulitis.

Eating the right diet may be able to help prevent and treat diverticular disease. And for those of us who have it, the right diet includes lots of fiber. In a study of nearly 48,000 men, researchers from Harvard University and Brigham and Women's Hospital in Boston found that those who got the most fiber in their diets were 42 percent less likely to have diverticulosis than those eating the least.

Try not to overindulge in red meat and high-fat foods, which contain little or no fiber. Researchers in the same study found that people who ate low-fiber diets and also ate high-fat foods or 4 ounces of red meat a day were significantly more likely to get diverticulosis than those who just skimped on the fiber.

POWER-EATING TIP

Aim for 20 to 35 grams of fiber a day, mostly from fruits, vegetables, high-fiber cereals, beans, and whole grains. While you're eating all that fiber, remember to drink enough water and other fluids—at least nine 8-ounce glasses a day. Fiber attracts fluid like a 5-year-old boy attracts dirt, so you'll need it.

Fatigue

The Power Foods: Tuna, beef, chicken, eggs and other low-fat sources of protein; sweet red peppers, kiwifruit, oranges, broccoli, and tomatoes and other foods high in vitamin C; fortified cereals, oysters, mussels, Swiss chard, lean meats, beans, and baked potatoes, for iron.

We're not talking about chronic fatigue syndrome, an illness with no known cause or cure. We're talking about garden-variety fatigue, a complaint of half of all adults who seek medical treatment. And there's no doubt that being female can be exhausting. Stress, lack of sleep, couch potato syndrome, crash dieting—all of which we fall prey to at one time or another—can trigger that I-must-take-a-nap-*now* feeling.

Your diet can be an energy drainer, too. There's evidence that changes in the levels of certain neurotransmitters—brain chemicals shown to affect mood and feelings—also affect our energy levels. For example, studies show that people think more quickly and feel more motivated when their brains are producing a lot of the neurotransmitters dopamine and norepinephrine.

To increase your brain's production of these "wake-up chemicals," try eating something high in protein, such as a 3- to 4-ounce broiled chicken breast or a hard-boiled egg. Just that amount of a high-protein food helps the brain make tyrosine, an amino acid essential to the production of dopamine and norepinephrine. Just don't overload the tuna or lean roast beef with high-fat cheese or mayo. Foods high in protein also tend to be equally high in fat. And a high-fat meal can leave a woman feeling sluggish instead of supercharged.

Try eating more fruits and vegetables rich in vitamin C, too. There's some evidence that fatigue is more common in women who don't get enough of this antioxidant. In a study of 411 men and women, those who consumed at least 400 milligrams of vitamin C a day said that they felt less tired than those consuming less than 100 milligrams. Excellent sources of C include broccoli, papayas, cantaloupe, and tomatoes.

If you're always too pooped to pop, you may be deficient in iron. As many as 20 percent of premenopausal women are. The result is fatigue and poor concentration. Among the best sources of iron are fortified cereals (12 milligrams), 3 ounces of oysters (6.6 milligrams), and 3 ounces of blue mussels (5.7 milligrams). Other good sources of iron include top round or top sirloin, baked potatoes, and navy beans or black beans.

POWER-EATING TIP

Here's what *not* to eat when you're tired.

- High-fat foods. Fat takes a long time to digest, leaving your brain feeling sluggish.

- High-carbohydrate foods. They cause production of tryptophan. This amino acid is the building block for serotonin, a neurotransmitter often dubbed the calm-down chemical because it regulates mood.

- Sugar. A candy bar or jelly doughnut causes your blood sugar levels to spike, igniting your energy. But that initial sugar buzz is often followed by a crash, as blood sugar levels plummet, leaving you more exhausted than before.

- Coffee. While a cup or two early in the day has been shown to boost alertness, drinking cup after cup day after day can cause fatigue.

Fibrocystic Breast Changes

The Power Foods: Foods low in fat (especially low in saturated fat); foods and beverages free of caffeine

A condition affecting half of all women at some point in their lives, fibrocystic breast changes occur when fluid-filled sacs form in the breast's milk-producing glands. Relax; this condition does not increase your risk of breast cancer. Still, the pain and lumpiness, which often intensifies before menstruation, can be frustrating and uncomfortable. While experts aren't sure what causes these breast changes, some suspect higher-than-normal amounts of estrogen and prolactin, the milk-release hormone.

There seems to be little solid information about the relationship between diet and fibrocystic breast changes—and the jury's still out on the evidence that one does exist. But some women report that changing their diets eases or completely eliminates their symptoms.

Some evidence suggests that women who consume a lot of dietary fat—especially the saturated fat in butter, bacon, and other animal foods—are more likely to develop fibrocystic breast changes. This is probably because a high-fat diet increases the amount of estrogen circulating in a woman's body, which can fuel the growth of breast lumps. In one small study, 10 women with these changes reduced their intake of dietary fat to 20 percent of their total daily calories. Three months later, all of them said that their pain was gone.

Researchers at Yale University School of Medicine found that women who drink about two cups of coffee a day (containing from 31 to 250 milligrams of caffeine) were 150 percent more likely to develop fibrocystic changes than women getting no caffeine. That may be due to coffee's content of methylxanthines, compounds that can cause breast lumps to become inflamed and tender. In a study at Ohio State University in Columbus, 45 women who drank an average of four cups of coffee a day quit cold turkey. After 2 months, 37 of the women—82 percent—said that their lumps were gone.

POWER-EATING TIP

Reduce the amount of fat in your diet to less than 20 percent. Cut back on coffee and other sources of caffeine to one cup or less a day.

Fibroids

The Power Foods: Green vegetables such as spinach, kale, turnip and mustard greens, and broccoli

An estimated 20 to 40 percent of all women have fibroids—noncancerous tumors that grow on the inside or outside lining of the uterus, or within its muscular wall. These growths can be as small as a pea or as large as a grapefruit. While experts aren't exactly sure what causes fibroids, they do know that they occur most often when a woman's estrogen levels are high—when she's pregnant, for example, or if she's taking the Pill.

Not all fibroids cause symptoms or need treatment. But some women experience a variety of bothersome or uncomfortable symptoms, including heavy bleeding, pressure in the abdomen, abdominal or lower-back pain, and frequent urination.

Preliminary evidence suggests that fibroids are linked to a meat-heavy diet and that eating lots of green veggies seems to be protective. Researchers in Italy compared 843 women with fibroids to 1,557 women without. Those with fibroids reported eating significantly more red meat and fewer servings of green vegetables. It's known that a diet high in meat raises a woman's levels of estrogen—which seems to increase the risk of developing fibroids—and that premenopausal vegetarian women have blood estrogen levels that are 15 to 20 percent lower than that of their meat-eating sisters.

POWER-EATING TIP

Shoot for one serving a day of broccoli, asparagus, spinach, and kale or other greens, which counts toward the recommended three to five daily servings.

Gallstones

The Power Foods: Foods high in fiber and low in fat, sugar, and cholesterol: fruits, veggies, high-fiber cereals, whole grains, and beans.

Each year, more than a million Americans are diagnosed with gallstones. Women are twice as likely to develop them as men.

These crystals of fat and cholesterol, which can be as small as grains of sand or as big as golf balls, form in your gallbladder, an organ about the size and shape of a pear. It's your holding tank for bile, a liquid that helps you digest food. The symptoms of gallstones are episodes of intense pain in the upper abdomen, continuous upper abdominal pain that lasts from 30 minutes to several hours, and pain that may spread to the right shoulder blade or back, often with nausea or sometimes vomiting.

While gallstones run in families, other factors, such as age and weight, taking birth control pills, or undergoing hormone-replacement therapy, may also increase risk. Both increase the amount of cholesterol in your bile, which makes it harder for the gallbladder to get rid of it quickly.

Since gallstones are petrified slivers of fat and cholesterol, it makes sense to switch to a low-fat, low-cholesterol diet. This means eating fewer bacon-and-egg breakfasts and replacing full-fat dairy products, such as whole milk and cheese, with low-fat or fat-free varieties. Consuming more fiber may also help. Fiber binds with bile salts, a major component of bile, and with cholesterol in your intestines, preventing your body from absorbing them.

Drinking coffee—in moderation—may also guard against gallstones. Researchers from Harvard polled 46,008 men over a 10-year period and

Waistline

The average American consumes about 45 pounds of sugar a year.

found that those who drank two to three cups of coffee per day had a 40 percent lower risk of gallstones than men who didn't drink coffee. Since decaffeinated coffee didn't reduce risk, it may be that caffeine somehow stimulates the gallbladder to decrease the amount of stone-forming cholesterol.

To prevent gallstones, limit your consumption of sugar and saturated fat, found primarily in meats and full-fat dairy products. Both appear to increase the likelihood of gallstones. Researchers in Italy compared 100 people with gallstones to 290 without. They found that those who ate more refined sugars—found in such foods as cookies, cake, and soda— were more likely to develop gallstones.

In the same study, folks who consumed more saturated fat each day were more likely to develop gallstones.

POWER-EATING TIP

Get no more than 25 percent of your total daily calories from fat, with no more than 10 percent of those calories coming from saturated fat. Consume at least 20 to 35 grams of fiber a day from fruits, veggies, high-fiber cereals, whole grains and beans. Drink no more than two to three cups of coffee a day.

Headaches and Migraines

The Power Foods: A high-carbohydrate diet; a low-fat diet; coffee (in moderation)

If you suffer chronic, recurring headaches, you have plenty of company: So do more than 45 million other Americans. Across the board, women get more headaches than men, and they tend to be more frequent and severe.

Waistline

Among the weirder things linked to headaches: frequent cellular phone use and eating ice cream.

Women are particularly prone to migraines, which are associated with changes in the size of the arteries inside and around the skull. Occurring three times more often in women than in men, migraines are often accompanied by nausea, vomiting, and sensitivity to bright light or sound. It's known that the hormonal changes that occur during the menstrual cycle, pregnancy and childbirth, and menopause affect migraines, as does taking oral contraceptives. Migraines may also be caused by a low concentration of serotonin, a brain chemical that plays a vital role in the regulation of sleep, appetite, and mood.

Women seek treatment more often than men for tension-type headaches—felt on both sides of the head, often described as pressing or tightening, and of mild or moderate intensity. On the other hand, far fewer women than men get cluster headaches, which occur daily or almost daily for 4 to 8 weeks and are about as painful as headaches can get.

When it comes to headaches, what you *don't* eat is more important than what you do eat. However, some dietary changes (along with stress-reduction techniques and adequate sleep and exercise) can help prevent those head pounders, especially migraines.

A low-fat diet may help reduce the frequency, severity, and duration of migraines. Researchers had 54 men and women prone to migraines reduce their mean fat intake from 65.9 grams to 27.8 grams per day. After 12 weeks, 35 of the 54 said that their symptoms improved from 85 to 100 percent. And 51 of the 54 reported a 40 percent improvement. Researchers think that a low-fat diet may reduce synthesis of a substance called PGI2, which causes blood vessels to expand. What's more, when people eat less fat, they tend to eat more carbohydrates. A high-carbohydrate diet has been shown to increase the availability of the amino acid tryptophan and vitamin B_6. Both are building blocks of serotonin production.

The next time you feel a headache coming on, try sipping a cup of coffee. The caffeine it contains temporarily constricts painfully dilated blood vessels. Caffeine has also been shown to boost the effectiveness of over-the-counter pain relievers. Just don't overdo the java. Too much will cause those constricted vessels to expand once again.

POWER-EATING TIP

Fat should account for no more than 25 percent of your daily calories. Drink no more than two 5-ounce cups of coffee a day, the equivalent of 200 to 300 milligrams of caffeine.

Avoid these trigger foods.

- Chocolate, alcohol (such as red wine, brandy, and sherry), and aged cheeses. These foods and beverages contain tyramine. This amino acid prompts the body to release prostaglandins, hormones that cause blood vessels to constrict. When the constricted vessels eventually dilate again, you'll experience that dreaded throb.

- Preserved meats, including canned ham, corned beef, pepperoni, salami, bacon, and the good old American hot dog. They contain nitrites, which also seem to painfully dilate blood vessels in the head.

- Monosodium glutamate (MSG). Long associated with Chinese food, this food additive is also found in foods that you eat every day: TV dinners, canned soups, instant gravy, dry-roasted nuts, and tenderizers and seasoned salt.

Heart Disease

The Power Foods: Olive oil, nuts, and other monounsaturated fats; cold-water fish; soy; whole grains; greens; garlic

Heart disease kills more women in this country than any other malady. Astonishingly, 80 percent of us (and one-third of our primary-care doctors) don't know it. But now you do. And as any devotee of Dean Ornish's "reversal diet" can attest, diet can heal a broken heart—or prevent it from breaking in the first place.

Mother Nature's pantry is stocked with heart healers.

Plant foods. Fruits, vegetables, legumes, and whole grains are loaded with fiber, the tough, indigestible part of plant foods that helps keep blood cholesterol levels in check, reducing heart disease risk. Plant foods are also rich in heart-loving phytonutrients, such as flavonoids, which, like beta-carotene and vitamins C and E, are antioxidants. These substances may keep "bad" LDL cholesterol from undergoing oxidation. Many scientists think that this harmful chemical process, caused by unchecked free-radical damage, leads to sticky fatty plaque buildup on blood vessel walls.

Bonus: Plant foods contain nary a trace of saturated fat, perhaps the heart's most treacherous dietary foe. (That's the fat found primarily in red meats, butter, cheese, and other animal foods.)

Even though it's a good idea to reduce the amount of fat in your diet, one type of fat you can feel good about eating is monounsaturated fat. It's well-known that replacing saturated fats with monounsaturated fats helps lower total and LDL cholesterol while leaving protective high-density lipoprotein (HDL) cholesterol alone. Olive oil, avocados, and nuts are brimming with monounsaturated fats. In an ongoing study of 86,016 women, those who ate more than 5 ounces of nuts a week had about a 35 percent lower risk of heart disease than women who rarely or never ate nuts. (But enjoy them a small palmful at a time. Nuts are exorbitantly high in calories and fat.)

Fish. Cold-water fish such as salmon, mackerel, and tuna are brimming with omega-3 fatty acids, another group of heart-loving fats. Omega-3's hinder the formation of compounds that may cause blood vessels to constrict, pushing up blood pressure. They also reduce the formation of clots that can block bloodflow to the heart and reduce the incidence of arrhythmias—abnormalities in heart rhythm that may lead to cardiac arrest, in which the heart stops beating entirely. Researchers who tracked a group of 1,822 men for 30 years found that men who ate an average of 1 ounce of fish a day were 38 percent less likely to die from heart disease and 50 percent less likely to die from a sudden heart attack than men who never ate fish.

Soy. The FDA recently agreed that soy protein—found in tofu and many meat substitutes—can reduce the risk of heart disease by lowering total and LDL cholesterol. Scientists believe that the therapeutic compounds are isoflavones, compounds that act as a weaker version of the estrogen women produce naturally. Experts think that the phytoestrogens in soy also may prevent LDL cholesterol from undergoing harmful oxidation. In a study conducted at the Wake Forest University School of

Medicine in Winston-Salem, North Carolina, 51 perimenopausal women consumed about 4 teaspoons of soy protein (containing 34 milligrams of isoflavones) a day and reduced their heart disease risk by about 12 percent.

Whole grains. Wheat, corn, barley, oatmeal, and other whole grains are nutritionally superior to refined grains such as white flour because they contain higher amounts of fiber as well as antioxidants, phyto-nutrients, and vitamins. In a study of 34,492 postmenopausal women, those who ate two or more servings of whole grains a day were 30 percent less likely to die from heart disease than those who ate three servings a week or less.

Certain greens—and garlic. Spinach and turnip greens are excellent sources of folate, which has been shown to lower blood levels of homocysteine, the amino acid linked to heart disease. In one study, women who consumed the most of this B vitamin (about 696 micrograms a day) were 31 percent less likely to die from heart disease or a heart attack than those who consumed the least (about 158 micrograms a day).

Sauté those greens in garlic. The "stinking rose" contains blood-thinning compounds that protect against heart-stopping clots and help prevent LDL from oxidizing in lab studies. Scientists added 900 milligrams of garlic powder to the diets of 61 people. After 4 years, the plaque buildup in their arteries had declined significantly—in some cases by as much as 18 percent.

POWER-EATING TIP

Consume at least 1 teaspoon a day of olive or canola oil among your daily 5 to 10 servings of healthy fats. Eat 2 tablespoons of nuts five times a week. Help yourself to one to two servings of cold-water fish a week—anchovies, tuna, herring, or salmon. Aim for 25 milligrams of isoflavones from soy foods a day. Look for foods that contain at least 6 grams of soy protein per serving. Substitute whole grains (at least three servings a day) for foods made with white flour (one slice of whole grain bread, ½ cup of whole grain pasta, ½ to 1 cup of cold cereal—check labels for the amount that will provide approximately 70 to 90 calories—or ½ cup of hot cereal). Be sure to get two servings of greens a day (1 cup raw or ½ cup cooked). Add one-half to one clove of garlic to your food each day.

Hemorrhoids

The Power Foods: Cereal brans, beans, whole grains and other fiber-rich foods, water and other fluids

Hemorrhoids are varicose veins. Only they don't develop on your legs; they develop in your anus, often in response to chronic constipation (with straining), the extra weight of pregnancy, childbirth, or obesity.

The best way to prevent and treat hemorrhoids is to consume enough insoluble fiber, found in cereal brans, fruits, and vegetables. Insoluble fiber bulks up stools, keeping them moving through the digestive tract, and retains water, keeping stools soft and easy to pass.

POWER-EATING TIP

Aim for 20 to 35 grams of fiber a day, mainly from high-fiber cereals, beans, and whole grains but also from fruits and vegetables. Increase fiber intake gradually, to give your digestive system time to adapt. Drink nine 8-ounce glasses of water and other healthy beverages such as fat-free milk, juice, soup, and herbal teas. These steps help keep stools soft, which eliminates the need to strain. If you already have hemorrhoids, avoid caffeine and alcohol during flare-ups. Both are diuretics, substances that cause the body to lose water. And when hemorrhoids act up, your digestive tract needs all the water it can get to help stools pass comfortably.

High Blood Pressure

The Power Foods: Fruits, vegetables, low-fat dairy products, fish, celery

If you have high blood pressure, and about 50 million Americans do, your heart must work harder than normal to pump blood through your arteries. And this condition quietly devastates the entire cardiovascular system. It strains the heart as it scars and hardens the linings of blood vessels (especially in the heart, kidneys, and eyes) and arteries. You have hypertension when your blood pressure is greater than or equal to 140/90 most of the time.

DISEASE "GENDER DISCRIMINATION"

It's not enough that women are far more likely than men to suffer from urinary tract infections, fatigue, and PMS. (Although some men may argue that PMS afflicts them, too.) We're also more prone to other conditions—some merely bothersome, others quite serious.

- Arthritis
- Alzheimer's disease
- Cardiovascular disease
- Constipation
- Depression

- Gallstones
- Macular degeneration
- Osteoporosis
- Overweight
- Urinary incontinence

The higher your blood pressure, the higher your risk of heart disease and stroke. Among the factors that may lead to high blood pressure are kidney disease, overweight, and taking some medications, including some cold and sinus medications, birth control pills, and estrogen-replacement therapy.

Fortunately, research has found that diet can have a significant impact on elevated blood pressure. The landmark Dietary Approaches to Stop Hypertension (DASH) study shows that a diet high in fruits and vegetables and low-fat dairy products can lower blood pressure as much as medication can—and in as little as 2 weeks. In this study, 459 men and women followed one of three diets for 8 weeks. The first diet matched the average American diet (37 percent of calories as fat), the second was rich in fruits and vegetables and almost as high in fat, and the third was a combination diet low in total and saturated fats and rich in fruits, vegetables, and low-fat dairy products. All three contained about 3,000 milligrams of sodium a day. The combination diet also contained three times as much calcium—a mineral found to help lower blood pressure—than the average American diet (443 milligrams versus 1,265 milligrams). While the fruit-and-vegetable and combination diets both lowered blood pressure, the combination diet was most effective. In people with high blood pressure, it reduced systolic blood pressure by 11.4 points and diastolic pressure by 5.5 points more than the control diet.

The DASH diet provides plenty of potassium (from the fruits and vegetables) as well as calcium (from low-fat dairy products). Both of these minerals help the arteries dilate, giving blood the room it needs to move easily through the arteries.

Including fish as part of a low-fat diet has also been shown to send blood pressure south. In one study at the University of Western Australia in Perth, researchers compared the effects of four diets—a low-fat diet; a high-fat diet; a combination low-fat, high-fish diet; and a regular diet—on the blood pressures of 63 people who took. While eating either less fat or more fish significantly reduced blood pressure, pairing the two diets dropped pressures even more.

The Chinese have used celery to treat high blood pressure for centuries. And modern-day tests on animals show that this stringy, pale green veggie works. Experts hypothesize that its pressure-lowering benefits are due to a compound called 3-n-butylphthalide.

Researchers at Tulane University in New Orleans studying 875 people found that half were able to stop taking blood pressure medication by reducing their salt intake by 25 percent and losing between 7 and 8 pounds.

POWER-EATING TIP

Include nine servings of fruits and vegetables a day in your diet. Include the equivalent of 1 cup of celery stalks. Eat two to three servings of low-fat or fat-free dairy foods per day. Eat one to two servings of cold-water fish a week—anchovies, tuna, herring, and salmon. Limit salt intake to no more than 2,400 milligrams of salt a day (about 1 teaspoon) if you have normal blood pressure, and no more than 2,000 milligrams a day if you have or are at risk for heart disease or high blood pressure.

High Cholesterol

The Power Foods: Orange juice, beans, garlic, soy, tuna, mackerel, salmon

Homocysteine, the amino acid that research links to increased risk of heart disease, may be the new villain on the heart disease front. But high blood cholesterol remains homocysteine's partner in crime. As LDL cholesterol circulates in the bloodstream, it undergoes oxidation. Essentially,

BREAK OUT THE BONBONS

This from the strange-but-true file: To safeguard your body against heart disease and cancer, pop a piece of dark chocolate. (Do we hear the faint sound of cheers?)

Dark chocolate contains a mother lode of catechins, a member of the flavonoid family of phytonutrients. Catechins are potent antioxidants, which help shield cells from the harmful effects of free radicals, cell-damaging molecules thought to contribute to the development of heart disease, cancer, and other chronic ills.

Researchers from the Netherlands measured the amount of catechins in dark and milk chocolate and tea. They found that dark chocolate contains more than three times the amount of catechins in milk chocolate (53.5 milligrams per 3.5 ounces versus 15.9 milligrams) and tea, another source of catechins. (White chocolate contains no catechins at all.)

Anyone for a chocolate cookie and a cup of tea?

it turns rancid. Your immune system quickly spots the decaying LDL and reacts to it as it would an invader. Immune cells gobble up the cholesterol. Once full, they stick to the walls of your arteries, hardening into a dense, fatty layer called plaque. When too much plaque accumulates, there's less room for blood to flow, which leads to a heart attack or stroke.

We all know that reducing intake of fat, particularly the saturated fats found in bacon, whole milk cheese, and butter, can lower cholesterol levels. So can eating plenty of whole grains, beans, and fresh fruits. They are rich in soluble fiber, which regulates the body's production and elimination of cholesterol. They also contain a mother lode of antioxidants and phytonutrients, believed to thwart oxidative damage to LDL.

Starting your morning with a glass of orange juice may be a good idea, too. In one small Canadian study, men and women with high cholesterol who drank three glasses a day saw their HDL increase by 21 percent and their ratio of HDL to LDL drop by 16 percent. The juice's cholesterol-lowering effects may be due to flavonoids such as hesperidin, limonoids, and vitamin C, which is one of the power trio of antioxidants.

POWER

CHOCOLATE CHEESECAKE

Build stronger bones with . . . cheesecake? Why not, when it's made from calcium-rich low-fat dairy products? Since every bit counts, the 5 percent of the Daily Value for calcium in each slice adds up. Serve with a frosty glass of milk to multiply the benefits.

CRUST

10	whole reduced-fat graham cracker rectangles
1	egg white

FILLING

2	cups 1% cottage cheese
1	package (8 ounces) reduced-fat cream cheese, softened
1	cup sugar
2	eggs, lightly beaten, or $\frac{1}{2}$ cup fat-free liquid egg substitute
$\frac{1}{2}$	cup fat-free sour cream
$\frac{1}{3}$	cup unsweetened cocoa powder
3	ounces semisweet chocolate, melted
1	tablespoon cornstarch
$\frac{1}{8}$	teaspoon salt
1	teaspoon vanilla extract
2	cups raspberries

Research shows that eating 1 cup of beans a day can lower cholesterol about 10 percent in 6 weeks. Beans are especially high in soluble fiber, which lowers cholesterol levels. Experts theorize that the soluble fiber in beans increases the amount of bile acid (a substance produced by the liver that helps you digest fats) excreted in bowel movements. Because your body uses cholesterol to make bile, reducing the amount of bile in your systems also reduces your cholesterol. Or it may be that as beans ferment

Preheat the oven to 325°F. Coat a 9" springform pan with cooking spray. Place on a square of foil and mold the foil around the outside of the pan.

To make the crust: In a food processor, grind the crackers into fine crumbs. Add the egg white and pulse to combine. Press evenly into the prepared pan.

To make the filling: In a food processor, process the cottage cheese for 2 minutes, or until very smooth. Add the cream cheese, sugar, eggs or egg substitute, sour cream, cocoa, chocolate, cornstarch, salt, and vanilla. Process until smooth. Pour into the pan.

Place the pan into a baking pan and set in the oven. Add enough hot tap water to the baking pan to come at least 1" up the side of the springform pan.

Bake for 1 hour, or until firm around the edge (the mixture will still be soft in the center). Transfer the springform pan to a wire rack. Immediately run a thin, wet knife around the edge of the cake to release it from the pan. Carefully remove the side of the pan. Let the cake cool completely. Replace the side of the pan, cover loosely with foil, and refrigerate for up to 2 days.

Arrange the raspberries in a single layer on top of the cheesecake, pressing gently to secure them.

Makes 12 slices

Per slice: 257 calories, 11 g protein, 33 g carbohydrates, 8.5 g fat, 50 mg cholesterol, 1 g dietary fiber, 340 mg sodium

Note: To make cutting easier and neater, dip a sharp knife into hot water and shake off the excess water before cutting each slice.

in your colon, they produce substances called short-chain fatty acids (SCFAs), substances that hinder the liver's production of cholesterol.

Another potent cholesterol buster is garlic. While a few studies have found that this pungent bulb did not lower cholesterol, dozens of others suggest otherwise. In one review article about garlic's cholesterol-lowering effects, researchers concluded that one-half to one clove of garlic daily reduced blood cholesterol by an average of 9 percent. It's thought that garlic's prodigious amount of antioxidant compounds, including S-allyl-cysteine, may be behind its significant cholesterol-lowering properties.

Stir-fry some tofu along with that clove. One study found that regularly consuming soy may reduce total cholesterol levels by up to 10 percent. It's thought that isoflavones—compounds in soy with weak estrogen-like activity—act like human hormones that regulate cholesterol levels. Soy isoflavones are also antioxidants, which may protect against LDL oxidation.

Good sources of soy protein include soy milk, tofu, and textured soy protein (TSP), the main ingredient in many meat substitutes.

Fish—particularly cold-water fish such as herring, mackerel, and salmon—is a rich source of a unique type of fat, omega-3 fatty acids. Besides lowering heart-harming fats called triglycerides, studies suggest that omega-3's also make blood more slippery, making it less likely to clot.

Researchers studied people in two villages in Africa, located 40 miles apart. While the lifestyles of both villages were similar, one village ate a diet high in fish; the other, a vegetarian diet. The villagers who ate lots of fish had lower cholesterol levels than the vegetarians.

POWER-EATING TIP

Drink three glasses of orange juice a day. Eat 1 cup of beans a day. Add one-half to one clove of garlic to your food each day. Help yourself to one or two servings of soy a day (½ cup of tofu, 1 cup of soy milk, 3 tablespoons of roasted soybeans, or a soy protein shake or bar with 30 to 50 milligrams of isoflavones). Eat cold-water fish twice a week.

Irritable Bowel Syndrome

The Power Foods: A high-fiber, low-fat diet

Irritable bowel syndrome, or IBS, is a disorder of the large intestine (colon) that keeps the bowels in a perpetual uproar: diarrhea, constipation, erratic swings from diarrhea to constipation, abdominal pain, bloating, and gas. For some reason, the colon reacts strongly to normal stimuli, such as eating or abdominal gas, with spasms—which may be where it got its other name, spastic colon. It's estimated that IBS affects one out of five Americans, and three times as many women as men.

Women with IBS may have more symptoms during their periods, suggesting a hormonal link to the condition.

A diet high in fiber is one of the most effective dietary remedies for IBS, whether for constipation, diarrhea, or both. High-fiber diets keep the colon slightly distended, which may help prevent spasms. Insoluble fiber, found in abundance in whole wheat products and certain vegetables such as sweet potatoes, is the most effective form of fiber for IBS. It helps keep water in the stools, making them easier to pass.

A common cause of IBS flare-ups is fat. Fat is hard to digest, and large amounts can cause your bowel to rebel. A low-fat diet can help reduce abdominal pain and diarrhea.

Fiber and water work together to regulate your bowels, so drink nine 8-ounce glasses of water and other healthy beverages a day. Avoid coffee, cola, and tea. The caffeine they contain can cause diarrhea and can increase painful bowel spasms.

POWER-EATING TIP

Consume 20 to 35 grams of fiber a day, avoiding gas-producing fruits and vegetables and beans. These include legumes, cruciferous vegetables (broccoli, brussels sprouts, cauliflower, and cabbage) even if they are cooked, corn, onions, nuts, and seeds. For the same reason, avoid beer, nuts, popcorn, wheat germ, cantaloupe, and honeydew melon. To get important vitamins such as beta-carotene, vitamin C, and folate, reach for sweet potatoes, spinach, and winter squash, citrus fruits and juices, and baked potatoes with the skin. Fat should account for no more than 25 percent of your daily calories. Drink plenty of water and other fluids: nine 8-ounce glasses a day. Two of the nine glasses can come from liquids other than water, such as juice, low-fat milk, herbal teas, or noncola sodas. Limit or avoid coffee and other caffeinated beverages.

With IBS, how you eat is as important as what you eat. For example, large meals can cause cramping and diarrhea. Eating smaller meals more often or just eating smaller portions may help. Also, no matter how hectic your schedule, don't skip meals. It can provoke symptoms, such as gas, bloating, abdominal pain, and irregular bowel movements.

Kidney Stones

The Power Foods: Orange juice, magnesium-rich foods, calcium-rich foods

Imagine a watermelon seed trying to pass through a tube the diameter of a strand of linguine—and getting stuck. That's what can happen when a large kidney stone tries to pass through one of your ureters, the thin tubes that transfer urine from your kidneys to your bladder. The result: Severe back pain, nausea and vomiting, and—despite the pain—an urgent need to urinate. In fact, the pain of passing a stone is reputed to be comparable to that of giving birth.

The simplest way to reduce your risk of oxalate-containing kidney stones? Drink up—at least ten 8-ounce glasses of fluids, preferably water. The fluid will dilute your urine and eliminate stone-forming oxalate, a form of salt normally excreted in the urine that is one of the main components of kidney stones. Also, limit your intake of foods shown to raise oxalate levels, such as spinach, beets, nuts, rhubarb, tea, wheat bran, strawberries, and, alas, chocolate.

Consider making orange juice a part of your anti-stone diet. It's loaded with citrate, a known stone inhibitor. In one study, men with a history of kidney stones were given either three 12-ounce glasses of orange juice a day or potassium citrate supplements. Turns out that the juice was nearly as effective as the supplements.

Good sources of magnesium, such as Swiss chard and beans, can help prevent stones by lowering the amount of oxalate in the urine. Researchers studied the association between diet and the development of kidney stones in 27,001 Finnish male smokers. They found that the men in the group who got the most magnesium in their diets (about 563 milligrams) had about half the risk that men in the group that ate the least (about 382 milligrams) had. The researchers believe that there would be similar results among nonsmokers (since smoking is not related to the formation of kidney stones), as well as among women.

While experts used to think that consuming too much dietary calcium increased the risk of kidney stones, more recent research has shown that the opposite is true. Researchers followed more than 91,731 women for 12 years and found that those with the highest intake of dietary calcium (1,119 milligrams per day), primarily from dairy foods, were 35 percent less likely to develop kidney stones than those who ate the least (about

430 milligrams per day). Dietary calcium keeps oxalates from being absorbed in the intestine and excreted by the kidney to form stones.

POWER-EATING TIP

Drink three 12-ounce glasses of orange juice a day. Shoot for 400 milligrams of magnesium a day from food. Include two to three servings of calcium-rich foods a day (fat-free or low-fat milk, low-fat yogurt, low-fat or reduced-fat cheese, calcium-fortified orange juice).

Osteoporosis

The Power Foods: Calcium-rich foods, especially low-fat dairy products; soy; fruits and vegetables

It's estimated that 10 million Americans have osteoporosis, in which bones become fragile and more likely to break. And 8 million of them are women.

That's hard to swallow, when virtually all of us know that getting enough calcium is vital to maintaining the strength and thickness of our bones. But apparently, calcium-rich foods are just as hard to swallow: The average American woman consumes about 750 milligrams of calcium a day, despite the recommended daily requirement of 1,000 milligrams for women under 50 and 1,500 milligrams for women 50 and over.

To bone up on calcium, add more calcium-rich foods to your diet. Dairy foods such as yogurt, milk, and cheese—even the low-fat versions—are the richest sources of calcium. Other excellent sources are calcium-fortified orange juice, breakfast cereals, and sardines. Good sources include collard and turnip greens.

Make sure to get enough vitamin D, too. Found in fortified milk, this vitamin is necessary for your body to absorb calcium. A good daily multivitamin will also provide what you need.

Consider adding tofu, soy milk, or other soy foods to your diet. While evidence is preliminary, scientists think that substances in soy called isoflavones may promote bone health. Isoflavones—one of a group of phytonutrients called phytoestrogens—mimic the estrogen women produce naturally. Estrogen encourages the calcium in bones to stay put. The theory is that by acting as a weak estrogen, isoflavones protect bone health. In one study of 66 postmenopausal women, researchers found that giving them 90 milligrams of soy isoflavones a day (in a soy protein powder) for 6 months increased their bone density by 2 percent. Women taking powdered milk experienced no such increase.

Fruits and vegetables may also help protect bones, by changing the body's acid/alkaline balance for the better. Here's the theory. The average American diet—heavy on meats, sugars, and fats—makes our bodies produce more acid. To neutralize this acid, the body "steals" calcium and other bone-protecting minerals from bone. By contrast, fruits and vegetables are a gold mine of potassium and magnesium. These minerals are thought to buffer the acid, which halts this grand larceny of minerals. In one study of older people, those who ate the most fruits and veggies every day had denser bones. What's more, every extra serving of a fruit or vegetable per day increased hipbone density (in men) by 1 percent. And every 1 percent increase means a 5 percent reduction in your risk of fracture.

No doubt about it: Chronic alcohol abuse weakens bones. But there's evidence that, consumed in moderation, alcohol may help keep them sturdy. In a study of 188 postmenopausal women, those who drank at least five alcoholic drinks a week had significantly higher bone densities than nondrinkers. That's even after researchers accounted for osteoporosis risk factors like exercise, hormone-replacement therapy, and daily intake of calcium and vitamin D. Researchers speculate that alcohol may increase the estrogen circulating in a woman's body or cause the body to produce extra calcitonin, a hormone that curtails the release of calcium from bone.

MASKED DISASTER

Nondairy Desserts

Some nondairy frozen desserts are so high in fat, calories, and sugar that you might as well just buy the Häagen-Dazs and be done with it. One brand's premium variety (Chocolate Supreme) packs 190 calories, 11 grams of fat, and 15 grams of sugar per ½-cup serving. By comparison, ½ cup of chocolate ice cream contains 142 calories and 7 grams of fat.

If quantity is more important than quality, opt for the fat- or sugar-free varieties of nondairy desserts. Or use ¼ cup of the good stuff to top fresh fruit, such as berries or grapes. You'll get all the creamy goodness with less fat, calories, and sugar. Plus, you'll get a dose of protective fiber and phytonutrients from the fruit.

Power-EATING TIP

Eat two to three servings of calcium-rich foods a day (fat-free or low-fat milk, low-fat yogurt, low-fat or reduced-fat cheese, and calcium-fortified orange juice). Don't let the day go by without eating or drinking a serving or two of soy (½ cup of tofu, 1 cup of soy milk, 3 tablespoons of roasted soybeans, or a soy protein shake or bar with 30 to 50 milligrams of isoflavones). Aim for nine servings of fruits and vegetables a day.

Premenstrual Syndrome

The Power Foods: Whole grain bread, brown rice, potatoes, and other complex carbohydrates; calcium-rich foods

Perhaps the only nice thing to say about a condition that plagues 30 to 40 percent of women with bloating, achy breasts, depression, restlessness, and weepiness is this: A poll found that 79 percent of men surveyed felt that we are not malingering—PMS is a bona fide health condition.

And there's convincing evidence that what you eat (or don't eat) during this touchy 7 to 14 days can make a significant difference in how you feel, both physically and emotionally.

For example, eating more carbohydrates before your period may help relieve PMS symptoms by elevating levels of serotonin, a brain chemical that plays a vital role in the regulation of sleep, appetite, and mood. But choose your carbs wisely. Complex carbohydrates in whole grain bread, brown rice, and potatoes are higher in nutrients and lower in fat than the simple carbohydrates found in sweets. Just as important, there's evidence that a diet high in simple carbohydrates may actually aggravate PMS symptoms in the long run.

Getting more calcium into your diet may also help ease premenstrual moodiness and discomfort. Researchers had 466 women with documented PMS take either 1,200 milligrams of calcium (in supplement form) or placebos. By the second menstrual cycle, the pain, foul moods, food cravings, and bloating of the women taking calcium began to improve. By their third cycle, their symptoms were reduced by 48 percent, compared with 30 percent in the placebo group. It's possible to get this

PERIMENOPAUSE: EAT TO CALM THE SYMPTOMS

If hot flashes or other harbingers of menopause bother you, fight back with your knife and fork. Simple dietary changes may make you feel more comfortable. Here are some perimenopausal "plate rules" from the experts.

EAT SMALL MEALS. Waistband-stretching meals take more energy to digest and metabolize. The extra heat this process generates can raise your body temperature. Plus, you may feel faint and sluggish after a large meal because a lot of blood is diverted to the stomach.

AVOID "FLASH" FOODS. In case you haven't noticed, hot and spicy foods, alcohol, and caffeinated drinks such as coffee, tea, and cola can likewise jack up your body temperature.

CARBO-LOAD AT DINNERTIME. Some women going through perimenopause experience insomnia. If you're having trouble sleeping, make dinner a high-carbohydrate meal, such as a plate of pasta and a slice of bread. Tryptophan, the amino acid in many high-carbohydrate foods, is essential in the production of serotonin, a brain chemical that helps regulate sleep.

STAY THE COURSE WITH SOY. Until recently, it was thought that tofu and other soy foods could help relieve perimenopausal symptoms such as hot flashes. More current research suggests otherwise. But there's still a compelling reason to eat soy foods. While they may not cool hot flashes, soy protein does reduce the risk of heart disease by lowering total and LDL cholesterol and, perhaps, by preventing LDL cholesterol from undergoing harmful oxidation. And since our odds of developing heart disease rise once we hit menopause, get those recommended one or two servings of soy a day—for your heart, if not for your heat.

amount of calcium through food. One cup of calcium-enriched orange juice contains 300 milligrams of calcium, the same amount as in 1 cup of milk and 25 percent of the amount used in the study for premenopausal symptoms.

What about chocolate? On the one hand, it's known to aggravate mood swings and breast tenderness. On the other, it's the premenstrual woman's best friend. A scientific review of the sweet and creamy delight suggests that chocolate cravings kick into high gear before a woman's period and may be related, among other things, to fluctuating hormone levels. So if you crave chocolate, indulge—in moderation.

POWER-EATING TIP

The week before your period, try eating at least 100 carbohydrate calories every 3 hours, while cutting back on fat and protein. (Protein inhibits serotonin production.) Choose whole grains such as whole wheat bread or pasta or brown rice. Eat two or three calcium-rich foods a day (fat-free or low-fat milk, low-fat yogurt, low-fat or reduced-fat cheese, or calcium-fortified orange juice). Consider limiting your intake of caffeine and salt 1 to 2 weeks before your period is due. Research links caffeine to premenstrual depression, irritability, and breast pain, while consuming too much salt is associated with premenstrual bloating, water retention, and weight gain. To help minimize moodiness and depression, avoid alcohol prior to your period, too.

Stroke

The Power Foods: Fruits and vegetables (particularly citrus fruit, broccoli, cabbage, cauliflower, and brussels sprouts), spinach, tea

Every 60 seconds, someone in the United States suffers a stroke, a condition in which the brain is literally starved of oxygen. The main causes are fatty deposits that clog the vessels that bring blood to your brain, a blood clot that lodges in one of the brain's vessels, or a burst blood artery in the brain (aneurysm). Fortunately, the same low-fat, healthy diet that can prevent or treat heart disease can also protect you against stroke.

Fruits and vegetables are brimming with potassium, a mineral linked to a reduced risk of stroke. In one study of 75,596 women ages 34 to 59, those eating the most fruits and vegetables (about 10 servings a day) had a 30 percent lower risk of stroke than those who consumed the least (less than 3 servings a day). What's more, every additional serving a day reduced stroke risk by 6 percent. The most potent stroke blasters? Citrus fruits and cruciferous vegetables such as broccoli, cabbage, cauliflower, and brussels sprouts.

Eat your spinach, too—along with your asparagus and beans. They're all excellent sources of the B vitamin folate, found to lower blood levels of homocysteine, an amino acid linked to a higher risk of heart disease and stroke. In a study of 167 women under 45, researchers found that women with the highest levels of homocysteine had double the risk of stroke compared to women with lower levels.

There's also evidence to suggest that flavonoids, a group of antioxidants found in tea, may cut stroke risk. In one study, researchers tracked the diets of 552 men for 15 years. They found that those who got most of their flavonoids from tea (about five cups a day) reduced their risk of stroke by 69 percent, compared to those who consumed the least (less than three cups).

POWER-EATING TIP

Eat no fewer than nine servings of fruits and vegetables a day, particularly those listed above. Drink up to five cups of tea a day.

Ulcers

The Power Foods: Cabbage, yogurt, garlic

At some point, 1 in every 10 Americans will experience the dull, gnawing ache of an ulcer. And not because they're fans of spicy food or chronic stress, for decades thought to be the root causes of ulcers. Now it's known that in 80 percent of cases, the culprit is a bacterium named *Helicobacter pylori*. This bacterium, which infects 20 percent of people under 40 and half of those over 60, can live on the delicate lining of your stomach and small intestine, damaging it along with the mucous layer that protects it from stomach acids. Ulcers can also be caused by daily use of nonsteroidal anti-inflammatory drugs (NSAIDs), such as aspirin and ibuprofen. Smoking and having a close relative with ulcers increase your risk.

It used to be that doctors prescribed a bland diet for people with ulcers. Now, they prescribe antibiotics to kill *H. pylori* and drugs to reduce stomach acid. Still, several foods may inhibit the growth of *H. pylori* or speed the healing of an ulcer itself.

Cabbage is the classic home remedy to soothe a burning stomach.

Back in 1949, a group of researchers at Stanford University School of Medicine had 13 people with ulcers drink about 1 quart of raw cabbage juice a day. Their ulcers healed six times faster than people whose only treatment was the standard bland diet. At that time, researchers attributed this vegetable's healing qualities to an unknown factor they dubbed

WHAT TO EAT WHEN YOU'RE TAKING ANTIBIOTICS

Antibiotics are good at killing the nasty bacteria that cause sinus and urinary tract infections. Unfortunately, they're also good at wiping out the friendly bacteria that live in your gastrointestinal tract and vagina and keep them healthy. Antibiotics often cause diarrhea and—yuck—yeast infections.

Fortunately, you can eat to avoid these bothersome side effects without weakening the effectiveness of your antibiotic.

YOGURT. You've probably heard that you should eat yogurt if you're taking antibiotics. And for good reason. Studies suggest that 1 cup of yogurt a day can help prevent antibiotic-induced diarrhea. It may be that the "good" bacteria in yogurt replenish some of the helpful bacteria in your gastrointestinal tract wiped out by the antibiotic.

Eating 1 cup of yogurt a day while you're taking antibiotics may also help restore the natural balance of good bacteria in your vagina, preventing yeast infections. A small study found that such yogurt consumption decreased yeast infections threefold.

GARLIC. Dubbed poor man's penicillin, garlic has been shown to kill *Candida albicans*, the fungus that causes yeast infections, on contact. What's more, garlic appears to stimulate the activity of neutrophils and macrophages, immune cells that fight infection.

Women who suffer from frequent yeast infections should consume one or two cloves of raw garlic a day, recommends Andrew Weil, M.D., director of the program in integrative medicine of the College of Medicine at the University of Arizona in Tucson. To make raw garlic more palatable, finely mince it and mix it into food. (When cooked, garlic loses its antibiotic properties.)

Vitamin U. Now it's known that cabbage contains glutamine, an amino acid that increases bloodflow to the stomach and helps strengthen its protective lining.

While milk can aggravate an ulcer, research suggests that fermented milk—also known as yogurt—can actually soothe one. Researchers from Sweden analyzed the diets of 764 people with ulcers and 229 people without. They found that men and women who ate the most yogurt reduced their risk of ulcers by 18 percent, compared with those who ate the least. The "friendly" bacteria in yogurt, such as *Lactobacillus bulgaricus* and *L. acidophilus*, may be the therapeutic substance.

Long known as a natural antibiotic, garlic may also inhibit the growth of *H. pylori*. In one laboratory study, the extract from the equivalent of two cloves of garlic was able to stop the growth of this ulcer-causing bacterium.

POWER-EATING TIP

When an ulcer flares, drink the juice from half a head (about 2 cups) of cabbage a day. Or simply eat 2 cups of raw cabbage. Don't cook the cabbage. Heat destroys its therapeutic powers. Or eat 1 cup of yogurt three or four times a day. Choose yogurt with live or active cultures, which contain beneficial bacteria. Add two cloves of raw garlic a day to your diet. Mince the raw bulb and mix it into food—it will go down more easily.

Urinary Tract Infections

The Power Foods: Cranberry juice, blueberries

Each year, an estimated 26 million women endure the frustrating symptoms of urinary tract infections (UTIs). Usually caused when bacteria take up residence in the urethra (the tube through which urine flows), the symptoms of a UTI include an urgent need to urinate and pain or burning upon urination. Women are 25 times more likely to get UTIs than men because our urethras are shorter, making it easier for bacteria to migrate there from the nearby rectal area.

Cranberry juice has long been a home remedy for urinary tract infections, and for good reason. In one study, researchers in Boston gave 153

older women 10 ounces of sweetened cranberry juice a day. After 6
months, the cranberry juice drinkers were 42 percent less likely to have
urinary tract bacteria in their urine than women who drank a look-alike
juice. Cranberries' healing power may come from proanthocyanidins.
These compounds may coat the walls of the urinary tract, preventing the
bacteria responsible for UTIs from sticking to the walls of the urethra.

Blueberries have also been found to stave off UTIs. Like cranberries,
they contain condensed tannins, compounds that also give bladder walls
a Teflon-like coating.

To prevent bladder infections, drink 10 ounces of cranberry juice a
day. (Because cranberry juice packs a lot of calories, you may want to opt
for artificially sweetened cranberry juice.) Research suggests that it takes
about 1 cup of blueberries a day, fresh or frozen, to prevent recurrent
UTIs.

Vaginal Infections

The Power Foods: Yogurt, garlic

Yeast infection is the second most common vaginal infection in North
America—an itchy, miserable affliction that plagues 45 percent of women
more than once. Most often, yeast infections are caused by the organism
Candida albicans. Normally, *Candida*, which lives mostly in the intestines
and the vagina, coexists peacefully with other microorganisms. But any
number of factors can destroy the so-called friendly bacteria in the vagina
that normally keep yeast in check, causing *Candida* to grow out of control. These include antibiotics, poor diet, and pregnancy.

Most women have heard that yogurt—specifically, the live bacteria in
yogurt called *Lactobacillus acidophilus*—is a potent home remedy for yeast

infections. In addition, research suggests that it works for another common type of vaginal infection, called bacterial vaginitis (BV). In one study of 46 women, 28 had bacterial vaginitis. Half of the women began eating yogurt that contained *L. acidophilus*, and the other half ate yogurt with no bacteria. After 1 month of eating ½ cup of yogurt that contained *L. acidophilus* a day, the percentage of women with BV fell from 60 percent to 25 percent. Among the women who ate yogurt without bacteria, the percentage of those with BV dropped only from 70 percent to 50 percent after 2 months.

Garlic contains a crew of chemical compounds, among them ajoene, allicin/alliin, and diallyl sulfide, all proven to fight fungal infections. In one animal study, mice with yeast infections were given either a solution made with aged garlic extract or an inactive solution. Two days later, the rats given saline were still infected. But those in the garlic group were completely fungus-free.

POWER-EATING TIP

Eat 1 cup of plain low-fat or fat-free yogurt a day. Eat a clove or two of garlic a day, minced into food.

Anti-Aging Foods from Your Pantry

Power Maker #26: For extra decades of sharp memory, clear vision, powerful immunity, and strong bones, make sure your weekly menu includes anti-aging Power Foods like berries, spinach, orange juice, and soy.

The latest discoveries about aging indicate that simply by choosing the right foods, you can enjoy years of active, pain-free living well into your seventies, eighties, and nineties. And it's a lot more fun than cryogenics.

Aging doesn't necessarily just happen, say experts. It's the result of things that occur at the cellular level. And researchers are finding again and again that one of those activities—oxidation—is a leading culprit in changes we normally associate with advancing age, such as memory loss, impaired vision, lower immunity, and weaker bones.

Here's why. Your body uses oxygen to burn food into energy. The process creates highly reactive molecules called free radicals. Some free radicals do important cleanup work, but excess free radicals flit around like sparks, damaging cells and tissue.

Strange as it may sound, the discovery that such "oxidative stress" is a major body-aging factor is a welcome one, since we have available to us enzymes and other chemicals that exist solely to reduce oxidation by neutralizing free radicals. They're called, logically, antioxidants. Some antioxidants are made in the body, but we get most through nutrients in some foods.

"Our oxidative stress load seems to increase as we age," says James Joseph, Ph.D., a researcher at the Jean Mayer USDA Human Nutrition Research Center on Aging at Tufts University in Boston. "So if certain fruits and vegetables have the potent antioxidant properties that we think they do, they'll go a long way toward providing protection."

Vitamins C and E and beta-carotene are antioxidants. So are many minerals, such as selenium, manganese, copper, and zinc. But an impressive array of antioxidant plant substances known as phytochemicals, or phytonutrients, grouped into families like the carotenoids and the flavonoids, also play a big role.

Many of the same Power Foods you eat to stay healthy—fruits and vegetables—also fight aging. Add to them specific eating strategies for preserving memory, vision, resistance to disease, and bone health—four hallmarks of youthfulness for women. In other words, you can eat certain foods right now—in your thirties, forties, and fifties—that may help usher in healthier and more vital years ahead without the declines long associated with getting on in years.

Chief Memory-Enhancing Foods

Admittedly, a certain amount of cognitive deficit is part of aging. It's not so much that you lose cells as that you lose connections among the neurons in your brain, leaving fewer pathways for information. Next thing you know, your memory isn't what it used to be.

But what oxidation can cause, antioxidants can correct. "Nutrition becomes even more important when you consider brain function," Dr. Joseph says. "We've shown that with certain berries and other antioxidant foods, we can help reverse the decline."

And there's a second food front for offsetting cognition decline. The vitamin B_{12} found in mackerel and tuna and the folate (another B vitamin) in lentils, spinach, chickpeas, baby lima beans, red kidney beans, and asparagus can help, too. (Folate is the naturally occurring form of folic acid.)

"Both vitamin B_{12} and folate are necessary for proper brain function,"

POWER

B R E A K F A S T

ORANGE FRENCH TOAST WITH WALNUTS

Here's a fun way to get age-defying nutrients like vitamin C and folate at breakfast. (The toasted walnuts help keep your heart young.)

1	cup 1% milk
3	eggs or ¾ cup fat-free liquid egg substitute
¼	cup orange juice
3	tablespoons sugar
1	teaspoon vanilla extract
12	slices whole wheat cinnamon raisin bread
3	oranges, peeled, seeded, and coarsely chopped
½	cup chopped toasted walnuts

In a medium bowl, whisk together the milk, eggs or egg substitute, orange juice, sugar, and vanilla. Pour into a 13" × 9" baking dish.

Working in batches, dip the bread into the mixture for about 30 seconds per side. Place a large nonstick skillet over medium heat until hot. Add the bread and cook for 4 minutes per side, or until golden. Serve sprinkled with the oranges and walnuts.

Makes 6 servings

Per serving: 379 calories, 12 g protein, 59 g carbohydrates, 12 g fat, 108 mg cholesterol, 7 g dietary fiber, 205 mg sodium

says Paul Jacques, Sc.D., associate professor in the School of Nutrition Science and Policy at Tufts University. "People with deficiencies may develop problems in this area."

For preventing memory loss and other age-related cognitive problems, blueberries may be the most effective, as well as the best-tasting, food there is. We know this because researchers fed healthy pre-middle-aged laboratory rats a steady diet of blueberries and found that they did much better than their nonberry-eating fellow rats on a variety of mental acuity tests as they reached middle age and beyond.

True, most human beings aren't rats. But Dr. Joseph, who led the study, is convinced that the findings suggest that such antioxidant-rich foods as blueberries may be beneficial in reversing the course of neuronal and behavioral aging. Says Dr. Joseph, "There are a lot of parallels to the way a rat ages and the way a human ages. They both show moderate cognitive deficits at about the same time—that is, in middle age, which is 15 months old for a rat and in their forties and fifties for humans. And they both lose similar kinds of receptors in the brain."

That the precise antioxidant phytonutrients responsible for slowing age-related cognitive decline haven't been isolated may actually be an indication of blueberries' potency. "Blueberries seem to contain a lot more of these compounds than most fruits and vegetables," Dr. Joseph says.

What's more, it appears that blueberries' memory protection may be the result of more than just their antioxidant action. They also produce an anti-inflammatory effect by loosening up rigid brain cell membranes. That's key, since it's precisely that kind of inflammation that plays a major role in such brain diseases as Parkinson's and Alzheimer's.

POWER-EATING TIP

Blend up some blueberries. Besides fresh blueberries for dessert—or blueberries topped with low-fat yogurt, whole grain blueberry muffins, or blueberries with your breakfast cereal—you can go for authenticity and duplicate the "extract" that a research team used to improve the mental performance of lab rats. If you want to make the extract, get a blender and throw in some blueberries.

Add some strawberries. Strawberries showed the same anti-aging effects as blueberries in Dr. Joseph's study. And another study at the USDA Human Nutrition Research Center on Aging—this time using humans—confirmed that eating strawberries increases the body's antioxidant capacity. Which is more good news for women who want to eat now and remember later. As Dr. Joseph puts it, "Who doesn't like strawberries?"

The Vision-Saving Nutrients

If you want to know why visual acuity so often degenerates with age, just look at where your eyes are. "They're in a very oxidative environment," Dr. Jacques says. "A lot of damage results from so much exposure to sunlight."

Indeed, oxidation is the probable cause of one of the most common age-related eye problems (cataracts) and a likely suspect in the other one (macular degeneration). "You look at cataracts, you see oxidized protein," Dr. Jacques says. "That suggests that getting antioxidants into the lens through eating the right foods will protect the lens."

THE VEGETARIAN ADVANTAGE

With just a few exceptions, the best anti-aging foods could make themselves right at home on any vegetarian's plate. Maybe that's why studies show that vegetarians are less prone to such notorious lifespan-reducers as heart disease, diabetes, and many kinds of cancers.

Most eating strategies to offset the physical and mental declines of aging emphasize antioxidants, so vegetarians have a clear advantage. Their diets tend to be higher in folate (the naturally occurring form of folic acid) as well as key antioxidants such as vitamins C and E, carotenoids, and phytonutrients.

Research on populations that are meatless by religious conviction tend to confirm the link with longer, healthier lives. "Some of the healthiest people in the country are Seventh-Day Adventists, and they are strict vegetarians," says James Joseph, Ph.D., a researcher at the Jean Mayer USDA Human Nutrition Research Center on Aging at Tufts University in Boston.

But Dr. Joseph also points out that Seventh-Day Adventists don't smoke, don't drink, and generally lead pretty conservative lives. That confuses the issue a bit. "It may be that people who have the sense to eat vegetarian diets are also the people who have the sense to take care of their lives in other ways," says Michael Fossel, M.D., Ph.D., clinical professor of medicine and a longevity researcher at Michigan State University in East Lansing. But, he adds, the plant-based diet itself still deserves most of the credit.

POWER

CAKE

BLUEBERRY-YOGURT SNACKING CAKE

Who doesn't love blueberries? And you'll adore them all the more when you realize that their antioxidants help prevent age-related memory loss. Bake them into this luscious low-fat cake, which is perfect for afternoon snacks and suppertime dessert. (A bonus: The yogurt in the cake not only keeps it moist but also supplements your calcium intake.)

1	cup whole wheat flour
1	cup unbleached or all-purpose flour
1	teaspoon baking powder
½	teaspoon baking soda
½	teaspoon salt
1	cup sugar
2	eggs or ½ cup fat-free liquid egg substitute
1½	cups low-fat plain yogurt
½	cup orange juice
2	tablespoons canola oil

Foods rich in vitamin C, vitamin E, and carotenoids will do just that. And they'll also help your eyes help themselves. "The lens and the retina have their own mechanisms to repair oxidative damage," Dr. Jacques says. "But those mechanisms age themselves, so proper nutrition, especially vitamin C, may help protect eye components involved in repairing oxidative damage."

Your Immune-Boosting Arsenal

"A good immune system is associated with living longer," says John Bogden, Ph.D., professor in the department of preventive medicine and community health at the New Jersey Medical School in Newark.

Grated rind of 1 orange

1½   cups blueberries

Preheat the oven to 350°F. Coat a 9" × 9" metal baking pan with cooking spray.

In a small bowl, mix the whole wheat flour, unbleached or all-purpose flour, baking powder, baking soda, and salt.

In a large bowl, whisk together the sugar and eggs or egg substitute until blended. Stir in the yogurt, orange juice, oil, and orange rind. Add the flour mixture and stir to mix well. Gently stir in the blueberries. Pour the batter into the prepared pan.

Bake for 1 hour, or until a toothpick inserted in the center comes out clean. Cover with foil for the last 10 minutes of baking to prevent over-browning. Remove to a wire rack to cool.

Makes 9 servings

Per serving: 259 calories, 7 g protein, 49 g carbohydrates, 5.5 g fat, 50 mg cholesterol, 3 g dietary fiber, 244 mg sodium

The connection between what you eat and how well your immune system holds up has a lot to do with the actual *size* of your immune system, which includes millions of cells in your bloodstream, and other organs like the spleen. "It's a large system with a high cellular turnover," says Dr. Bogden. "That combination makes it a big user of nutrients."

There's nothing like antioxidants, especially vitamins E and C, to neutralize those free radicals and keep them from harming the cells of that immense immune system of yours. Richest sources of vitamin E are nuts (like almonds and walnuts) and fresh vegetable oils (like olive oil and canola oil). Richest sources of vitamin C are sweet red peppers, cantaloupe, strawberries, and citrus fruit.

ANTI-AGING FONDUE?

Lots of anti-aging foods, like strawberries, are pretty darn delicious. But is it possible that chocolate, the ultimate feel-good taste treat, helps you live longer?

Maybe so, say Harvard researchers who gathered information on the candy bar–consuming habits—as well as death certificates—of thousands of Harvard graduates who entered college between 1916 and 1950. They found that those who ate candy one to three times a month had the lowest mortality rate, while those who never ate candy had the highest.

Now, this study was done with men, not women, and included candy that wasn't chocolate-based. But still, as the researchers note, the pro-candy results of the study may be explained by how rich chocolate is in phenols, the same antioxidants found in red wine. They are known to lower the risk of heart disease and cancer and boost your body's overall antioxidant capacity to protect you against all kinds of age-related problems.

So, should you dip those strawberries in hot melted chocolate for an anti-aging fondue? Sure, as long as it's an occasional treat. Chocolate is a high-calorie food, even without the added milk and sugar. The cocoa bean itself has more than twice as much fat as it has carbohydrate and more than three times as much fat as protein. "Chocolate is loaded with antioxidants, but I wouldn't make it a part of my daily diet," says James Joseph, Ph.D., a researcher at the Jean Mayer USDA Human Nutrition Research Center on Aging at Tufts University in Boston.

Build Bone with Dairy

Food will strengthen your bones with two important nutrients. Simply eat a lot of the bone-building mineral calcium, along with vitamin D, mostly via low-fat dairy products. "One message any woman cannot hear enough is the need for calcium and vitamin D," says William Evans, Ph.D., director of the nutrition, metabolism, and exercise laboratory at the University of Arkansas for Medical Sciences/Veterans Affairs Medical Center in Little Rock.

POWER-EATING TIP

Reach for the yogurt. Low-fat yogurt is one of the best sources of the dairy foods you need for bone-saving calcium and the vitamin D needed to absorb it. Low-fat or fat-free milk and low-fat cheese will also do the trick. Recommended calcium intake for women goes up from 1,000 to 1,500 milligrams a day after age 50. But to avoid the brittle bones that plague so many women in the later years of life, experts suggest that you do less counting and more eating. Consume as much low-fat dairy food as possible, starting right now. Low-fat dairy products are much more bioavailable sources of calcium than supplements.

Spinach: The All-Purpose Rejuvenator

Spinach is packed with such a variety of phytonutrients that eating it regularly can help discourage at least three kinds of age-related declines.

For vision. Lutein and zeaxanthin are antioxidant carotenoids abundant in two places: spinach and the lens of your eyes. Coincidence? Dr. Jacques doesn't think so. "Since lutein and zeaxanthin are in the lens in such high concentrations, you have to assume that they're playing a critical role," he says. "Our bodies don't make them, so vegetables high in lutein and zeaxanthin must be important."

While Dr. Jacques points out that there is still no direct evidence that the carotenoids in spinach can prevent age-related vision loss, observational studies certainly indicate that they do. One that followed female nurses over decades found that those with the highest intake of lutein and zeaxanthin had a 22 percent decreased risk of cataracts. Another found beneficial changes—even reversal—in a group of veterans with early signs of macular degeneration after they ate three to four portions of spinach for 12 weeks.

That's about one every other day, a doable spinach load in exchange for better vision in the years to come. But there are other foods rich in lutein and zeaxanthin that you can turn to for variety, including corn, orange peppers, egg yolk, kiwifruit, orange juice, grapes, and zucchini.

For immunity. As the quintessential dark leafy green (romaine lettuce and kale are others), spinach is one of the best ways to eat vitamin E as food without the fat concerns of other E sources such as nuts or vegetable oils. A potent antioxidant, vitamin E is thought to be an immune system enhancer whose free-radical scavenging helps keep your immunity up as you age.

For memory. The vitamin E in spinach may also help limit brain cell damage that can lead to memory loss as you age. But more important, spinach is a rich source of folate, the B vitamin that is essential for proper brain function.

Orange Juice Does Double Duty

Oranges are the best easy-to-find food source of the antioxidant vitamin C, and orange juice is the best way of getting lots of it into you. Vitamin C, as mentioned, helps protect the immune system, but its outstanding anti-aging benefits may be more for vision and memory than for immunity.

The lens protector. Just like the carotenoids lutein and zeaxanthin (which are also found in orange juice, by the way), vitamin C is concentrated in the lens—up to 50 times more than in the blood. That suggests that it's needed there. And indeed, in a study of 247 women, those who were given vitamin C supplements had a 75 percent lower risk of cataracts than those who didn't.

The fact that the decreased risk of cataracts showed up after 10 years of observation underscores the possible advantages of upping your vitamin C intake right now, no matter what your age, for later benefits. And you can get enough with foods, not pills. "From your diet, you can actually obtain the amount of vitamin C needed to raise the levels of vitamin C in the lens and eye tissues," Dr. Jacques says. "You don't need to get into supplements to see the potential benefits."

The trick, experts agree, is to drink orange juice every day. Then up the ante by treating yourself to at least one serving a day of another good vitamin C food. Other C-loaded fruits are guava, cranberries, papaya, kiwifruit, mango, and strawberries as well as the rest of the citrus fruits. For vegetables, get C in red and green peppers, tomatoes, kale, broccoli, and brussels sprouts.

The "smart juice." When you think of orange juice, you think of vita-

POWER

LENTILS

INDIAN-STYLE SPINACH, LENTILS, AND POTATOES

Look to spinach for phytonutrients that safeguard vision, build immunity, and preserve memory. Here, it's paired with nutrient-dense potatoes and lentils, bone-building yogurt, and savory spices to make an exotic dish your whole family will love.

1	tablespoon canola oil
1	large onion, finely chopped
8	ounces potatoes, peeled and cut into ½" cubes
1	teaspoon curry powder
½	teaspoon ground cumin
2½	cups water
1	cup brown lentils
½	teaspoon salt
¼	teaspoon ground black pepper
1	box (10 ounces) frozen chopped spinach, thawed and drained
¼	cup fat-free plain yogurt
1	tomato, finely chopped

Warm the oil in a large nonstick skillet over medium heat. Add the onion and cook, stirring, for 5 minutes. Stir in the potatoes, curry powder, and cumin. Cook for 1 minute longer.

Stir in the water, lentils, salt, and pepper. Bring to a boil. Reduce the heat to medium-low, cover, and simmer for 30 minutes, or until the lentils and potatoes are tender. Stir in the spinach and cook for 5 minutes. Serve topped with the yogurt and tomatoes.

Makes 4 servings

Per serving: 298 calories, 18 g protein, 50 g carbohydrates, 5 g fat, 1 mg cholesterol, 11 g dietary fiber, 348 mg sodium

min C. But it's also a super source of folate, the B vitamin that's key to maintaining a good memory.

Soy: The Four-Star Food

Isoflavones, the natural estrogens in certain plant foods, especially soy, can go a long way to offset the bone-weakening effects of post-menopause. "There's a whole body of emerging literature showing that soy protein may be protective against bone loss because it is rich in phy-toestrogens," Dr. Evans says.

In addition, research is not yet conclusive, but the isoflavones in soy probably work much like vitamin E in cleansing your body of cell-damaging free radicals, Dr. Evans says.

As a bonus, soy is a complete, quality protein source—that is, it provides all of the amino acids you need in your diet and is easily digestible in most forms. And it's much lower in saturated fats than meat. So by substituting soy protein for animal protein as often as you wish, you can increase the anti-aging power of your meals without going over your calorie limit. Such nutrient-rich eating—choosing foods that deliver more nutrients in fewer calories—becomes more important as you age, Dr. Joseph says.

POWER-EATING TIP

Seek out some soy. Besides the now-familiar Asian foods such as tofu, tempeh, and miso, your soy options can include soy milk and an array of flavored soy beverages; breads, muffins, crackers, biscuits, and pastas made wholly or partially from soy flour; and all kinds of meat substitutes made from soy proteins that can impersonate hamburger, bacon bits, turkey—even sliced beef and breakfast sausages.

Round Out Your Anti-Aging Menu

Here are some other foods to keep in mind as you plan your meals.

Red wine. For many, even an anti-aging meal isn't complete without a glass of wine. Make it red wine, which has been shown to

EAT LESS, LIVE LONGER?

Cutting down on food not only helps you fit into your jeans. It may also expand your life.

"In every single mammal species in which it has been tried, cutting 30 percent of their total calories means they tend to live a lot longer—as much as 50 percent longer," says Michael Fossel, M.D., Ph.D., a longevity researcher at Michigan State University in East Lansing. "For humans, we could conceivably live to be 130 to 150."

Why does calorie restriction work? Nobody knows yet, Dr. Fossel says, though less free-radical production is probably a part of the reason. Researchers do know that the risk of some deadly diseases—like heart disease and cancer—drop along with calorie intake.

For now, much of this work is being done on monkeys fed nutritionally complete, low-calorie diets. "The early data shows that these monkeys don't have the same incidence of heart disease and of cancer," Dr. Fossel says. "It's totally consistent: You eat less, and you're healthier."

There's no such work being done on humans, but history reveals an interesting side effect of food rationing in occupied Holland during World War II. "The rate of getting shot went way up, but the rate of heart disease just plummeted through the floor."

Don't start crash-dieting yet, however. When you consistently eat drastically reduced amounts of food, you starve yourself of vitamins, minerals, and other nutrients essential for good health.

"Caloric restriction for longevity is a complicated issue," says James Joseph, Ph.D., a researcher at the Jean Mayer USDA Human Nutrition Research Center on Aging at Tufts University in Boston. "You need a balanced diet with enough vitamins and minerals and lots of other things, as well as a certain amount of calories. To just start eating a lot less can be very dangerous."

deliver antioxidant phytonutrients in the form of phenolic compounds. So aside from the heart benefits of moderate alcohol consumption, red wine in moderation boosts your body's protective antioxidant capacity. If wine is not for you, try Concord grape juice for the antioxidants in grapes.

Salmon. Two servings a week of a fatty fish like salmon may help protect your future cognition by providing generous amounts of the omega-3 essential fatty acid DHA, which is thought to improve the brain's nerve cell function. Other choices are Atlantic mackerel, anchovies, and albacore tuna, which throw in as a bonus vitamin B_{12}, essential for brain function. And all of these fatty fish (herring is another one) are good sources of vitamin D to help your bones through the upcoming years.

Olive oil. Extra-virgin olive oil is the vegetable oil richest in monounsaturated fat, as well as one of the lowest in cholesterol-raising saturated fat—hence a good vegetable oil choice. Now there's evidence that those monounsaturated fats help your brain stay sharp into old age. Researchers studying the eating habits of southern Italians came up with this head-turning conclusion: The more monounsaturated fats that participants consumed, the more protected they were against age-related decline.

Up-and-comers. Once the Pandora's box of antioxidants popped open and all those phytonutrients began flying out, research began to take off. As a result, a number of offbeat foods have been named as candidates for your anti-aging meals by virtue of their apparently abundant antioxidant content.

• Seaweed. Some edible seaweeds—or more politely, sea vegetables— are loaded with a carotenoid called fucoxanthin that's been the focus of much scientific interest in Japan. The most promising appear to be brown seaweeds, especially hijiki. Your local Japanese restaurant or grocery store can help you out.

• Wasabi. This Japanese horseradish that looks like green toothpaste on your sushi plate is being studied for possible strong antioxidant content, Dr. Joseph says.

• Sesame seed oil. Rat studies already indicate that the phytonutrients called lignans in sesame seed oil provide protection against the negative effects of free radicals.

• Onions. Increasing bone mass may be another benefit of onions. At least, that's the preliminary conclusion based on studies using rats.

• Thyme and other spices. A number of kitchen spices, notably thyme, are being looked at for their antioxidant activity. "We could be talking about spices and foods working together to create a potent package against the harmful effects of free radicals and aging," Dr. Joseph says.

Think (and Eat) Positive

Working foods that fight aging into your diet is easy. Here's how.

Go fruit-and-vegetable-crazy. One vegetable as a side dish with lunch and dinner isn't going to get the anti-aging job done. While campaigns are underway to encourage Americans to eat five servings of fruits and vegetables a day, women who want to fight aging (and who doesn't?) should eat twice that. "Unless you have some sort of medical condition like diverticulitis, it's pretty hard to overdo it with fruits and vegetables," Dr. Joseph says.

Do a variety act. Eating 9 or 10 reasonably sized servings of fruits and vegetables a day leaves you lots of room for variety. The foods described in Almonds to Yogurt: 101 Power Foods on page 480 give you enough variety to last for months. But even then you should mix things up.

"No one of them is a magic bullet," says Dr. Joseph. "Eat lots of different kinds of fruits and vegetables."

Eat your antioxidants, don't "take" them. True, much of the research is done with supplements. And true, even some pretty exotic nutrients are available in capsule form these days. But your best benefits come from eating the foods that contain the good stuff. "We cannot mimic with multivitamins and supplements all of the complex ingredients that are in foods," Dr. Bogden says. "There are phytochemicals present in small amounts that may be a part of the protection these foods offer."

The exception is vitamin E, which is hard to get in food in the amounts thought to be beneficial. The usual recommendation is supplementing with 100 to 400 IU of E daily, Dr. Bogden says.

Put These High-Energy Foods on the Menu

Power Maker #27: No food can make up for a lack of sleep or overwork. But a little protein and, yes, even fat, combined with the right carbohydrates interspersed throughout the day can jump-start your inner battery.

You don't need a Ph.D. in biochemistry to know that food is fuel and that it affects our energy levels. But not just any food will do. "Certain eating strategies will definitely help you ward off fatigue," says Stacey Whittle, R.D., a registered dietitian in the department of hospitality services at the University of Southern California in Los Angeles.

Ironically, the very foods we so often rely on for quick energy—concentrated sources of sugar, like candy bars or soda—are the very foods that you should avoid if you want enduring energy, say experts.

Here's why. Your body uses food for energy by turning it into blood sugar, or glucose. Carbohydrates convert most easily into this ready-to-burn fuel, making them your macronutrient of choice for energy eating. The problem is that some simple carbohydrates, like sugar, tend to break down so fast that, after providing a short-lived burst of energy, they leave your blood sugar levels low, your energy inadequate, and your plans for the day unaccomplished. Complex carbohydrates, like grains, replace this spike-and-dip act with a steady energy supply that keeps you going at full throttle.

Striking the Optimal Energy Balance

You don't have to radically change your diet to ratchet up your energy levels. Chances are, you're already eating many of the foods best suited for daylong energy. It's simply a matter of eating them at the right time, in the right amounts, and in the right combinations.

POWER - EATING TIP

Combine carbohydrates with protein and fat. Don't make the mistake of eating too many carbs at any one meal, even if they're complex carbohydrates, because a high-carb meal can actually make you drowsy by altering brain chemistry. That is, it raises levels of serotonin, a neurotransmitter responsible for creating a sense of calm. But if you're *too* relaxed, you're not as alert and energetic as you need to be.

What's the ideal mix? High (but not exclusively) carbohydrates, moderate protein, low (but not no) fat. Think of a turkey sandwich with low-fat mayo, a small serving of spaghetti and meatballs, or a bowl of chili.

Distribute your calories equally among breakfast, lunch, and dinner. A skimpy breakfast, a hurried lunch, and a huge evening feast is about the least energy-efficient eating schedule imaginable. "What do you need all those calories for if you're going to bed?" says Debra Wein, R.D., cofounder of Sensible Nutrition Connection in Hingham, Massachusetts.

"Anybody who's ever done justice to a Thanksgiving dinner knows that you get tired when you overstuff," says Ann Grandjean, Ed.D., director of the International Center for Sports Nutrition in Omaha, Nebraska.

NOT ALL ENERGY BARS ARE CREATED EQUAL

For antifatigue snacks, you'll do a lot better with energy bars—also called power bars or sports bars—than with typical candy bars. Unlike most candy bars, a power bar's energy-giving carbohydrates might typically include whole grains and cereals (such as rolled oats and brown rice) and dried fruit, as well as a variety of sugars. They'll also provide useful amounts of vitamins, minerals, and other nutrients. And they're often lower in fat.

The ingredients—and the ratio of carbohydrates to protein and fat—vary wildly among the energy bars sold. What's best for you depends on when you'll be eating it.

AS A SNACK BEFORE EXERCISING. If you want your energy bar to fuel your workout, choose one that's almost all carbohydrates, says Debra Wein, R.D., co-founder of Sensible Nutrition Connection in Hingham, Massachusetts. For example, the apple-cherry flavored Clif bar packs 52 grams of carbs, with just 4 grams of protein and 2 grams of fat (a quarter of it saturated fat). And there are plenty more bars to fill that bill.

"You don't want a lot of protein or fat in the bar you choose to eat before exercise because they'll slow down your digestion," Wein says. "What you're looking for is quick energy."

AS A MIDMORNING OR MIDAFTERNOON SNACK. Energy bars can be a mini-meal unto themselves occasionally. But here you want long-lasting sta-

Never, ever skip a meal. "Many women skip breakfast," Wein says. "And some may even skip lunch because they think it will help them lose weight." But by skipping breakfast or lunch—or both—not only are you depriving your body of calories just when it needs them the most, you're also likely to compensate with a lethargy-inducing pig-out when you do eat. So much for weight loss! "And if you keep skipping meals, the result over time is a general malaise," Wein says.

Eat five meals a day. The experts favor adding a midmorning and midafternoon snack to your daily meal schedule, and downgrading your other three meals accordingly to keep your total calories where you want them. This mini-meal plan is a super energy booster because you're get-

mina—not quick energy—so choose a better balanced bar than you would for a preworkout snack. "Look for the same thing you look for in a meal," says Stacey Whittle, R.D., a registered dietitian at the University of Southern California in Los Angeles. "You need a good balance of carbohydrates, protein, and fat so you get energy but your blood sugar remains stable."

That is, look for mostly carbohydrates (for energy), but enough protein (and some fat) to meter the release of that energy. One yogurt-honey-peanut bar, for instance, includes protein from soy, peanut, and whey sources totaling 14 grams, along with 22 grams of carbohydrates and 6 grams of fat (half of it saturated fat). Shoot for those kinds of proportions.

AS A LUNCH REPLACEMENT. Keeping a well-balanced—as opposed to ultra–high-carb—energy bar handy in your purse or briefcase can save the day (and your energy supply) when something unexpected puts the kibosh on your lunch plans. But as a meal replacement, energy bars are for emergency use only.

Not only are regular meals more likely to deliver the nutrients you need for all-around health, an energy bar just isn't enough to satisfy you. A typical bar might deliver 200 to 250 calories (though you can find them with less or more) That's about the right amount for a snack, but too low for a meal, where you're looking for 400 to 500 calories, Whittle says.

ting energy into your body right when you need it, you won't be going too long between meals, and you're less likely to overeat or undereat. "If you watch your portion size and take time for that midmorning and midafternoon snack, you'll be surprised at how positively your energy levels are affected," Whittle says.

Wein suggests the following energizing calorie allotments: If you're a fairly typical weight-watching woman, your calorie count per day will probably fall between 1,400 and 2,000. If you're at the higher number, shoot for 500 calories at breakfast, lunch, and dinner, with midmorning and midafternoon snacks at 250. If you're down at 1,400 total calories, your meals should be 400 calories each, with two 100-calorie snacks.

If you're overweight, slim down. "Carrying around 10 or 20 pounds of excess weight in the form of body fat is like dragging an anchor," says Wayne Askew, Ph.D., professor of nutrition and director of the division of foods and nutrition at the University of Utah in Salt Lake City. "The best way to feel energetic is to maintain a proper body weight for your height and frame size."

Forget crash-dieting. It's pretty hard not to get enough calories in our food-privileged country, but lots of women go out of their way to do just that. Low-calorie diets—fewer than 1,200 calories a day, depending on your size—can sap your energy. For one thing, it's more challenging to get the nutrients you need once you go below 1,800 calories a day. And, though every woman has different calorie needs, consuming fewer than 10 calories per pound of body weight is clearly too low, Dr. Grandjean says. "The body compensates by going into a lower gear."

The Power Duo

Vitamins and minerals don't provide energy directly, but they're big-time players in processing energy. So if you don't get enough of them, you may find yourself waking up tired and staying that way. Lots of variety in fruits and vegetables is the best way to get the whole array of micronutrients, from vitamin A to zinc. But for energy, two foods are standouts.

Drink lots of fresh orange juice. Believe it or not, perhaps one out of three women isn't getting enough vitamin C, says Carol Johnston, Ph.D., assistant professor of food and nutrition in the family resources department at Arizona State University in Tempe. A shame, since women she studied who were low in vitamin C did much better on treadmill tests after they were given extra C daily. "They felt better and they had more energy," she says.

Dr. Johnston suspects that the connection between vitamin C and how energetic you feel has to do with its role in producing carnitine, a molecule that helps your body burn fat for energy. "People likely have up to a 50 percent drop in muscle carnitine levels when they're vitamin C–depleted," she says.

Although 500 milligrams of C was used in the research, Dr. Johnston thinks 200 to 300 milligrams daily is enough for you to feel more energy, assuming that you were short on C. You can get that much without supplementing if you drink plenty of orange juice (two 8-ounce glasses a day) and eat a diet high in vitamin C–rich foods. "But you have to do it every day," she says. She suggests adding another vitamin C–rich food each day, such as broccoli, peppers, brussels sprouts, kale, or strawberries.

Benefit from iron. Iron is a must mineral for energy because of its role in transporting oxygen via red blood cells to wherever it's needed in the body. Too little iron creates a cascade of problems that end up lowering your metabolic rate—and your energy levels.

A lot of women aren't getting in their diets the 18 milligrams a day of iron they need. "And women who are deficient in iron often feel lethargic," Dr. Askew says.

If you suspect that mildly low iron (rather than serious anemia-level deficiencies) is slowing you down, eat for iron by choosing legumes (soy, beans, and lentils) dark leafy greens (like spinach or kale), tofu, steamed clams, and red meat. A small cut of lean beef with spinach and lentils, washed down with orange juice (for better absorption) would be a great iron-rich meal.

If you think that you are anemic or have significantly low iron levels, see your primary-care physician before taking iron supplements.

Power Breakfasts: Wake-Up Foods for Your Whole Body

"When you wake up in the morning, you've gone for 6 to 8 hours without taking in any calories," Wein points out. "That is the time to wake up your body by providing it with the right kind of calories to burn for energy."

So if you skimp on breakfast, you run the risk of a lackluster morning, since your blood sugar will probably be low and stay low, depriving your brain of the glucose it needs. Here's how to eat a true power breakfast.

Hold the pancake syrup. Sweet breakfasts are an energy disaster, since nothing plummets your blood sugar faster (after an initial boost) than concentrated forms of simple carbohydrates like corn or maple syrup. Pouring one of them over refined carbohydrates like white flour pancakes or waffles exaggerates the effect.

Whittle warns that any sweet topping with corn syrup in it—like the typical maple-flavored syrup or a lot of jellies—is an especially good bet to spike-and-dip your blood sugar to lethargic levels.

SIX TOP ENERGY FOODS

The most energizing foods don't necessarily have the zingiest reputation. But experts suggest that these mostly unsexy foods are some of your best bets for energetic eating.

1. APPLES. Like most fruits, apples have simple sugars, like fructose for energy, and fiber to spread that energy out over time. Moreover, the fiber in an unpeeled apple has been associated with improved regularity and the prevention of colon cancer.

2. ORANGE JUICE. It's a great source of energy-essential vitamin C, and it helps absorption of energy-essential iron.

3. OATMEAL. This whole grain, unrefined cereal is rich in energy-metering soluble fiber. In tests, oatmeal eaters could exercise longer than those fed other carbs.

4. BEANS. These fiber-filled legumes have been shown to improve endurance performance. And they're a great source of iron, the most important mineral for fighting fatigue.

5. COFFEE. In moderation, it works as a pick-me-up by making energy stores more available and increasing "muscle fiber recruitment," that is, by helping the fiberlike cells in your muscles work together for maximum efficiency. But the boost from caffeine is unsustainable, so coffee should never replace eating.

6. WATER. This vital liquid prevents acute dehydration, which forces your cells to borrow water from the bloodstream, reducing your feeling of vitality. At least nine glasses a day also prevent cumulative dehydration, which could build during the week and end up as Friday fatigue. And it's still the best antidote to hot-day lethargy.

So try some healthier and more energizing alternatives, she suggests. Go for French toast made with whole grain bread and egg substitute, or use a whole grain flour like buckwheat in your pancake or waffle mix. Top them off with your favorite fruit instead of syrup. (The fructose in fruit is also a simple sugar, but it takes longer to digest, and the fiber in fruit helps slow the absorption of sugar, blunting the effect on blood sugar.)

Reach for some protein. While fruit and whole grain cereal are fine morning choices, your breakfast carbohydrates still need to be balanced with some protein foods for more enduring energy, Whittle says. The fat-free milk or low-fat yogurt you add to the cereal will work. Or go for eggs or egg substitutes with an English muffin or a slice of whole grain toast. When you eat a meal high in carbohydrates with very little protein, your body starts producing insulin. That insulin causes most of the large amino acids in the bloodstream to be transported to the muscles, effectively energizing them, she explains. An exception to this is the amino acid tryptophan, the precursor of serotonin. With the other, competing amino acids cleared out of the bloodstream, more tryptophan can get carried to the brain. The more tryptophan the brain receives, the more serotonin it produces. Since serotonin is the calming chemical that makes you feel sleepy, that's why a pure carb meal will tend to trigger drowsiness.

Shoot for 3 grams of fiber per serving. Whole grains, unlike refined flour products, deliver energy laced with fiber, which slows down the digestion so that the energy is released over a longer period of time.

That's why whole grain, high-fiber cereals are an excellent breakfast selection for all-morning energy. "Look for one with at least 3 grams of fiber per serving," Wein says. "Some have 8 grams or more. Eat it with fat-free milk, and you have a perfect balance."

Stock up on oatmeal. A fiber-packed whole grain cereal, oatmeal is your best breakfast choice for long-lasting energy, says William Evans, Ph.D., director of the nutrition, metabolism, and exercise laboratory at the University of Arkansas for Medical Sciences/Veterans Affairs Medical Center in Little Rock.

Dr. Evans fed a group of volunteers oatmeal and others another type of high-carbohydrate cereal and then put everybody on exercise bikes. "There's no doubt that eating oatmeal allowed both men and women to exercise for a significantly longer time," he says.

Dr. Evans gives the credit for oatmeal's energy boost to its soluble fiber content. Much more than the insoluble fiber in, say, wheat bran, the soluble fiber in oatmeal slows down carbohydrate absorption, thus keeping your blood sugar levels more constant.

Both oat bran and rolled oats are high in soluble fiber, so on mornings when you don't feel like eating oatmeal, try oat bran muffins.

Ace Those Midmorning Meetings

Faced with an interminable meeting, it's all to easy too rely on the doughnut-Danish-bagel axis: low-fiber, protein-free, high-refined-carb foods that yo-yo your glucose levels. Instead, reach for steady-energy allies. Here are some suggestions from the experts.

A peanut butter sandwich. Make it with whole wheat bread, and it will have the macronutrient mix that will keep your eyes open and your brain humming. That's because the fiber in the whole wheat and the protein (and fat) in the peanut butter will ration out the energy over time.

"Even if you'd like to add a little jelly, it's going to be absorbed slowly because of the peanuts, which have fat and fiber, so your blood sugar won't plummet," says Whittle.

Or, she says, prepare your own peanut butter crackers with natural peanut butter (without questionable hydrogenated trans fatty acids that resemble saturated fat) and crackers made from whole grain.

Another good option is peanut butter on apple slices. An apple is almost pure carbohydrate, with simple sugars, but the energy it provides will be metered over time by its own fiber and by the peanut butter.

Fruit and cheese. Chop up half an apple (for carbohydrates) and mix it with 1% cottage cheese (for its protein and some fat) and bring it to work for balanced midmorning fortification, suggests Whittle. Equally healthy variations are low-fat cheese on whole grain bread or a small salad with tuna and chopped apples.

Vim in the Afternoon

Lunch should leave you invigorated, not asleep at your workstation. Make these adjustments to come back strong for the day's second act.

Take it easy. Hefty lunches of 1,000 calories or more are proven energy sappers. "Portion size is key," says Whittle. "Most people overeat at lunch."

Pass on pure pasta. Unless you're planning to run a marathon after lunch, it's probably not a good idea to overemphasize pasta or any other refined carbohydrate at lunchtime. "Susceptibility to grogginess after a high-carbohydrate lunch is more common in women than men, and in people over 40," Dr. Grandjean says.

Better carb choices are fiber-rich whole grain bread, brown rice, and beans or lentils instead of white bread, white rice, or white pasta. "Just making those choices is going to balance your blood sugar levels and benefit your energy," Wein says.

Push the protein. Along with choosing fiber-rich unrefined complex carbohydrates, the next best thing you can do to ramp up your afternoon energy levels is to offset your lunch carbohydrates with a high-protein food, Whittle says. Excellent midday protein choices are soy burgers, seafood, tuna, turkey, or cottage cheese.

Build a high-energy salad. "Just a salad" is a common lunch request by weight-watching women, but a plateful of not much more than lettuce hardly qualifies as energy food even for rabbits. "A typical lunch should be 400 to 500 calories, so salads usually just aren't enough," Wein says. "You'll never be satisfied after a 150-calorie lettuce salad, so you won't stick to your meal plan over the long run."

Instead, she suggests making your own lunch salads with energy in mind. "Choose dark leafy greens, which are higher in nutrients and fiber," she says. "Add a variety of colorful vegetables such as carrots, peppers, or

PROTEIN POWDER AND DRINKS: FOOD WILL DO

Those muscled folks you see in the protein drink ads sure look energized. Can you, too, rally by mixing powder and water?

Probably not. Protein drinks are intended to help build muscle through resistance exercise, not to help you burn energy. Your body uses amino acids, the basic components of protein, to create muscle mass. Protein drinks supply those amino acids, usually isolated from soy or dairy sources, to make sure muscle-building efforts won't be limited by an insufficient amino acid supply.

Not only does all this have little to do with your energy levels, but it's probably overkill even for your muscle-toning goals. Unless you're planning on qualifying for a bodybuilding competition, you probably don't need the extra amino acids in protein drinks to get the most out of your weight work, says Debra Wein, R.D., cofounder of Sensible Nutrition Connection in Hingham, Massachusetts. "Extra protein doesn't build more muscle," she says. "Working hard builds more muscle." Ordinary protein from real foods will suffice.

broccoli. And always include a low-fat source of protein such as chick-peas or grilled chicken to round it out."

Power Up for Lunchtime Workouts

If you're going to be exercising at lunchtime, make your midmorning snack higher in carbohydrates than you otherwise would. If you exercise after work, up the carbohydrate content of your midafternoon snack. "Those carbohydrates an hour or so before exercising will serve directly as energy to burn for your workout," Wein says. It is also a great way to provide energy to your muscles during your workout, she adds.

And eat your next meal soon after you finish your workout. Exercise itself lowers blood sugar, so enjoying a balanced meal afterward will help stabilize glucose levels and keep you going for the rest of the day.

Beat Afternoon Slump

As any woman knows, the workday doesn't end when you leave the office. After-hours errands, or what have you, put extended demands on your stamina. A midafternoon snack can help see you through. Plus, you won't get home so hungry that you inhale the first thing that you get your hands on, or overeat at dinner.

The ideal midafternoon snack consists of the same mix of components as a good breakfast or midmorning snack: a mini-meal that includes protein and some fat as well as carbohydrates—say, the other half of a turkey sandwich, or a couple more peanut butter crackers.

Eat to Beat the Heat

If you notice that you tire more easily in the summer, heat itself isn't necessarily to blame. "Dehydration is what makes you tired," Dr. Grandjean says. That's because your body will keep its cells hydrated at all costs, she says, so if you don't replace water lost through perspiration, it will simply take water out of the circulating blood, reducing your blood volume. "As your blood volume goes down, your heart has to work a little harder," she says. "Your body adapts to that by slowing down, and that affects your general feeling of vitality." So your daily nine glasses of water become more important on hot days, and, in fact, may not be enough on some days.

Beauty Foods: Nurture Your Skin, Hair, and Nails

It makes perfect sense: If eating the right Power Foods and nutrients can help keep your heart, bones, immune system, and other inner workings at their best, they can also keep your outer wrappings looking their best. Conversely, eating too much of the wrong foods will make your skin, hair, and nails suffer visibly.

Of course, diet isn't the only factor in great-looking skin. Basking in the sun speeds the breakdown of collagen and elastin, the structural proteins that give skin its youthful plumpness and pliability, resulting in premature aging, wrinkles, roughness, age spots, and blotches. So does smoking cigarettes. As with anything else, genetics also plays a role. Some of us simply have better skin than others.

Using moisturizers and sunscreen protects your skin from dryness and sun damage. Eating the right foods—and moisturizing your skin from the inside out—affords further protection. Even if you've yet to spot your first wrinkle, you still have good reason to treat your skin right. "The earlier you start to care for your skin, the bigger the difference you'll see as you age," says Francesca J. Fusco, M.D., a dermatologist in New York City.

475

CAN SUGAR GIVE YOU WRINKLES?

You probably limit your intake of sugary treats for the good of your teeth and waistline. Here's a new incentive: After a yearlong study, researchers at the Israel Institute of Technology in Haifa found that rats given high levels of the natural sugar fructose experienced changes in their skin and bone collagen. These changes reduced the rats' skin elasticity, making it stiff and rigid—which could lead to wrinkles.

"This doesn't mean that the same thing will happen in humans, but in theory it is possible," explains Edward Masoro, Ph.D., a physiologist and professor emeritus at the University of Texas Health Science Center in San Antonio. (The rats in the study were fed much higher amounts of fructose than an average woman typically would eat in a day.)

Sugar consumption from junk food has increased steadily over the past 2 decades, with Americans now eating an average of 20 teaspoons a day. So curbing intake of fructose is a good idea (particularly for people with diabetes) for overall health. Pay particular attention to high-sugar "carriers" such as soda, ice cream, frozen yogurt, baked goods, and sweet desserts.

Don't reduce your intake of honey or of fruits that naturally contain high levels of fructose, such as figs, dates, grapes, oranges, apples, and berries. Besides containing antioxidants, which help in the fight against aging, fruits offer scads of essential nutrients and have far fewer grams of fructose than sweets of little nutritional value.

A Skin-Friendly Eating Plan

Power up with fruits and vegetables rich in the antioxidant nutrients vitamins C and E and beta-carotene, says Dr. Fusco. Antioxidants help protect skin from the damaging effects of free radicals, unstable oxygen molecules that are generated after exposure to the sun.

Strawberries, papaya, kiwifruit, navel oranges, and sweet red peppers are especially rich sources of vitamin C. You'll find vitamin E—another powerfully protective antioxidant—in salad and cooking oils, wheat germ, nuts, and seeds. For beta-carotene, load up on Power Foods like spinach

FOOD CULPRITS TO WATCH FOR

Eating a diet high in Power Foods can make your skin glow, but certain foods may trigger a rash or pimples in some people. Harvey Arbesman, M.D., clinical assistant professor of dermatology at the State University of New York at Buffalo School of Medicine and Biomedical Sciences, offers this list of foods that can improve—or aggravate—different skin conditions.

PROBLEM	POWER FOODS	FOODS TO AVOID	CONNECTION
Acne (at times triggered by hormones)	None	Dairy products, fast food, shellfish, kelp, chocolate	Foods high in iodine can trigger breakouts. Iodine cleansers are used on milking machines and cow udders, and a fast-food meal may contain 30 times the Recommended Dietary Allowance for iodine. Chocolate can trouble some people.
Eczema (atopic dermatitis)	Salmon, mackerel, tuna, flaxseed oil	Dairy products, eggs, soy, peanuts, wheat	Eczema may be helped by a diet sufficient in essential fatty acids, such as omega-3's. Certain foods can trigger allergic reactions.
Hives	None	Strawberries, some fish, some nuts, food colorings	Hives are an allergic reaction. Some people are sensitive to yellow dye #5, found in many processed foods.
Skin cancer (basal and squamous cell carcinoma) and other sun damage	Various fruits and veggies, whole wheat, low-fat diet	High-fat foods may increase risk	Antioxidant-rich foods may help prevent nonmelanoma skin cancers by scavenging free radicals. Getting fewer than 20% of calories from fat may reduce risk of certain precancerous and cancerous skin conditions.

and other dark leafy greens, along with deep orange fruits and vegetables such as carrots, sweet potatoes, cantaloupe, and pumpkin.

POWER-EATING TIP

Consider taking extra vitamin C, since your skin needs it to build collagen. Aim for 1,000 milligrams a day from a vitamin C supplement or from a combination of a multivitamin and a separate supplement.

Also, say no to yo-yo dieting and starvation diets. To avoid saggy jowls and flabby upper arms, avoid gaining and losing weight over and over. "It leads to wear and tear on collagen and elastin," says Debra Jaliman, M.D., a dermatologist in New York City. And very low calorie diets deprive your skin of the nutrients it needs to thrive, she says.

Besides needing nutrients, your skin needs fluids. You've heard it a million times, but the advice, well, holds water: "Drink, drink, drink— eight glasses a day, at least," says Linda K. Franks, M.D., a dermatologist in New York City. Drink more during the winter, when the indoor air is dry. "Skin continually loses moisture to the air, so it draws on the reserve of water that's in the skin's deeper layers.

Although drinking more liquids is good for your skin, back off the booze. Alcohol dilates blood vessels. In some women, consuming more than moderate amounts of alcohol will cause their vessels to continually dilate and constrict, stretching them like rubber bands until they have no more snap, says Dr. Franks. Eventually, vessels just stay dilated, leading to spider veins and broken capillaries. Alcohol also causes the skin to lose water, and dehydrated skin is more sensitive to sun damage.

POWER-EATING TIP

Nix the high-fructose corn syrup. An 8-ounce glass of pure orange juice, for example, contains about 5.5 grams of fructose; 12 ounces of cola, which contains high-fructose corn syrup, has about 22.5 grams.

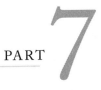

THE ULTIMATE
POWER-EATING PLAN

Almonds to Yogurt: 101 Power Foods

BY JANIS JIBRIN, M.S., R.D. No need to become a one-woman encyclopedia of nutrition facts in order to put Power Eating into action. Just make sure that your pantry is stocked with Power Foods, and you can make almost any recipe in this book. Build your weekly shopping list around the 101 Power Foods listed here with capsule summaries of their key healing powers. What could be simpler?

You'll notice that some of the studies cited were done on mice, rats, or men, not women. Not to worry: The results apply to women. And it's nice to know that the foods you serve yourself will also help keep the man in your life healthy.

In Your Day-to-Day Power-Eating Plan on page 541, you'll find a handy table outlining the suggested number of servings and tips to help you plan and prepare meals using these foods.

1. Almonds

Almonds are a treasure trove of protective compounds, particularly for the heart. When 18 men and women added 3½ ounces of almonds to their regular diets, their total blood cholesterol fell 12 percent during 4 weeks—and their "bad" LDL cholesterol fell 17 percent. These cholesterol drops were even more impressive than those of another group in the same study who added olive oil to their diets. Both almonds and olive oil are high in monounsaturated fat, which is kind to cholesterol levels.

"The fact that almonds sent cholesterol down even lower than olive oil makes us think that there are other things at work here, such as fiber, phytosterols, and maybe other phytochemicals," says study leader Gene Spiller, Ph.D., director at the Health Research and Studies Center in Los Altos, California. Plus, almonds are a good source of two other pro-heart minerals: magnesium and copper.

How much/how often: Count ¼ cup of almonds (a little over an ounce) as one of your five nut or seed servings per week.

2. Apples

Just a few years ago, when the nutritional yardstick was limited to vitamins and minerals, apples looked pretty shabby (except for fiber), and apple juice might as well have been sugar water. With the research explosion into other healing plant compounds—phytonutrients, or phytochemicals—apples started looking a whole lot better. It turns out that they are a rich source of flavonoids, antioxidant compounds that fight both heart disease and cancer. Flavonoids zap free radicals, destructive molecules that initiate heart disease, cancer, eye diseases, and general aging. And once cancer has set in, flavonoids help stop its spread. By preventing the oxidation of LDL cholesterol, flavonoids halt the process that clogs arteries. Researchers at the University of California, Davis, put extracts from six commercial apple juice brands to the test, along with extracts from fresh apples. In test-tube experiments, the apple juice prevented up to 34 percent of LDL oxidation; the flesh and peel, up to 38 percent.

How much/how often: Count an apple as one of your two or more daily fruit servings.

3. Apricots

If you are looking for beta-carotene, the plant version of vitamin A, you have most of the vegetable world at your feet. But when it comes to fruits, the pickings get a little slimmer, especially if you're dealing with the average supermarket fare. So when summer hits and apricots are at their peak, indulge. Three apricots, for a puny 50 calories, provide 55 percent of the Daily Value (DV) for vitamin A in the form of beta-carotene.

How much/how often: Count three raw or dried apricots as one of your daily fruit servings.

4. Artichokes

Even when you throw out the 60 percent of an artichoke that's tough and inedible, you still wind up with a whopping 6½ grams of fiber, plus 20 percent of the DV for vitamin C and a healthy 5 to 18 percent of most minerals. But scientists didn't stop with that discovery: They uncovered a powerful cancer fighter in artichokes called silymarin. Researchers have shown that applying silymarin to the skin of mice exposed to a carcinogen prevented skin cancer at various stages in the cancer process. In other research, giving mice a single dose of silymarin before they were given a liver toxin completely protected them from the toxin.

A British study found that artichoke extract acted as an antioxidant, preventing dangerous LDL cholesterol from oxidizing and leading to clogged arteries. Researchers suspect that a compound in artichokes called luteolin is behind the protection because studies show similar results with pure luteolin extracted from artichokes.

How much/how often: Count one-half to one artichoke as one of your four or more daily servings of vegetables.

5. Arugula

The sharp taste that livens up salads is a telltale sign that arugula belongs to the crucifer family of vegetables, which includes cabbage. That means that it is dousing you with compounds called indoles, which deactivate cancer-causing agents. There's more: One cup of raw arugula has only 5 calories but manages to squeeze in 32 milligrams of calcium and about 10 percent of a day's worth of cancer-fighting vitamin A (in the form of beta-carotene and other antioxidant carotenoids).

How much/how often: Count 2 cups of raw arugula as one of your one or more daily servings of greens.

6. Asparagus

That elegant and delicious touch to your meal is also helping fight cancer. A series of test-tube experiments at Rutgers University in New

Brunswick, New Jersey, found that compounds extracted from asparagus called saponins halted the growth of leukemia tumor cells. Saponins not only kill cancer cells but also lower blood cholesterol. In addition, 1 cup of asparagus squeezes in an impressive array of other disease fighters: 19 percent of the DV for vitamin A (from beta-carotene), 32 percent of vitamin C, and 65 percent of folate (the naturally occurring form of folic acid), the B vitamin that helps prevent birth defects and is linked to a reduced risk of heart disease and cancer.

How much/how often: Count ½ cup of cooked asparagus as one of your one or more daily servings of greens.

7. Avocados

You wouldn't think a fruit (yes, it's technically a fruit) containing 80 percent of calories from fat could lower two types of blood fats: cholesterol and triglycerides. But that's what a number of studies show—including a Mexican one where researchers compared the effects of two diets, both deriving about half of their calories from fat. In one, men and women ate about 1½ of the small, dark green, pebble-skinned type of avocados a day; in the other, fat came from a variety of sources. On the avocado-enriched diet, both people with normal cholesterol and those with high cholesterol lowered their levels about 17 percent. Even better, the LDL cholesterol fell by 23 percent. Triglycerides, another heart-disease-promoting blood fat, fell about 20 percent. People on the diet without avocados had virtually no changes in their cholesterol or triglycerides.

Between 55 and 65 percent of the fat in an avocado is monounsaturated fat, which has been shown repeatedly to lower LDL cholesterol and raise beneficial HDLs. Avocados also contain compounds called phytosterols, which play a role in lowering cholesterol. Avocados are excellent sources of the B vitamin folate, which helps lower levels of homocysteine, a substance that increases heart disease risk. Half a Florida avocado covers 20 percent of your daily folic acid needs; half a California avocado takes care of 14 percent. Half a cup of pureed avocado also supplies a whopping 6.8 grams of fiber.

How much/how often: If you're watching your weight, stick to half an avocado, at 162 calories per half, as one fruit serving. If you are exercising intensely, burning lots of calories, and maintaining a normal weight, a whole avocado is fine.

8. Bananas

Among the many assaults lobbed at our bodies by the modern diet is a huge increase in sodium and a decrease in potassium. Many Americans consume more sodium than potassium, when it should be the other way around. But we love bananas, and they're available year-round, so we eat lots of them and get lots of potassium (467 milligrams per medium banana). You can also feel good about the 3 grams of fiber per fruit.

How much/how often: Count one medium banana toward your daily fruit servings.

9. Barley

If you're like many women, you automatically put rice or pasta on to boil at dinnertime. Why not try barley instead? This grain helps lower blood cholesterol and evens out levels of insulin and blood sugar. In a study at the University of California, Davis, researchers watched what happened when 11 men ate meals based on either regular pasta or pasta made of a combination of barley and wheat flours. Barley eaters had a smaller rise in insulin than wheat eaters, and 4 hours later, their blood cholesterol was slightly lower (with the wheat eaters, cholesterol was slightly raised). And good news for weight watchers: Levels of cholecystokinin—a hormone that keeps you feeling full—were elevated for a longer period after the barley meal.

In another barley-versus-wheat standoff, published in the *American Journal of Clinical Nutrition*, 21 men with high cholesterol knocked it 6 percent lower on a barley-rich diet compared with a diet high in whole wheat. And LDL cholesterol fell 7 percent. What's at work is the same substance that gives barley its creamy texture: beta-glucans, a type of soluble fiber. Beta-glucans draw in water, creating a gel in the intestines that slows the absorption of glucose from both the barley and the rest of the meal. This appears to be the way it lowers cholesterol as well, trapping a fraction of the fat and cholesterol from the meal and from the body's bile acids and sending it out of the body before it can be absorbed.

How much/how often: Research shows that 3 or more grams of beta-glucans daily lowers cholesterol; ⅓ cup of cooked barley provides 3 grams. Count ½ cup of cooked barley as one of your 5 to 10 daily servings of whole grains.

10. Basil

There's nothing like the smell of fresh basil, thanks in large part to its monoterpenoids, flavor and aroma compounds that fight cancer in a number of ways. Because basil is an important spice in Thai cuisine, Thailand's National Cancer Institute included it in a study of the health benefits of common Thai foods. The study found that basil was a particularly potent stimulator of enzymes that detoxify carcinogens. Monoterpenoids also kill cancer tumor cells.

Basil also supplies some carotenes and minerals. But the teaspoon or so that we get in most recipes doesn't provide much of these things. That's the beauty of Basil Pesto on page 58; you get about ½ cup of basil per serving.

How much/how often: Have basil as often as you like, the more the better. One teaspoon of fresh or ¼ teaspoon of dried counts as one serving.

11. Beans

In many societies, cooked dried beans are a staple food among the poor; only the rich eat meat for protein. So nutritionally first-rate beans acquired second-class status, and perhaps that is the reason that less than a third of Americans eat any beans at all, according to a large-scale USDA survey. It's not surprising, then, that there aren't enough bean eaters around to make statistically significant comparisons of disease risks between those who eat the most and those who consume the least amounts of this food. Numerous studies show, however, that vegetarians have lower risks of chronic diseases, and it is assumed that they are eating a lot of beans. Here's what you get when you eat more beans.

Lowered cholesterol. Since the mid-1980s, University of Kentucky fiber researcher James W. Anderson, M.D., has been documenting the benefits of beans. In one study, he gave 20 men with high cholesterol a diet supplemented with 1 cup of cooked beans for 21 days. On this diet, cholesterol fell by 19 percent. Even better, LDL cholesterol dropped a heart-saving 24 percent. Other studies indicate that ½ cup of cooked beans will lower serum cholesterol about 10 percent.

Researchers at the Veterans Affairs Medical Center in Minneapolis may have figured out how beans do it. They discovered that when people eat ½ cup of cooked beans daily, they excrete more cholesterol in the form of bile acids than on a similar diet without beans. Bile acids are the body's detergent, breaking down fat particles for absorption. They are made from cholesterol and usually get recycled back into the body. By excreting them, people reduced their bodies' cholesterol load.

Steadier blood sugar. Beans help keep blood sugar and insulin—a hormone that regulates blood sugar—on an even keel, making beans an excellent food for women with diabetes. Unlike many high-carbohydrate foods, beans do not raise blood sugar quickly, thanks to the blunting effects of fiber and tannins. Foods that don't spike blood sugar have a low glycemic index, and a Harvard study found that women who eat more of these types of foods are less likely to develop diabetes.

Low-fat protein. You can rely on beans for protein, and you don't have to combine them with grains at the same meal to get a "complete" protein, as was previously believed. As long as you get both grains and beans over the course of the day, you'll get the full complement of amino acids. Rice and wheat are rich in just the amino acids (building blocks of protein) that beans are a little low in.

The type of protein in beans is healthier than animal protein. For instance, numerous studies indicate that animal protein causes the body to lose calcium; the type in beans doesn't.

Disease protection. One-half cup of beans gives you 25 percent of the DV for folate, the B vitamin that reduces the risk of birth defects and is linked to a lower risk of heart disease and certain cancers. Iron, zinc, and calcium have strong showings on beans' nutrition profiles. Several less-familiar components of beans have a role in cancer prevention. Phytic acid, for instance, prevents colon cancer in lab animals.

How much/how often: Have ½ cup of cooked beans at least three times a week. As a vegetarian substitute, count ½ cup of cooked beans for 1 ounce of animal protein (the fish/poultry/meat group). If flatulence is a problem, get Beano, a product containing an enzyme that digests the gas-producing sugars in beans.

12. Beef and Lamb

After decades of beef-bashing, scientists are finding something nice to say about this meat. It turns out that beef and lamb actually contain a type of fat that fights cancer. It's called conjugated linoleic acid (CLA) and is in the fat of animals like cows and lambs. Much of the CLA research has taken place at the University of Wisconsin in Madison and has been led by Michael Pariza, Ph.D., distinguished professor and director of the food research institute. In the 1980s, Dr. Pariza found that CLA helped prevent skin cancer in mice, and since then, numerous animal and test-tube studies confirm CLA's anti-cancer power.

CLA also enhances the immune system in studies on lab animals. Dr. Pariza linked up with David Kritchevsky, Ph.D., of the Wistar Institute in Philadelphia, for a study showing that rabbits fed CLA had lower levels of artery-clogging blood cholesterol and triglycerides than rabbits that didn't get CLA.

The problem is that you have to eat the fattier cuts of beef and lamb as well as full-fat dairy products to get CLA. That means unhealthy doses of saturated fat, which raises blood cholesterol and heart disease risk.

On another front, beef and lamb are good sources of minerals, particularly iron and zinc, and the B vitamin niacin.

How much/how often: The amount of CLA in beef and lamb isn't worth loading yourself up with these high-saturated-fat foods, so limit them to about 3 ounces three times a week or less.

13. Beets

Like so many of the compounds that pigment deeply colored fruits and vegetables, the ones in beets are health promoters. The principal pigment is betacyanin, and it's probably the reason that beets were rated high on a list of foods that test-tube experiments show may protect against chromosome damage, a first step on the road to cancer. Betacyanin is an antioxidant, so it has the potential to protect cells against chromosome damage by free radicals. Beets are also a good source of fiber (nearly 3 grams per cooked cupful) and magnesium (16 percent of the DV in the same amount).

How much/how often: One-half cup of cooked beets counts as one of your four or more daily servings of vegetables.

14. Blackberries

If you want lots of fiber fast, eat blackberries. A mere ½ cup packs in 4 grams of fiber, more than most bran-flake cereals. Blackberries contain a mix of soluble fiber (to lower cholesterol) and insoluble fiber (to prevent constipation and ward off cancer). Three of these fibers are chlorogenic acid, ellagic acid, and catechins. A German test-tube study ranked blackberries among the top 10 most powerful carcinogen-busting fruits and vegetables.

How much/how often: Count ¾ cup as one of your one or more servings of citrus/berries per day.

15. Blueberries

The 1990s were good years for blueberries. First, it turned out that they help prevent urinary tract infections, for the same reason that cranberries do. Then they ranked among the top three fruits and vegetables in antioxidant power in a study at the Jean Mayer USDA Human Nutrition Research Center on Aging at Tufts University in Boston. One study showed that blueberry extract helped antioxidants do their job more efficiently.

A study done on rats showed that supplementing the diet for 8 weeks with blueberry extract improved two big age-related concerns: loss of memory and loss of coordination. Older rats given blueberry extract learned and remembered better and performed better on a balance beam than rats taking other fruit or vegetable extracts.

Tufts researchers think that blueberries' anti-aging effects might be due to the pigments that give the fruit their blue color: anthocyanins, flavonoids that are powerful antioxidants. "In general, the darker the color, the more anthocyanins in fruits and vegetables. Blueberries have 18 to 20 active anthocyanins," says study leader and scientist Ronald Prior, Ph.D. Known for their ability to zap compounds that damage the heart and trigger cancer, anthocyanins may also protect brain cells from age-related damage.

How much/how often: Count ¾ cup as one of your one or more servings of citrus/berries per day.

16. Brazil Nuts

With their stratospheric levels of selenium, Brazil nuts are a nutritional wonder. Just one nut covers 171 percent of the DV for selenium; 1 ounce of Brazil nuts—about seven nuts—offers 1,200 percent. Selenium is part of glutathione peroxidase, a powerful antioxidant enzyme in the body that destroys cancer-causing free radicals. Test-tube studies on human cancer cells show that selenium also destroys tumors and thwarts their growth. In lab animal research, supplementing the diet with selenium reduces cancers of the skin, colon, liver, and breast. Researchers at Roswell Park Cancer Institute in Buffalo, New York, found that mixing Brazil nuts into rats' diets reduced breast cancer risk just as effectively as did plain selenium.

Dozens of surveys of dietary habits link higher selenium intake to lower risk of cancer, but these epidemiological studies aren't considered as accurate as clinical trials that give one group selenium and another a placebo. That's why a University of Arizona in Tucson clinical trial made headlines. For 4½ years, 947 men took either 200 micrograms of selenium or a placebo daily. Men on selenium were 63 percent less likely to develop prostate cancer 6½ years after starting supplementation.

Surveys of dietary habits show that people who eat more selenium have lower risk of heart disease. And a Yugoslavian study found that, compared with healthy people, those with high blood pressure had 19 percent less selenium in their blood. Those with heart disease had 33 percent less.

How much/how often: Have one Brazil nut every other day, and your selenium levels will be fully stocked. Doses above this amount must be taken under medical supervision.

17. Broccoli

Unless you've been hiding out in a jungle for the past 15 years, you know that broccoli is exceptionally good for you. It pops up in the dozens of studies linking diet to disease protection. For instance, a UCLA study found that men and women who ate the most broccoli (averaging 2 cups per week) had half the risk of developing colon cancer as those who reported never eating broccoli. A Harvard study tracking nearly 48,000 male health professionals found that those eating at least 1 cup of broccoli weekly had about half the risk of developing bladder cancer as men eating less than ½ cup.

While broccoli offers an arsenal of protective compounds, the research buzz is all about sulforaphane. Broccoli is one of the richest sources. Sulforaphane is an isothiocyanate, a compound that stimulates our cells to produce detoxification enzymes. These enzymes zap cancer-causing chemicals before they can wreak havoc in our bodies. Other disease fighters in a cup of cooked broccoli include about 6 grams of fiber and about 10 percent of the DV of calcium, 8 percent of selenium, 70 percent of vitamin A (from beta-carotene), 123 percent of vitamin C, and 26 percent of folate. Broccoli is also a great source of the carotenoids lutein and zeaxanthin, which help protect against macular degeneration, a cause of blindness.

How much/how often: Count ½ cup of cooked or 1 cup of raw broccoli as one of your five or more cruciferous vegetables per week.

18. Broccoli Sprouts

You thought broccoli was healthy? Get a load of this: Johns Hopkins University researchers in Baltimore were stunned to find that young broccoli sprouts contain 10 to 100 times more cancer-fighting sulforaphane as broccoli. When lab animals were exposed to carcinogens, those on a sprout-enriched diet developed only half the number of breast cancer tumors as those who didn't get the sprouts. The same sprouts used in the research are available in markets under the name BroccoSprouts.

How much/how often: A serving is considered ½ cup of sprouts, and they're equal in cancer-fighting ability to about 9½ cups of broccoli. Extrapolating from the research on broccoli, just a few tablespoons of the sprouts a few days a week should be protective. (Since that's such a small amount, you don't need to count it toward any of the daily or weekly foods.)

19. Brussels Sprouts

Both human and animal studies have shown that eating brussels sprouts thwarts a major cancer-causing event: DNA damage. A Dutch study giving people 10½ ounces of cooked brussels sprouts daily for 3 weeks found a 28 percent decline in DNA damage, as measured by a compound excreted in the urine. The Dutch researchers then turned their microscopes to colon cancer and found that the same amount of brussels sprouts hiked up levels of carcinogen-zapping enzymes in the colon and rectal area, an indication that this vegetable helps prevent colon cancer.

Like cruciferous vegetables, brussels sprouts contain cancer-fighting indoles. And they're particularly rich in indole-3-carbinol, which helps block the cancer process at its inception by boosting levels of carcinogen-busting enzymes. Brussels sprouts are also a good source of phenethyl isothiocyanate (PEITC), a tongue twister that also deactivates carcinogens.

This vegetable is a fantastic source of more familiar nutrients. One cup cooked provides 22 percent of the DV of vitamin A (through beta-carotene), 23 percent of folate, and 161 percent of vitamin C. Plus, it has a generous sprinkling of minerals and B vitamins.

How much/how often: Count ½ cup of cooked brussels sprouts toward your five-times-a-week or more cruciferous quota.

20. Butternut Squash

Its orange color tips you off to the presence of the antioxidant beta-carotene. One cup of squash cubes supplies a very generous 287 percent of the DV for vitamin A, mainly in the form of beta-carotene, and also throws in loads of alpha-carotene, another antioxidant. Piles of research papers show that beta-carotene protects against various cancers in lab animals. Human studies consistently find a link between diets (or blood levels) high in beta-carotene and a decreased risk for cancer, heart disease, and cataracts.

Butternut squash is a great source of fiber (another heart disease and cancer fighter) with about 6 grams per cup.

How much/how often: Count ½ cup of cooked squash toward your one or more daily servings of deep yellow, orange, or red vegetables.

21. Cabbage

Wrinkling your nose at cabbage? There's nothing wrong with coleslaw, sauerkraut, and Chinese stir-fries! But what's best about cabbage is that it's a crucifer, a family of vegetables linked to reduced cancer risk in dozens of studies. For instance, a Harvard study tracking nearly 48,000 male health professionals found that men who ate ½ cup of cabbage at least once a week were half as likely to develop bladder cancer as men who ate cabbage less than once a month.

In a series of studies at Rockefeller University Hospital in New York City, a compound called indole-3-carbinol was extracted from cabbage and given to men and women for 1 to 8 weeks. The compound reduced their levels of estrogen—a stimulant of breast and prostate cancers. A University of Illinois at Chicago study found that another cabbage compound in the same chemical class—indoles—reduced numbers of breast and skin cancer tumors in mice exposed to a carcinogen. Indoles raise levels of enzymes in the body that destroy carcinogens before they can trigger cancer and also help halt the cancer process once it's begun.

Cabbage is also a good source of the familiar antioxidant vitamin C. Depending on the variety, a cup of cooked cabbage provides 50 to 67 percent of the DV for C. Savoy and bok choy are good sources of folate, (about 20 percent of the DV in 1 cup), a B vitamin that helps reduce risk of both heart disease and cancer.

How much/how often: Count ½ cup of cooked or 1 cup of raw cabbage toward your five or more weekly servings of cruciferous vegetables.

22. Canola Oil

While not as rich in monounsaturates as olive oil, canola oil is a good source of this healthy fat. Canola's vital statistics: 59 percent monounsaturates, 30 percent polyunsaturates, and 7 percent saturated fat. And although nothing can beat olive oil's all-around healthfulness, there are times when you just don't want olive oil's distinctive taste. That's where canola oil steps in. And unlike virgin and extra-virgin olive oils, which smoke easily at high temperatures, canola has a high smoke point, so it's excellent for stir-frying.

How much/how often: One teaspoon of canola oil counts toward your daily quota of 5 to 10 servings of healthful oils.

23. Cantaloupe

Besides being one of the best-tasting foods on Earth, cantaloupe offers superhigh levels of vitamin C and beta-carotene, both linked to decreased risk of heart disease and cancer. One cup of sliced cantaloupe covers 100 percent of the DV for vitamin A (mainly in the form of beta-carotene) and 110 percent of the vitamin C.

How much/how often: Count 1 cup of cantaloupe cubes toward your two or more daily servings of fruits.

24. Carrots

Carrots have become synonymous with beta-carotene, since they're loaded with the antioxidant. Many studies in many different countries consistently show that people who eat the most beta-carotene (or have the most in their blood) are less likely to develop the diseases that kill most Americans: heart disease and cancer. Extensive animal research supports the cancer connection. Carrots are also exceptionally high in another carotenoid: alpha-carotene.

These carotenoids disarm destructive compounds that attack cells and alter their DNA in a cancer-promoting fashion. Beta- and alpha-carotene also help prevent plaque from forming in the arteries by protecting cholesterol from oxidation (rancidity). Further, they convert to vitamin A in the body as needed, and vitamin A protects against cancer and heart disease. A medium carrot supplies $3\frac{1}{2}$ times the DV for vitamin A.

A study supported by the National Cancer Institute compared the eating habits of 3,543 women with breast cancer and 9,406 women without the disease. Those who ate cooked carrots more than twice a week had a 38 percent lower risk of developing breast cancer than those who never ate carrots. (Eating raw carrots more than twice a week brought a 19 percent lower risk.) An Italian study found that people who ate three servings of raw or cooked carrots weekly had a 30 percent lower risk of rectal cancer and a 20 percent lower risk of breast cancer.

When it comes to heart disease, an Australian study showed that 3 weeks of drinking carrot juice and orange juice partially protected LDL cholesterol from oxidation.

Besides carotenoids, carrots contribute 2 grams of fiber apiece to a healthy diet.

How much/how often: Count one medium carrot or $\frac{1}{2}$ cup of cooked or 1 cup of raw slices as one of your one or more daily servings of deep yellow, orange, or red vegetables.

25. Cauliflower

Loaded with the standard cruciferous arsenal of nutrients, cauliflower has the potential to help prevent a variety of cancers, including those of the breast and colon. American Health Foundation researchers gave rats a compound extracted from cauliflower called S-methylmethane thio-sulfonate (S-MMTS) along with the anti-inflammatory drug sulindac. The combo reduced the number of colon cancer tumors in rats exposed to a carcinogen. S-MMTS helps suppress cancer once it has already taken hold; so do a variety of indoles in cauliflower. As antioxidant icing on the cake, 1 cup of cauliflower covers 92 percent of the DV of another disease fighter—vitamin C—and provides 3 grams of fiber.

How much/how often: Count ½ cup of cooked or 1 cup of raw cauli-flower florets toward your five-times-a-week crucifer minimum.

26. Celery

Celery contains phthalides, compounds that reduce blood pressure and cholesterol. The Chinese figured it out long ago; their traditional medicine used celery to treat high blood pressure—a treatment now sup-ported by animal research and preliminary human studies. A study on rats fed a cholesterol-raising high-fat diet also showed that extracts from fresh celery lower undesirable LDL cholesterol. And a study published in *Nu-trition and Cancer* found that feeding mice celery seed oil helped prevent stomach cancer.

How much/how often: Count 1 cup of sliced raw celery or ½ cup of cooked as one of your four or more daily vegetable servings.

27. Cheese

Cheese presents nutritionists with a considerable dilemma. On the one hand, it's a great source of calcium that's easier for lactose-intolerant people to digest than milk. (An ounce of Cheddar, for instance, has 20 percent of the DV for calcium.) But on the other hand, there's all that saturated fat, proven to raise blood cholesterol. A good compromise, therefore, is reduced-fat cheese. You just might need a little trial and error to find a brand you like. Incidentally, the fat in cheese isn't all bad for you. Cheese is a good source of conjugated linoleic acid (CLA), a type of fat that actually fights cancer and high cholesterol.

Cheese offers another bonus: It protects your teeth from cavities. Test-tube, animal, and human studies all support that link. A study at Tufts University School of Dental Medicine in Boston probed the diets of 274 men and women, looking for links with dental health. As expected, the more sugar eaten, the higher the rate of cavities. But those who ate the most cheese (five servings a week) had only half the risk of developing cavities as those who ate no cheese. Researchers speculate that cheese lowers the pH of the mouth to the point that plaque-causing bacteria can't bear to live there.

How much/how often: Count 1 ounce of reduced-fat cheese (5 grams or less of fat per ounce) as one of your daily two to three dairy servings. For men and women over 50: Even with three dairy servings daily, you may need to take a calcium supplement to meet the recommended amount of 1,500 milligrams.

28. Cherries

Cherries' phytonutrient claim to fame is a cancer-fighting agent called perillyl alcohol, which prevents—and treats—pancreatic and liver cancer in lab animals. Perillyl alcohol is currently being tested as a cancer treatment in humans. "Cherries probably contain the most perillyl alcohol of any fruit or vegetable," says researcher Pamela Crowell, Ph.D., associate professor of biology at Indiana University–Purdue University in Indianapolis. The amounts used in the research studies, however, far exceed the amount of cherries you can eat, she says.

Phytonutrients tend to work synergistically, meaning that they help each other in the body so that their combined protective effect is greater than the sum of their individual efforts. "So it's very possible that—in combination with other phytochemicals, vitamins, and minerals in the diet—the small doses of perillyl alcohol you'd get in a serving of cherries could be quite protective," Dr. Crowell speculates.

How much/how often: Three-quarters cup of cherries covers one of your two or more daily fruit servings.

29. Cinnamon

This apple pie spice offers a surprising health benefit: It helps regulate your blood sugar. And it does so by improving the body's responsiveness (or sensitivity) to insulin, according to studies led by Richard Anderson, Ph.D., a biochemist and lead scientist at the USDA Beltsville Human Nutrition Research Center in Maryland. Insulin is a hormone released by the pancreas that allows cells to take up their favorite fuel—

glucose—from the blood. In diabetes, the body's cells are insensitive to insulin, meaning that insulin can't usher glucose into cells. Glucose floats around in the blood and, over the long run, harms organs.

In test-tube research at the USDA, a cinnamon extract caused insulin to be 20 times more effective. How could an everyday spice perform such a feat? The theory is that one or more of cinnamon's ingredients make a cell's insulin receptor (the landing site for insulin) a more welcoming place for this important hormone. "There are beneficial compounds in cinnamon and other natural products that make your insulin work better," says Dr. Anderson.

Cinnamon even battles the dreaded *Escherichia coli* bacteria, a potentially fatal form of food poisoning.

In one study, 1 teaspoon of cinnamon killed 99.5 percent of the bacteria in apple juice samples over a 3-day period. Adding cinnamon to food could help prevent the growth of this dangerous bug, although researchers say that this doesn't ensure that the product is absolutely safe. In addition, this versatile spice has been shown to have some antifungal effects. In a test tube, cinnamon oil destroyed respiratory tract mycoses, a growth of fungi in the lungs. Another study determined that cinnamon is also effective against overgrowth of oral candidiasis (yeast infection).

How much/how often: With so many beneficial effects, start sprinkling on the cinnamon. While researchers don't know the minimum amount it takes to improve insulin sensitivity, they suggest ½ to 1 teaspoon daily. Try it in your cereal, coffee, oatmeal, yogurt, and other foods throughout the day as part of your one or more daily servings of herbs and spices.

30. Citrus Rind

Nothing livens up fruit salad, salsa, desserts, or most any other dish like a little grated lemon rind. Lemon and other citrus rinds also liven up your body's defenses against disease. More than 90 percent of the oils in orange, tangerine, and lemon rinds are made up of a potent anti-cancer compound called d-limonene. This compound raises levels of enzymes that destroy cancer-causing chemicals before they can do harm. In addition, a study done on rats found that adding tangerine rind to the diet lowered cholesterol. And this compound has even been used to dissolve gallstones.

How much/how often: Enjoy as much as you'd like as often as you'd like; it doesn't count toward any of the food groups.

31. Clams and Mussels

Beef is always touted as a great source of iron, but clams and mussels have it beat. Three ounces of cooked clams have 74 percent of the DV, and mussels have 34 percent (compared with 14 percent in cooked beef). While too much iron is linked to heart disease and possibly cancer, too little produces the dull, fatigued feeling characteristic of iron-deficiency anemia. This condition is most common in women who are still menstruating, because of monthly blood—and iron—losses. With a decent dusting of other minerals, clams and mussels make a great low-fat, high-nutrient source of protein.

How much/how often: Count 3 ounces of cooked clams or mussels as one of your two to three servings a day of the fish/poultry/meat group.

32. Cranberries and Cranberry Juice

If you've ever suffered through the agony of a urinary tract infection, or worse, if the condition turned into a bladder infection, you'll appreciate what cranberry juice has to offer. A number of studies show that it helps prevent urinary tract infections. One published in the *Journal of the American Medical Association* followed older women (average age 78) who drank 1¼ cups of sweetened cranberry juice daily for 6 months. Compared with a group of women drinking an artificial look-alike, the cranberry juice drinkers were 42 percent less likely to have urinary tract bacteria in their urine.

Cranberries may even help prevent gum disease, according to an Israeli study. In 58 percent of the test-tube experiments, extracts from cranberries prevented bacteria from congregating (which is how they form destructive dental plaque). The type of bacteria that cranberries worked best against cause the leading gum diseases (gingival and periodontal diseases). It's important to note that, unlike the urinary tract study, this one used cranberry extracts, not the sweetened juice. The researchers say that the sugar in the juice would probably negate the gum-saving effects, and they are trying to figure out a way for people to get just the protective extracts.

Pigments that give cranberries their beautiful red color—proantho-cyanidins—may also be what's helping prevent both the urinary tract infections and the dental plaque. These compounds create an environment so slippery that bacteria just can't stick, either to each other or to the walls of the urinary tract.

How much/how often: Three-quarters cup of cranberries or 6 ounces of cranberry juice counts toward your one or more daily citrus/berries servings. To ward off urinary tract infections, start with ¾ cup of juice daily. If this isn't enough, go with the 1¼ cups used in the study. Start with less because sweetened cranberry juice is high in calories; unsweetened is unbearable. You could also try artificially sweetened juice.

33. Dry-Roasted Soybeans

Cooked and dried soybeans taste pretty awful unless they're dry-roasted. Then they can be eaten like nuts. At 152 calories and 8 grams of fat per 3 tablespoon serving size, these are not diet food. But with all those isoflavones, that healthy soy protein, and 8 grams of fiber, they're a much better alternative to other snacks.

How much/how often: Three tablespoons of dry-roasted soybeans has 41 milligrams of isoflavones; you need one serving daily of 30 to 50 milligrams.

34. Fish

Scientists became fascinated with the health effects of fish when they looked into the diets of Greenland Eskimos. How could these people have such low rates of heart disease yet eat so much fat in the form of seal blubber and fatty fish? This seeming paradox launched a wealth of rewarding research into the type of fat in fish: omega-3 fatty acids. In particular, fish are rich in two types of omega-3's: eicosapentaenoic acid (EPA) and docosahexaenoic acid (DHA). Here are some of fish oil's benefits.

Heart health. After the Eskimo observations, other large-scale studies fortified the theory that fish protects against heart disease. For instance, 1,822 men in Chicago were tracked for 30 years. Those who averaged more than 1 ounce of fish daily were 38 percent less likely to die of heart disease and about half as likely to die of a sudden heart attack as the men who didn't eat fish. In an Indian study, people who took fish-oil capsules for the year following their heart attacks were only half as likely to die of a second heart attack as those taking a placebo. The fish-oil group also had fewer heart disease complications and symptoms.

Decades of test-tube, animal, and human studies have pinpointed many of the ways that fish helps the heart. While other attributes of fish could be at work, it is the fish oils that seem to be the main protectors. Fish oils help prevent arrhythmia (irregular heartbeat), which can lead to sudden death; reduce the risk of a blood clot by thinning the blood; and help prevent high blood pressure by enhancing the production of two substances that dilate blood vessels. They may also help keep arteries clear by preventing damage to artery walls, and they may lower two types of blood fats linked with heart disease: cholesterol and triglycerides.

Brainpower. The DHA in fish oil is also the predominant fat in the brain and the retina. In premature infants, a DHA deficiency causes weakened vision and may even lower IQ. For this reason, manufacturers in Europe and Japan have added DHA to infant formulas (U.S. manufacturers are still debating it). Preliminary research also shows that fish oils may help treat certain types of psychiatric conditions. A study of people with bipolar (manic-depressive) illness showed that a 9.6-gram daily supplement of fish oil caused longer remission periods and fewer symptoms than a placebo supplement.

Arthritis relief. A University of Washington study comparing women with and without rheumatoid arthritis (RA) found that women who ate two or more servings of fish weekly were only half as likely to get RA as women who ate less than one serving per week. A number of studies have found that taking fish-oil supplements alleviates arthritis symptoms. A review of 10 studies concluded that, after 3 months of fish-oil supplementation, people experience fewer tender joints and less morning stiffness. Fish oil helps alleviate RA by producing fewer inflammation-causing by-products than omega-6 fatty acids, the fat that predominates in corn, safflower, and sunflower oils.

How much/how often: Have fish at least twice a week. The fattier the fish—like salmon, mackerel, sardines, and halibut—the better. A 3-ounce fish fillet counts as one of your two to three daily servings of the fish/poultry/meat group, depending on its size.

35. Flaxseed

If you went looking for flaxseed a few years ago, you were lucky if your local health food store carried a packet. But as the news of flaxseed's astonishing disease-fighting potential traveled from research labs to consumers, the food industry responded with an increasing choice of products made from the seeds: frozen waffles, breads, and cereals. These are some of the main reasons flaxseed belongs in your diet.

Cancer prevention. Animal research shows that flaxseed helps prevent cancers of the breast and colon as well as skin cancer that has spread to the lungs. Mice injected with cancer cells were studied at the Creighton University School of Medicine in Omaha. They were on diets that were 2.5, 5, or 10 percent flaxseed. They developed, respectively, 32, 54, or 63 percent fewer lung cancer tumors than mice on a control diet.

A study at the University of Toronto showed that feeding rats diets enriched with either flaxseed or some of flaxseed's active ingredients reduced the number and size of breast cancer tumors. When 28 postmenopausal women added 5 or 10 grams of ground flaxseed to their diets each day, they had less estrogen in their systems than when they did not consume flaxseed. Lower estrogen is linked to a reduced risk for breast and endometrial cancers.

Two disease fighters in flaxseed that have researchers abuzz are plant lignans and a type of fat called alpha-linolenic acid. Flaxseed is the highest source of lignans, estrogen copycats that act as weak hormones and thwart the harmful, cancer-causing effects of the real hormone.

Prostate cancer is linked to testosterone. Lignans may help reduce the risk of this cancer in your husband by interfering with an enzyme that triggers the production of testosterone.

It gets better: Lignans are also antioxidants, which deter cancer from ever taking hold. "There's no direct evidence yet in humans, but studies indicate that people who excrete the most lignans in their urine—signaling a high lignan production in the body—have lower risk for cancer," sums up lignan researcher Lillian Thompson, Ph.D., professor in the department of nutritional sciences at the University of Toronto.

Heart protection. In two animal studies at the University of Saskatchewan, supplementing the diet with flaxseed reduced atherosclerosis (clogging of the arteries) by 46 and 69 percent. Human studies show similar promise. In a University of Toronto study, people with high cholesterol ate either wheat bran or flaxseed muffins along with a low-fat diet. The flaxseed muffins brought cholesterol down 5 percent lower than wheat bran muffins did, and brought down LDL cholesterol by an extra 8 percent compared to the wheat bran.

Flaxseed is also one of the richest plant sources of omega-3 fatty acids (of fish-oil fame). The type of omega-3 in flaxseed is alpha-linolenic acid. Like the fish oils EPA and DHA, it helps fight heart disease on a number of fronts. It seems to have its own powers to reduce heart disease risk factors, such as lowering blood cholesterol and inflammation (both precursors to clogged arteries). A fraction of it gets transformed into EPA, a known heart disease fighter. But there appears to be something else protecting the heart. Even a type of flaxseed very low in alpha-linolenic acid reduced the risk of atherosclerosis in lab animal research. It could be flaxseed's antioxidant properties, which can nip atherosclerosis in the bud by preventing the oxidation of LDL cholesterol.

Constipation control. As for digestive health, flaxseed has amazing laxative effects. But that's no mystery. At 3 grams of fiber per tablespoon, it's one of the highest sources around.

How much/how often: Flaxseed comes as whole or ground seeds. You can easily add the ground seeds (flaxseed meal) to recipes. (Use a little trial and error to determine the right amount for various recipes.) A rule of thumb for muffins and fruit breads: Replace one-quarter of the flour with flaxseed meal. The meal also works as a partial fat substitute; use 3 tablespoons in place of each tablespoon of oil or shortening. Dr. Thompson suggests including 1 to 2½ tablespoons of flaxseed per day in your meals to get its beneficial effects. If you're taking medication or have a bowel obstruction, ask your doctor before adding flaxseed to your daily eating plan—it can affect absorption of medications.

36. Flaxseed Oil

One of the many alarming dietary trends of the latter half of the 20th century was the shift in the types of fat we eat. It's not just that we eat too much artery-clogging saturated fat in burgers and other fatty animal foods. We're also getting too much of a fat everyone thought was healthy: polyunsaturated omega-6 fatty acids, the base of corn, safflower, sunflower, and other popular vegetable oils and many salad dressings. Sure, this type of fat doesn't raise blood cholesterol. But in excess, it has been linked to cancer.

What's missing from this picture is the polyunsaturated omega-3 fatty acids. Omega-3's may actually protect against cancer, while defending against heart disease in more ways than omega-6's. Our diets contain almost 10 times more omega-6's than omega-3's. Experts recommend a ratio of three parts omega-6's to two parts omega-3's. Flaxseed is the richest plant source of a type of omega-3 called alpha-linolenic acid. Fish oils are the other main source of omega-3's.

Both flaxseed oil and alpha-linolenic acid come with strong research credentials as heart protectors. In an Australian study of obese men and women, 4 weeks on a low-fat diet supplemented with ⅔ ounce of flaxseed oil per day caused their arteries to become more elastic, an important indicator of heart health. An ongoing Harvard study tracking male health professionals found that over a 6-year period, those who took in the most alpha-linolenic acid were the least likely to have a heart attack.

A French study gave men and women who had had a heart attack either a Mediterranean-style diet enriched with alpha-linolenic acid (in the form of a flaxseed-oil margarine) or a standard low-fat diet. Two years later, only 14 of the 302 people on the alpha-linoleic diet wound up with a worse case of heart disease or a second heart attack compared with 59 of the 303 people on the other diet. That's a risk reduction of 76 percent. Four years later, the risk reduction was 53 percent.

Alpha-linolenic acid uses a number of tricks to work its heart magic. By reducing blood "stickiness," it reduces the chance of a blood clot causing a heart attack. It also helps bring down blood cholesterol. The body converts a fraction of alpha-linolenic acid into two other potent omega-3's found in fish oils: DHA and EPA. So your body gets some of the heart (and other) benefits of increased levels of EPA and DHA.

How much/how often: One teaspoon of flaxseed oil counts as one of your daily quota of 5 to 10 servings of healthful oils.

37. Garlic

Garlic has inspired hundreds of studies because it casts such a wide healing net. It protects against cancer, heart disease, bacterial infections, and maybe more. On the heart disease front, garlic battles a number of risk factors: high cholesterol, high blood pressure, and sticky blood platelets that cause blood clots. After reviewing five of the best studies, researchers at New York Medical College in Valhalla concluded that one-half to one clove of garlic daily (or the powdered equivalent) lowers blood cholesterol by about 9 percent. Over the years, a few well-publicized studies questioned garlic's cholesterol-lowering ability, but the bulk of the evidence strongly supports the link.

Studies from China, Europe, the United States, and other countries show that people who eat the most garlic are less likely to develop cancer. The research is especially strong for stomach cancer.

There are dozens of therapeutic compounds in garlic. Here are the ones you're most likely to find on supplement labels.

- Allicin, which has been shown to wipe out disease-causing micro-organisms

- Ajoene (named for the Spanish word for garlic), which plays a role in lowering cholesterol and preventing clots

- S-allylcysteine and gamma-glutamyl-S-allylcysteine, sulfur-containing amino acids that rev up the activity of antioxidant systems and lower cholesterol production in the body

- Diallyl disulfide and allyl methyl sulfide, organic sulfide compounds that have anti-cancer and anti-cholesterol properties

How much/how often: Count one-half to one clove toward your one or more daily servings of the onion/garlic group. In conjunction with a diet low in saturated fat, this amount helps lower blood cholesterol and may help stave off stomach and other cancers.

38. Ginger

Since antiquity, this herb has been a staple of healers from China, India, and the Middle East. A scientific review of the research named 20 different medicinal functions for ginger. The herb helps relieve pain, nausea, and constipation; and it fights infection, cancer, and heart disease. The anti-nausea benefit is particularly important for pregnant women, because stronger medication can harm the fetus. A review of 10 studies into alternative therapies for nausea published in *Obstetrics and Gynecology* concluded that ginger is effective.

On other research fronts, extracts from ginger have reduced cholesterol and artery-clogging plaque. In a study of rabbits on a high-cholesterol diet, those given supplements of ginger extracts had about half the level of blood cholesterol as rabbits not getting ginger. Ginger also reduces blood clot risk by thinning the blood. In addition, test-tube research shows that ginger extracts wipe out leukemia cells. And an animal study found that ginger extracts applied as an ointment reduced skin cancer tumors.

When researchers aren't using ginger itself, they usually test gingerol, paradol, and shogaol, compounds that give ginger its unique pungent bite. These compounds have proven effective against cancer, cholesterol, and blood clotting.

How much/how often: Have 1 teaspoon or more of fresh or ¼ teaspoon or more of dried ginger every day, if possible, as part of your one or more daily servings of herbs and spices. For seasickness, adults and children over 6 years old should take ¼ to 1 teaspoon of powdered ginger 30 minutes before traveling and then that same amount every 4 hours during travel. If you have gallstones, check with your doctor before using ginger, since it can increase bile secretion.

39. Grains

When you commit to eating whole grains regularly, it's nice to switch around and keep things fresh. Not that there's anything wrong with the most common choices of brown rice, barley, whole wheat pasta, and whole grain couscous. But for variety, try quinoa, a tiny round seed with a pleasant, slightly nutty taste. While it's not a true cereal grain, quinoa can be substituted for almost any grain in most recipes. One-quarter cup dry (½ to ¾ cup cooked) provides 17 to 22 percent of the DV of two heart helpers: copper and magnesium.

Bulgur is another delicious whole grain. In fact, it's a form of whole wheat that comes in three degrees of coarseness. The finest one doesn't have to be cooked; you can merely soak it and use it for tabbouleh and other salads. Medium bulgur is good for mixing into casseroles, meat loaf, and stuffings. Coarse-textured bulgur makes an excellent substitute for rice. Like any whole wheat product, bulgur contains cancer-fighting lignans and lots of fiber (4 grams in ½ cup of cooked bulgur).

How much/how often: Count ½ cup of cooked quinoa or bulgur as one of your 5 to 10 daily whole grain servings.

40. Grapefruit and Grapefruit Juice

On the heart-disease-protection front, grapefruit has much to offer. It's an excellent source of potent cholesterol-lowering pectin, a type of dietary fiber. In a study at the University of Florida College of Medicine in Gainesville, men and women with high blood cholesterol supplemented their diets with pectin extracted from grapefruit. On average, their total cholesterol fell by about 8 percent, and more important, their LDL cholesterol fell by about 11 percent.

Grapefruit is one of the best sources of a cancer-fighting antioxidant called naringenin. A University of Western Ontario study showed that giving a naringenin supplement to rats exposed to a carcinogen reduced their number of breast cancer tumors. This fruit is also a serious source of the disease-fighting antioxidant vitamin C, with 148 percent of the DV in 1 cup of grapefruit juice and 72 percent in half a grapefruit. Pink and red grapefruit juice offer a bonus: beta-carotene and lycopene.

How much/how often: Have half a grapefruit (pink or red is best) or 6 ounces of grapefruit juice as one of your one or more daily servings of citrus/berries. Calcium-fortified grapefruit juice, which provides as much calcium as milk, is an even better choice.

41. Green Beans

Green beans aren't as dramatically endowed with disease-fighting compounds as cooked or dried beans, broccoli, or other vegetable superstars, but they plod along with respectable levels of many nutrients. And since green beans are fairly popular, the cumulative effects could be very protective for fans of this vegetable. One cup of green beans is a very good source of fiber (4 grams) and provides 20 percent of the DV of vitamin C and 17 percent of vitamin A, mainly through beta-carotene. Green beans are also a good source of two other carotenoids—lutein and zeaxanthin—which offer protection from blindness caused by macular degeneration.

How much/how often: One-half cup of cooked green beans counts as one of your four or more daily servings of vegetables.

42. Green Soybeans (Edamame)

Next time you're in a Japanese restaurant, order edamame as an appetizer. You'll see how delicious young, in-the-pod soybeans can be—much better than mature dried soybeans. The pods come salted, so don't eat them; just use your teeth to slip out the soybeans. You can also find edamame, fresh or frozen, in the pods or not, in some supermarkets and health food stores.

How much/how often: One-half cup of cooked, shelled fresh soybeans has 11 milligrams of isoflavones; you need one serving daily of 30 to 50 milligrams.

43. Horseradish

If you love this sharp-tasting condiment, pile it on for a dose of isothiocyanates, compounds that deactivate chemicals before they can turn into cancer triggers. That dollop of horseradish is also adding to your vitamin C supply; there's 27 percent of the DV in 4 teaspoons of fresh horseradish and 8 percent in prepared horseradish.

How much/how often: Since it's used mainly as a condiment, there is no recommended serving amount, and it doesn't count toward any of the food groups, so use it as often as you like.

44. Hot Peppers

You like it hot, hot, hot? Enjoy your pain—those peppers are also burning down destructive disease-causing chemicals. Capsaicin, the antioxidant compound that gives jalapeños and other peppers their fire, is also what fights cancer and heart disease. Capsaicin helps nip cancer in the bud by boosting enzymes that detoxify carcinogens, including one of the principal poisons in tobacco. It was once thought that hot peppers would encourage stomach cancer by irritating the stomach lining. But Mexicans, who are voracious hot pepper eaters, have one of the lower rates of stomach cancer. And animal studies show that capsaicin actually lowers stomach cancer risk. These studies also show that capsaicin helps suppress the growth of skin cancer.

Capsaicin protects the heart on a few levels. It reduces inflammation, one of the first steps in arterial plaque formation. It also makes blood less sticky, thereby discouraging blood clots.

Ironically, since hot peppers can cause pain when eaten and touched, capsaicin is used medically as a pain-relieving ointment. Studies in which people are administered it as an ointment show that it reduces the pain from osteoarthritis, diabetic neuropathy, and herpes flare-ups by up to 55 percent.

How much/how often: No dose has been determined, so add hot peppers to foods according to your tastebuds.

45. Kiwifruit

Kiwifruit has long been touted for its extravagant vitamin C levels (124 percent of the DV in just one) and its helpful dose of fiber (2.6 grams in each). A University of Texas at Galveston study found that kiwifruit is also a good source of the antioxidant eye protectors lutein and zeaxanthin, which fend off macular degeneration and cataracts.

How much/how often: One kiwifruit counts as one of your two or more daily fruit servings.

46. Leafy Greens

If you relish the strong taste of dark bitter greens like kale, chard, collards, and mustard greens, consider yourself fortunate. They're jam-packed with an extraordinary array of disease fighters. If your tastes run milder, spinach is no nutritional slouch. When scientists survey populations to see which foods are linked to disease prevention, greens stand out.

Harvard University studies tracking 75,596 female nurses for 14 years and 38,683 male health professionals for over 8 years found that those who ate the most fruits and vegetables (9 to 10 servings daily) had a 31 percent lower risk of suffering an ischemic stroke, the type caused by a blood clot in the brain, than those who ate the least. Among the fruits and vegetables that were most protective were leafy green vegetables.

An Italian study found that people who ate at least one serving of greens weekly were 20 percent less likely to develop colon cancer and 30 percent less likely to develop rectal cancer.

A study sponsored by the National Eye Institute compared 356 patients with macular degeneration (a leading cause of blindness) and 520 people without the disease. It found that those who ate spinach or collard greens two to four times weekly had about half the risk of developing the condition. Eating greens five or more times weekly had an even bigger payoff: an 86 percent drop in risk. Greens, particularly spinach and kale, also lower the risk of developing cataracts by about 20 percent, according to the Harvard studies.

Besides whopping doses of beta-carotene (1 cup of any of these greens covers your vitamin A needs for the day), many greens are loaded with two other types of carotenoids: lutein and zeaxanthin, the ones that protect against macular degeneration and cataracts. These two antioxidant carotenoids are abundant in the macula of the eye and protect eyes against destructive free radicals.

The bitter or peppery greens such as kale, collards, turnip greens, and mustard greens also contain cancer-fighting phenethyl isothiocyanate. Chlorophyll, which gives greens their color, is converted in the body to antioxidant compounds that have been shown to prevent cancer.

Most greens are excellent sources of another major health promoter: the B vitamin folate. One cup (two servings) of cooked spinach provides 66 percent of the DV of this vitamin; that amount of turnip or collard greens has about 43 percent. Harvard University's ongoing study of female nurses found that, over a 14-year period, women who took in the most folate (696 micrograms daily) were 31 percent less likely to have a heart attack or die of heart disease than those taking in only 158 micrograms. (The DV for folate is 400 micrograms.) This vitamin lowers levels of an amino acid called homocysteine, which is linked to heart disease.

That same Harvard nurses' study also found that women getting the most folate were at lower risk for colon cancer. And when given to pregnant women, supplements of folic acid lowered the risk of having a baby with neural tube defects by 72 percent, according to a seven-country study. Based on that and other research, the FDA now requires flour and several other grain products to be fortified with folate to guard against this birth defect.

Dark greens are also good sources of calcium (especially kale and bok choy), magnesium, vitamin C, and vitamin K. Dandelion greens are a good source of vitamin C and offer some calcium and magnesium as well.

How much/how often: One-half cup of cooked or 2 cups of raw greens counts toward your one or more daily servings of greens. Sautéing greens in a little oil (olive or canola is healthiest) makes it easier for your body to absorb the carotenoids.

47. Lobster

Sometimes you get a break, and a luxury food turns out to be good for you. A 3-ounce portion of lobster takes care of 52 percent of the DV of selenium and a smattering of other minerals. But lobster's true nutritional calling is copper: 82 percent of the DV is in 3 ounces. Indulge in an 8-ounce lobster tail, and you're getting 121 percent of this often neglected mineral. According to USDA surveys, most Americans get only 60 percent of the DV. That's too bad, because copper is a crucial component of enzymes, which are important to the heart, bones, brain, blood, and hair. Low levels of copper are linked to increased risk of heart disease and osteoporosis and may increase the risk for diabetes.

How much/how often: Two to 3 ounces of lobster counts as one of your two to three daily servings of the fish/poultry/meat group. You can eat it as often as you like.

48. Mangoes

You can't go wrong with a delicious fruit that provides 161 percent of the DV for vitamin A (through beta-carotene) and nearly 100 percent of the vitamin C requirement. These two antioxidants are champions against heart disease, cancer, and other chronic diseases. Half a mango also supplies 2.9 grams of fiber.

How much/how often: Count one mango toward your two or more daily fruits.

49. Milk

When we think of milk, we think calcium and protein. The average woman gets more protein than she needs, leaving calcium as the real nutritional advantage to milk. In recent years, nutrition experts have increased the amount of calcium recommended to 1,000 milligrams daily for adults up to age 50 and 1,500 milligrams for those 51 and older.

That's a lot of calcium. The major sources of calcium are dairy foods, calcium-fortified citrus juice, and certain greens, like kale. There are 300 milligrams of calcium in 1 cup of fat-free or low-fat milk (these are your best bets for keeping a lid on fat and calories).

Calcium is most famous for its role in building bones up until age 30. After that, it's best for stemming bone loss. But the research linking high levels of calcium to lower rates of osteoporosis in adult women is controversial. Unfortunately, supplementing with calcium tablets doesn't seem to help much during the time of life when women experience the most bone loss: menopause and 5 years afterward. Research does show, however, that supplementation helps 6 or more years after menopause, probably because the hormonal activity that stimulates bone loss has quieted down.

And the evidence for the role of dairy products is even more controversial. The ongoing Nurses' Health Study at Harvard University tracked 77,761 women for 12 years and found that women drinking two or more glasses of milk a day had the same, or even more, bone fractures as women drinking just one glass of milk per week. In a study at the University of Massachusetts in Worcester, however, premenopausal women were given enough dairy products to increase their calcium intake over their regular amount by 610 milligrams daily (the equivalent of two glasses of milk). Over a 3-year span, these women did not lose bone. Another group of women in this study who didn't increase dairy intake lost an average 3 percent of their bone.

Remember, calcium isn't the only factor in preventing osteoporosis: Bones need vitamins C, D, and K and the minerals phosphorus and magnesium. Vitamin D is an especially important player; without it, your body can't properly absorb calcium. Vitamin D–fortified milk may be your only good source of this vitamin in the winter months, when there isn't enough sunlight to trigger vitamin D production in the skin.

The Nurses' Health Study suggests that women who take in the most calcium and dairy foods are at lower risk for stroke than those who take in the fewest.

Blood pressure control is a controversial area. Some research shows that higher intakes of calcium reduce blood pressure; others don't. And some studies indicate that dairy foods may lower the risk for colon cancer, but not enough research has weighed in yet to make a clear connection.

How much/how often: At this stage in the research, experts are still recommending two to three dairy servings daily. Count one glass of milk as a serving. Fat-free and low-fat milk are best. For men and women over 50, even with three dairy servings daily, you may need to take a calcium supplement to get the recommended 1,500 milligrams.

50. Mint

Menthol, a flavoring in mint gum, really does come from mint. Besides acting as a flavoring, menthol does a number of good things for you: It fights bacteria and may also have anti-inflammatory properties. Anti-inflammatory agents help fight rheumatoid arthritis, asthma, and heart disease. And mint does more to your mouth than just freshen breath. A Swiss study found that peppermint oil also kills oral bacteria that cause plaque, and a study done on hamsters found that mint helps protect against oral cancer.

How much/how often: Have mint as often as you like. One teaspoon of fresh or ¼ teaspoon of dried counts as one of your one or more daily servings of herbs and spices.

51. Miso

If you've ever had the pleasure of eating a bowl of miso soup, you'd never guess that the paste used to make it is a mix of soybeans, grain, salt, and a mold culture aged for 6 months to 3 years.

How much/how often: Two tablespoons of miso—a standard serving for a bowl of soup—contains 15 milligrams of isoflavones; you need one serving daily of 30 to 50 milligrams.

52. Oat Bran

Oat bran mania probably peaked on the day that nutritional contradiction in terms—oat bran doughnuts—hit the market. In the mid-1980s, oat bran was sensationalized as the answer to high cholesterol, and people couldn't get enough. Later, the media turned on oat bran, pointing to one or two studies that showed no beneficial effect.

Fortunately, oat bran returned to grace, and a review of 20 studies published in the *Journal of the American Medical Association* said, "Incorporating oat products into the diet causes a modest reduction in blood cholesterol level." By modest, they mean a drop of 4 to 8 points in total cholesterol. But the authors also note that oat bran can cause more drastic reductions in people with higher blood cholesterol (equal to or more than 229 milligrams per deciliter).

Beta-glucan, a type of fiber plentiful in oat bran, seems to be the active ingredient. A Canadian study of men and women with high cholesterol showed that giving straight beta-glucan as a gum (the daily equivalent of ¾ cup of raw oat bran) lowered both total cholesterol and LDL by 9 percent after 4 weeks. Like a sponge, beta-glucan soaks up moisture, creating a gel in the intestines. This gel traps a number of substances (like dietary fat and cholesterol) and sends them out of the body before they can raise blood cholesterol. Beta-glucan also traps bile acids, the body's own detergent used to break down fat for absorption. Bile acids are made from cholesterol. After they're used, they usually get absorbed back into the liver, where they add to the body's cholesterol load. Beta-glucan prevents some of the bile acid resorption.

The beta-glucan gel may also ward off cancer by trapping and eliminating carcinogens.

Oat bran has another weapon against heart disease as well as diabetes and possibly obesity: a low glycemic index. That's the measure of how a food raises blood sugar. Low glycemic index diets minimally raise blood sugar; high ones do just the opposite. Low glycemic index diets make insulin more responsive or "sensitive," which helps diabetics keep blood sugar under control and helps reduce blood triglycerides (fats that can cause heart disease). A Harvard study of nearly 65,000 nurses suggests that low glycemic index diets help prevent diabetes.

In another study, obese teenage boys experienced higher blood glucose and insulin levels and ate 81 percent more calories after a high glycemic index breakfast than they did after finishing a low glycemic index breakfast. "Low glycemic index meals result in substantially lower insulin secretion, which helps the body access stored fat, decrease hunger, and potentially lower cardiovascular disease risk," concludes study leader David Ludwig, M.D., director of the obesity program in the division of endocrinology at Harvard Medical School.

How much/how often: One-half cup of raw oat bran or 1⅓ cups of cooked contains 3 grams of beta-glucan, the amount shown to lower blood cholesterol. Count 1 cup of cooked oat bran toward your daily 5 to 10 servings of whole grain foods. This will give you almost the same amount of beta-glucan used in the studies. Eat a little more if you can.

53. Oatmeal

In terms of lowering blood cholesterol, oatmeal is a less potent player than oat bran, but it's still important. Whereas oat bran is nearly pure beta-glucan, oatmeal contains other types of carbohydrates and some protein. A Harvard University study tracking nearly 69,000 nurses found that women who ate oatmeal at least five times a week lowered their risk for heart disease by 29 percent. In addition to some beta-glucan, 1 cup of oatmeal provides 27 percent of the DV for selenium, a mineral that is an integral part of a powerful antioxidant system in the body.

How much/how often: Two cups of cooked oatmeal provides 3 grams of beta-glucan, the amount shown to lower blood cholesterol. Count ½ cup of cooked oatmeal as one of your 5 to 10 daily whole grain servings. For cold oat breakfast cereals (like Cheerios), one serving consists of enough cereal to provide 70 to 90 calories.

54. Olive Oil

Olive oil got its legendary nutrition status because it is the main fat used in the Mediterranean diet, the traditional diet of people in Greece, southern Italy, and certain other Mediterranean countries. These people are blessed with low rates of heart disease and cancer as well as some of the highest life expectancy rates. It's hard to tease out the effects of olive oil from all the fruits, vegetables, whole grains, fish, and other healthful foods eaten in this region, but researchers are working on it. Much of olive oil's benefits are linked to its composition: 74 percent monounsaturated fat, 8 percent polyunsaturated, and 13 percent saturated.

One way scientists judge how effective a particular fat is at lowering blood cholesterol and other blood fats is by replacing a portion of the carbohydrates in the diet with the fat. In such experiments, monounsaturated fat lowers total cholesterol, LDL cholesterol, and triglycerides while raising beneficial HDL cholesterol.

Monounsaturated fat is roughly equivalent to polyunsaturated fat when it comes to lowering blood fats. When polyunsaturated fat is the major source of fat in the diet, however, it promotes cancer; monounsaturated fat protects against it. In studies, animals fed 40 percent of calories from polyunsaturated fat are at high risk for breast, colon, and pancreatic cancer. But diets high in monounsaturated fat don't raise cancer risk in similar animal research.

Surveys linking people's diets to disease risk mirror the animal research. For instance, in a joint Karolinska Institute/Harvard University study tracking nearly 62,000 Swedish women over a 4-year period, those who ate the most monounsaturated fat were 20 percent less likely to get breast cancer than those eating the least. Women taking in the most polyunsaturated fat, however, were 20 percent *more* likely to develop breast cancer. And in University of Milan research comparing 2,569 Italian women with breast cancer and 2,588 women without it, those who ate the most olive oil (more than 10 teaspoons daily) were 13 percent less likely to develop breast cancer than those eating 2 teaspoons or less.

How much/how often: One teaspoon of olive oil counts toward your daily quota of 5 to 10 servings of healthful oils.

55. Onions

Onions come up smelling like roses when it comes to research linking foods with disease protection. The studies are numerous. For example, in a French study comparing 345 women with breast cancer and 345 healthy women, eating onions (and garlic) 7 to 10 times weekly cut the risk of developing breast cancer by half. Eating them more than 16 times weekly plunged the risk 70 percent.

Swiss research suggests that onions may also protect the bones. Adding onions to rats' diets reduced bone resorption (calcium release from bones) by 20 to 25 percent. Bone resorption accelerates after menopause, contributing to the disabling bone-thinning disease osteoporosis.

While researchers aren't yet sure how onions affect bone, they're zeroing in on compounds that help ward off cancer and heart disease. Onions contain many of the same protective sulfur compounds as garlic and are also a rich source of quercetin. This compound helps zap carcinogens before they can cause cancer and also puts the brakes on cancer at all stages of the disease. Quercetin's heart protection is twofold: It thins the blood, reducing the risk of a blood clot, and it helps cut down on artery-clogging plaque by preventing LDL cholesterol from harmfully oxidizing. Red onions have an extra bonus: anthocyanins, a type of antioxidant shown to protect against cancer and the formation of artery-clogging plaque.

And you can add one more benefit to the ever-expanding list: a reduction in asthma symptoms, in part caused by compounds called thiosulfates and cepaenes, which quell histamine release and other inflammatory reactions of asthma.

How much/how often: Count ¼ cup of raw onion or 2 tablespoons of cooked or more at least every other day toward your one or more daily servings of the onion/garlic group.

56. Orange Juice

A cup of juice provides 161 percent of the DV for vitamin C and more than one-quarter of the DV for folate, the B vitamin that helps prevent heart disease, birth defects, and cancer. In fact, it has more of everything that's in oranges with one notable exception: fiber. (That's why it is always a good idea to have whole fruits as well as fruit juices.)

A study at the University of Western Ontario found that drinking orange juice caused a reduction in the amount of breast cancer tumors in rats exposed to a carcinogen. Researchers suspect the active ingredient is a compound in oranges called hesperidin. In a Michigan State University study of rats exposed to a carcinogen, those given orange juice as their only beverage had 22 percent fewer colon cancer tumors than rats drinking water. Research leader Maurice R. Bennink, Ph.D., professor of food science and nutrition at the university, suspects that hesperidin and another compound called limonin glucoside are the tumor fighters. "There are probably many things in the diet that will help prevent cancer, and this test shows that orange juice is one of these foods," he says.

Orange juice deserves its fame as a great source of vitamin C. This antioxidant vitamin seems to have a hand in fending off nearly every chronic disease. It fights heart disease in myriad ways: by helping prevent clogged arteries, by relaxing arteries (which lowers blood pressure), and by enhancing the potency of vitamin E, another heart protector. And that's just for starters. Vitamin C also shows promise as an anti-asthma agent, and numerous animal studies and population surveys link it to decreased cancer risk.

How much/how often: Count 6 ounces of orange juice as one of your one or more daily servings of citrus/berries. Calcium-fortified orange juice, which provides as much calcium as milk, is an even better choice.

57. Oranges

It's not just about vitamin C. Oranges are benefiting from research into phytonutrients (naturally occurring plant chemicals), and what's been uncovered is that our favorite winter fruit is one of the richest sources of hesperidin. That's a compound from a class of antioxidants called flavonoids, which help fight cancer and heart disease. In animal research, hesperidin fights breast cancer and is showing real potential as a cholesterol-lowering agent. Another flavonoid in oranges, d-limonene, has also been shown to reduce the number and size of cancerous tumors. d-limonene is currently being tested on women with breast cancer.

Of course, vitamin C is still a large part of the orange's allure. One orange has 116 percent of the DV of this vitamin, which has been linked to reduced risk of heart disease and cancer. One advantage to choosing a whole orange over the juice is the 3 grams of fiber it provides—a good start toward the 20 to 35 grams recommended each day to prevent constipation, heart disease, and certain types of cancer.

Oranges and other citrus also protect against stroke. Citrus fruits and juices were among the fruits and vegetables that stood out as most protective against ischemic stroke (the type caused by a blood clot in the brain) in a Harvard study.

How much/how often: Count an orange as one of your one or more daily servings of citrus/berries.

58. Oysters

Oysters' sexy reputation as aphrodisiacs may make you feel a little naughty, but nutritionally, they're nothing but virtuous. They're the world's greatest source of zinc: Three ounces of steamed Eastern oysters contain a phenomenal 645 to 1,029 percent of the DV for this mineral. Farm-raised oysters are on the lower end of this range; wild oysters, the higher end. Pacific oysters are also zinc-filled but not as dramatically so, with 188 percent of the DV in a 3-ounce serving.

Zinc is critical to dozens of enzymatic reactions in the body dealing with building protein, facilitating growth, maintaining healthy tissues (especially skin), and boosting immunity. The immunity angle is getting a lot of play in the research world. Probably the best-known research was the 1996 study that showed that zinc fights the common cold, although later research concluded that zinc's ability to treat colds is still questionable. The common cold aside, other studies show that zinc bolsters immunity. Researchers at Wayne State University School of Medicine in Detroit found that zinc increases immune defenses such as T-cells and natural killer cells. In a Tufts University study, elderly people who got less than the recommended levels of zinc showed depressed immune function.

Oysters' mineral bonanza doesn't end with zinc. In 3 ounces of cooked oysters, you get 114 to 322 percent of the DV of heart-preserving copper and 87 to 187 percent of the DV for cancer-fighting selenium. Oysters are also rich in iron and contain a sprinkling of B vitamins.

How much/how often: Count 3 ounces of cooked oysters as one of your two to three daily servings of the fish/poultry/meat group. Cooked oysters are safest; raw may be contaminated with bacteria.

59. Papaya

This gorgeous fruit is as good—and good for you—as it looks. Its deep reddish orange color screams beta-carotene, but actually a cup of cubed papaya covers only 8 percent of the DV for vitamin A in the form of beta-carotene. But papaya *is* a good source of another cancer-fighting carotenoid: beta-cryptoxanthin. And papaya really hit the vitamin C jackpot: 144 percent of the DV per cup. That same amount also donates a respectable 2.5 grams of fiber.

How much/how often: One cup of cubes or half of a medium papaya counts as one of your two or more daily fruit servings.

60. Parsley

If you want to take advantage of the wealth of disease-fighting compounds parsley has to offer, use this herb generously. It's not as strong-tasting as many other herbs, so add it by the ½-cupful to the family salad bowl and eat a lot of tabbouleh (in traditional Arab cooking, it's about 50 percent parsley).

Parsley is a rich source of vitamin K; just ¼ cup covers the DV for this important vitamin. Vitamin K helps blood clot (so you don't lose too much blood from a wound), and it works alongside a protein called osteocalcin that helps deposit calcium in bone. Harvard University's ongoing Nurses' Health Study found that women who took in the least vitamin K were 70 percent more likely to have hip fractures associated with osteoporosis. Parsley is also a great source of vitamin C and beta-carotene and a decent source of folate. In the phytonutrient department, parsley contains a number of beneficial compounds, such as terpenoids, which delay the onset of cancer, reduce the number of cancer tumors, and lower cholesterol.

How much/how often: Enjoy parsley as often as you like. One teaspoon of fresh parsley or ¼ teaspoon of dried is considered a serving. Since it's such a mild herb, feel free to have more. Parsley reduces in volume when it's chopped, so if you use ½ cup of parsley (as in a serving of tabbouleh), count it as half of your one or more daily greens servings.

6I. Peanuts and Peanut Butter

With 76 percent of peanut butter's calories coming from fat, you might feel a little guilty about your snack habit. Well, you're absolved. As long as your habit isn't out of hand and making you fat, peanut butter is worth every gram of fat. Same for peanuts themselves. Harvard University's ongoing study tracking 86,000 female nurses found that, over a 14-year period, women who ate more than 5 ounces of nuts a week were 35 percent less likely to get heart disease than those who never ate nuts or who ate less than 1 ounce of nuts per month. Those who specifically ate 2 to 4 ounces a week of peanuts cut their risk by half over those who rarely ate peanuts. Interestingly, peanut butter offered only minor protection; researchers blame the addition of cholesterol-raising hydrogenated fats in most brands.

The take-home message? Buy either natural peanut butter (that is, with nothing added, except maybe salt) or plain roasted peanuts. Besides containing cholesterol-lowering mono- and polyunsaturated fat, peanuts are rich in the amino acid arginine, which converts to nitric oxide, a substance that lowers blood pressure and helps prevent blood clots.

How much/how often: Count 1 ounce (3 tablespoons) of peanuts or 2 tablespoons of natural peanut butter with no hydrogenated oil as one of your five nut or seed servings per week.

62. Peas

Peas look like beans but count as greens—they have much less protein and more water than beans, and they offer some of the same nutrients supplied by greens, like vitamin K and beta-carotene. At 4 grams of fiber per ½ cup, peas are an excellent source of this health promoter. Yet another nutrition highlight is worthwhile amounts of lutein and zeaxanthin, two carotenoids that help ward off macular degeneration, a cause of blindness.

How much/how often: Count ½ cup of cooked peas as one of your one or more daily servings of greens. Since peas are not as high in some of the other nutrients that greens are known for, don't rely on them as a daily staple.

63. Potatoes

Potatoes are most notable for what they're *not*. They're not inherently high in fat or sodium. And potatoes can make up the bulk of your meal at a reasonable calorie expense. All bets are off, of course, if your spuds are french-fried, cream-smothered, hash-browned, or otherwise fattened up. Have them baked instead. A 7-ounce potato with skin has 220 calories, no fat, 43 percent of the DV for vitamin C, and 4 to 35 percent of the DV for most B vitamins.

Don't throw away the peel, which contains an anticarcinogenic compound called chlorogenic acid. In laboratory studies, this has been shown to help the fiber in potatoes absorb benzoapyrene, a potential carcinogen found in smoked foods such as grilled hamburgers. In one laboratory study, it almost completely prevented the carcinogen from being absorbed.

How much/how often: Eat them daily if you'd like. A medium baked potato with the skin still on counts as one of your four or more vegetable servings.

64. Prunes and Prune Juice

Your grandmother was onto something with her morning saucer of stewed prunes. Prunes' famed laxative effect comes partly from the 2.5 grams of fiber in just four prunes. There are 2 grams in 6 ounces of prune juice, and that's amazing since most juices have no fiber. Prunes and prune juice also contain dihydrophenyl isatin, which stimulates the intestinal contractions that are necessary for regular bowel movements. Prunes also contain tartaric acid, which acts as a natural laxative.

The type of fiber that predominates in prunes—soluble fiber—has been shown to lower cholesterol. In a study published in the *American Journal of Clinical Nutrition*, men with high blood cholesterol levels added either grape juice or 12 prunes a day to their usual diets. Four weeks later, prunes brought down LDL cholesterol 5 percent more than grape juice did. And while that may seem a small difference, even little dips in cholesterol pay off big when it comes to lowering heart disease risk. In addition to fiber, prunes are loaded with antioxidants, ranking number one in antioxidant power in a study at the Jean Mayer USDA Human Nutrition Research Center on Aging at Tufts University.

How much/how often: Three or four prunes or 6 ounces of prune juice counts as one of your two or more daily fruit servings. If you don't like prunes, you can get some of the same benefits from raisins.

65. Pumpkin

If Thanksgiving dinner is the first and last time you have pumpkin all year, you're missing out on a food chock-full of carotenoids. There are five times the DV of vitamin A (coming from both alpha- and beta-carotene) in ½ cup of canned pumpkin. These carotenoids have been shown over and over again to be protective against cancer. An American Institute for Cancer Research review of the medical literature concluded that carotenoids are strongly linked to a decreased risk of lung cancer. The research also shows a possible protective effect for cancers of the esophagus, stomach, colon, rectum, breast, and cervix. Carotenoids work their wonders by acting as antioxidants and destroying cancer-causing free radicals, and they also help slow down the cancer process once it's begun. A half-cup of pumpkin also supplies more than 3 grams of fiber.

As with all foods high in carotenoids, eating them with a little bit of fat greatly enhances absorption. Besides pumpkin pie, use pumpkin in risotto, stews, soups, pumpkin bread, and in other sweet and savory recipes.

How much/how often: Count ½ cup of cooked pumpkin as one of your one or more daily servings of deep yellow, orange, or red vegetables.

66. Pumpkin Seeds

Magnesium is one of those minerals sprinkled throughout foods in small to medium doses. It's unusual to find one food that really pours it on. Well, that food is pumpkin seeds; 1 ounce fulfills 38 percent of the DV for this mineral. Magnesium doesn't get as much press as other minerals like calcium, but it's a biggie, involved in more than 300 enzyme systems and critical to contraction of muscles—including the heart muscle. Magnesium helps prevent arrhythmias (irregular heartbeat) and helps keep blood pressure down.

This mineral is also critical to your skeleton. It's not only found in bone but also helps regulate calcium's movement in and out of bone. A magnesium deficiency has been linked to a higher risk for osteoporosis, and a few studies, including one from Tel Aviv University, have shown that magnesium supplements helped increase bone density in women with osteoporosis. Magnesium also helps make insulin (a hormone that regulates blood sugar) more effective and so may help prevent diabetes.

How much/how often: One ounce of pumpkin seeds counts as one of your 5 ounces of nuts or seeds per week.

67. Purple Grapes

Scientists are examining grapes to see whether these fruits can match the famous heart protection of red wine. And they like what they see. In fact, purple grape juice just might steal red wine's thunder. A number of animal and test-tube experiments show that purple grape juice (white grape juice doesn't appear to work) counteracts heart disease risk factors such as blood clotting and the oxidation of LDL cholesterol, which causes arterial plaque buildup. These studies also reveal that the juice causes arteries to relax, thus reducing blood pressure.

Studies on humans are turning up the same findings. In a University of Wisconsin study, 15 men and women with partially clogged heart arteries drank about 21 ounces of purple grape juice daily for 14 days. At the study's end, there were two promising signs of a decreased risk for heart disease: increased bloodflow (more relaxed arteries) and less LDL oxidation.

The researchers speculate that compounds called flavonoids—abundant in purple grape juice—are behind the heart-healthy effects. Purple grape juice is rich in the following flavonoids—quercetin, catechin, myricetin, kaempferol, and tannic acid—all known to be strong antioxidants or blood vessel relaxers. Resveratrol, a well-researched compound in grape juice and red wine, helps guard against blood clots by thinning the blood. Animal and test-tube research at the University of Illinois and in labs worldwide indicate that resveratrol also may help prevent a variety of cancers.

How much/how often: Count 6 ounces of purple (Concord) grape juice as one of your two or more daily fruits. (If you drink a glass of red wine with dinner, you're also covered.)

68. Purslane

A while back, it wouldn't have been worth listing this green because it was unavailable, except as a weed in your backyard. But it's now a feature in summer farmers' markets and gourmet stores. Researchers have taken a shine to this plant because it's unusually high in heart-healthy omega-3 fatty acids. Of course, since purslane is very low in total fat, you don't get a big dose of omega-3's in a serving. But if you were to eat about 3 cups, you'd get about a half-gram of omega-3's. Since our diets are so low in omega-3's, every bit helps.

An analysis done by the Center for Genetics, Nutrition, and Health in Washington, D.C., found that purslane is also a decent source of vitamin E and contains glutathione, a powerful cancer fighter. Purslane is also a good source of vitamin K; 2 cups provide four times the DV for this bone bolsterer.

How much/how often: When you can get it, mix it with other salad greens. Count 2 cups toward your one or more daily servings of greens.

69. Radishes

Bite into a radish and note how quickly your mouth goes from cool to hot. Chewing sets off a chain of chemical reactions that forms the sharp-tasting cancer-fighting compounds indoles and isothiocyanates. A Polish study found that people who eat radishes frequently are 35 percent less likely to develop stomach cancer than those who rarely or never eat the vegetable. Animal research backs up the link, demonstrating that isothiocyanates greatly reduce breast cancer.

How much/how often: Enjoy radishes as often as you like. One-half cup of radishes counts as one of your five or more cruciferous vegetables per week.

70. Raspberries

The next time you hesitate to spend $3 to $4 for ½ pint of raspberries, think of the taste . . . then think of the fiber. In that cup's worth, you'll get 8 grams, more than in a cup of bran flakes. Hundreds of studies have attested to fiber's role in the prevention of heart disease and cancer, and recent evidence points to a role in the prevention of diabetes. Raspberries contain a mix of soluble fiber (the type that helps reduce blood cholesterol) and insoluble fiber (which helps prevent constipation and possibly colon cancer). Another cancer fighter in raspberries is ellagic acid. These berries are also high in another soldier in the war against heart disease and cancer: vitamin C, with 51 percent of the DV per cup.

How much/how often: Count ¾ cup of raspberries as one of your one or more daily servings of citrus/berries.

71. Rice

The traditional Asian diet—linked to protection from heart disease, diabetes, and a number of cancers—is based on rice. Researchers aren't crediting rice alone for the disease protection; it works alongside other well-known risk reducers like a high intake of vegetables and fish and a low level of saturated fat. In addition, when rice is eaten in large quantities, it leaves little room for bad-for-you foods. But 1 cup of rice, especially brown rice, is no nutritional lightweight. You get 3.5 grams of insoluble fiber (the type similar to wheat bran), up to 15 percent of the DV for a variety of B vitamins, and 107 percent of the DV for manganese, a mineral that plays a role in bone health and blood sugar regulation.

How much/how often: Count each ½ cup of rice that you eat as one of your 5 to 10 daily servings of whole grain foods.

72. Rice Bran Oil

You've probably had rice bran oil if you've eaten in a Japanese restaurant. And you've surely passed it on the shelves of supermarkets and health food stores. A USDA/Tufts University study put rice bran oil on the nutritional map when their researchers showed that consuming two-thirds of total fat from it (as part of a 30 percent fat diet) lowered LDL cholesterol just as well as canola oil.

While rice bran oil isn't quite as rich in monounsaturated fat as olive and canola oils, it has a pretty good profile: 39 percent monounsaturated, 35 percent polyunsaturated, and 20 percent saturated fat. But researchers suspect it's more than the monounsaturates in rice bran oil that give it cholesterol-lowering power. They think it may be a compound unique to this oil—gamma-oryzanol—that's at work.

A University of California, Davis, study found that supplementing the diet with 3 ounces of rice bran every day for 6 weeks lowered LDL cholesterol by about 14 percent in people with high cholesterol. Even better, it didn't knock down levels of HDL cholesterol. Rice bran has a higher percentage of oil compared to other brans, and researchers believe that is what caused the cholesterol reduction.

How much/how often: One teaspoon of rice bran oil counts as one of your daily 5 to 10 servings of healthful oils. Since it's a little higher in polyunsaturates than olive or canola oil, don't make rice bran oil your principal fat.

73. Rye Bread and Crackers

Why, despite a diet high in saturated fat, are women in Finland less prone to breast and colon cancer than other Scandinavians or Americans? It could be the whole grain rye fiber they eat, suggests John Weisburger, M.D., Ph.D., of the American Health Foundation in Valhalla, New York. Rye flour has a few ways of dealing with these cancers. For one, it's high in dietary fiber, which, along with adequate fluid intake, pulls water into the stool, diluting the concentration of substances that are involved in the development of colon cancer and sending them out of the body more quickly. A study in the journal *Carcinogenesis* showed that rats on a high-fat diet supplemented with rye bran had only 12 percent as many tumors as rats on the same diet without rye bran. Intake of rye bread also eliminates constipation and other intestinal problems.

Breast, endometrial, and prostate cancers are triggered by estrogen and testosterone. Fiber helps pull them out of the intestines before they can be absorbed back into the system. Another compound plentiful in rye, lignans, also fights these hormone-triggered cancers by converting to a compound that looks like estrogen but doesn't act like it (called a phyto-estrogen). Phytoestrogens compete with real estrogens for landing sites on organs, reducing the amount of estrogen that comes into contact with the organs. Low lignan levels are associated with increased risk for breast cancer in Finland as well as in the United States, Sweden, and Australia. And lignans may also protect against heart disease, according to a review of the research by Finnish scientists.

Sorry—the white rye bread that comes with your pastrami doesn't cut it; most of the lignans have been processed out of it. Only whole grain rye flour is packed with healers. You get it in many rye crackers (like Finn Crisp, RyKrisp, and Wasa, which have 5 to 6 grams of fiber per ounce) and in dark rye breads that come thinly sliced and sealed in plastic for long shelf life.

How much/how often: Count one slice of whole grain rye bread or 70 to 90 calories' worth of whole grain rye crackers (3 or 4 crackers, or ¾ to 1 ounce) as one of your daily 5 to 10 servings of whole grains.

74. Sage

This herb shares some flavor compounds with rosemary: carnosol and carnosic acid, both antioxidants that help prevent cancer in lab animals. These compounds raise levels of enzymes that detoxify cancer-causing substances.

How much/how often: Eat sage as often as you like. One teaspoon of fresh sage or ¼ teaspoon of dried is considered one of your one or more daily servings of herbs and spices.

75. Salad Greens

Sorry, iceberg lovers, that's not what we're talking here. To get superfood status, your lettuce has to be dark green, like romaine or leaf lettuce. These darker leaves have seven times the cancer-fighting carotenoids of iceberg. And more than half of those carotenoids are lutein and zeaxanthin, which protect your eyes against macular degeneration.

How much/how often: Count 2 cups of mixed greens as one of your one or more daily servings of greens. Look for mixes that include mustard greens, curly endive, red oak leaf lettuce, and other dark greens.

76. Seaweed

It's a little unfair to lump the many varieties of seaweed into one category; this will change when there's more research on particular varieties. In a test of 68 foods, seaweed was ranked number two as a source of lignans, compounds that act as benign or weakened hormones, muting the cancer-causing effects of real hormones.

Research has turned up some more unusual protective compounds in seaweed. For instance, Japanese researchers uncovered a rare antioxidant called fucoxanthin in hijiki, which they suspect is behind the plant's ability to zap destructive free radicals. The dried types of seaweed, like the sushi wrapper nori, are very concentrated sources of nutrients. There's 88 percent of the DV for vitamin A in the form of carotenoids in 1 ounce of dried nori. The same amount of dried agar and kelp have between 34 and 55 percent of the DV of magnesium.

How much/how often: Count 1 cup of seaweed salad as one of your one or more daily servings of greens. It's available in Japanese restaurants (you can also make it yourself from ingredients found in health food and Asian specialty stores).

77. Sesame Oil

It takes just a teaspoon of sesame oil to give your stir-fries authentic Asian flavor. The compounds that give this oil its unique flavor—sesamin, sesamolin, and sesaminol—are also antioxidants. In a Japanese study, rats whose diets were spiked with sesamolin had more antioxidant activity going on in their bodies than rats eating an unsupplemented diet. Specifically, fats in their liver were spared from oxidation by the free radicals that initiate heart disease and cancer. Sesame oil also has a pretty good fat profile: 40 percent monounsaturated fat, 42 percent polyunsaturated, and 14 percent saturated.

How much/how often: One teaspoon counts as one of your daily 5 to 10 servings of healthful oils. Since it's a little higher in polys than olive or canola oil, don't make sesame seed oil your principal fat (since it's so strong-tasting, you wouldn't want to anyway).

78. Shiitake Mushrooms

Any way you slice them, shiitake mushrooms prove protective. Test-tube studies as well as studies on animals and humans show that extracts from the mushrooms fight cancer. In a Japanese study, mice received a carcinogen that causes bladder cancer; only half of the mice with shiitake-supplemented diets got the cancer compared with 100 percent of the mice who didn't get shiitakes. Test-tube studies show that a compound in shiitakes, lentinan, boosts the body's cancer-fighting defenses and helps destroy cancer tumors. Another Japanese study gave cancer patients lentinan and found that it prolonged the lives of some patients. Shiitakes are good sources of two other cancer fighters: fiber and selenium. Just four mushrooms contain 1.5 grams of fiber and 18 micrograms (about 26 percent of the DV) of selenium.

How much/how often: Count ½ cup of the cooked mushrooms as one of your daily four or more vegetable servings.

79. Soy

Americans have higher rates of breast cancer, prostate cancer, and heart disease than the Japanese. Is the Japanese diet making all the difference? The Japanese eat more fish, less fat, and something most Americans don't: soy foods. These include miso, dry-roasted or green soybeans, soy milk, soy protein, tempeh, textured vegetable protein, and tofu.

The Chinese are also big on soy. A University of South Carolina study of women in Shanghai found that they eat between 1 and 8 ounces of soy foods daily, with an average intake of 3½ ounces.

While it's not clear how large a role soy plays in the disease gap between the United States and Asian countries, it is clear that soy foods have remarkable disease-fighting powers. Compounds abundant in soy—isoflavones—impart some, if not all, of the health benefits. The two major isoflavones in soy are genistein and daidzein. Here are some of the ways soy can contribute to good health.

Preventing heart disease. There's something about soy protein that lowers levels of both total blood cholesterol and harmful LDL. And soy isoflavones are antioxidants, which have been shown to halt one of the first steps in the formation of artery-clogging plaque: the oxidation of LDL.

Blocking cancer. Soy isoflavones are also phytoestrogens: estrogen look-alikes found in plant foods that act as benign or weak estrogen. Estrogen is a trigger for cancers of the breast and endometrium. The theory is that phytoestrogens diminish estrogen's effects by competing with the hormone for landing sites on cells. So far, the breast cancer research is promising but inconclusive. Some test-tube experiments show that isoflavones help prevent breast cancer. And human studies indicate that eating soy foods may lower the risk of developing breast cancer before menopause but not after.

Building stronger bones. Both human and animal research shows that diets enriched with soy or soy isoflavones help improve bone density. In a University of Illinois study, women who took 90 milligrams of isoflavones daily in a soy protein powder increased their spinal bone density in 6 months; women using powdered milk experienced no increases. Bones become less dense and more brittle with age, particularly after menopause, increasing the risk for osteoporosis. That's because estrogen levels drop sharply after menopause. Unlike the situation with cancer, estrogen is a good guy when it comes to bones, encouraging calcium to stay put. The theory is that by acting as a weak estrogen, soy isoflavones improve bone density.

Making menopause easier. Since hot flashes and other symptoms of menopause are caused by dwindling estrogen, there's hope that soy's phytoestrogens can alleviate some of the symptoms. Several studies have hinted at a benefit. In one study, women took in 60 milligrams or more of isoflavones from three daily servings of soy foods, and their menopausal symptoms were cut in half.

How much/how often: No soy or isoflavone recommendation has been established; however, the FDA has approved a food label health claim stating that as part of a diet low in saturated fat and cholesterol, 25 grams of soy protein daily may reduce heart disease risk (by lowering cholesterol). Although research showed that 90 milligrams of isoflavones daily improved bone density and 60 milligrams daily reduced menopause symptoms, experts recommend consuming no more than 30 to 50 milligrams of isoflavones from soy foods daily (about one serving). Check package labels of the various soy products for their isoflavone concentration. Be aware that there are no isoflavones in soybean oil and barely any in soy sauce.

80. Soy Milk

Amazingly, this creamy-tasting liquid is made from cooked and ground soybeans. The calcium-fortified versions make a wonderful milk substitute, especially for the lactose-intolerant. And you get from 4 to 20 percent of the DV of other minerals, plus a sprinkling of B vitamins.

How much/how often: One cup of soy milk has 24 to 30 milligrams of isoflavones; you need one serving daily of 30 to 50 milligrams.

81. Soy Protein (Soy Protein Isolate)

This powder is the protein-only component of soy. Add it to shakes, soups, muffins, and other recipes.

How much/how often: One ounce (3 tablespoons) of soy protein has about 28 milligrams of isoflavones (products vary, so check nutrition labels). Get one serving daily of 30 to 50 milligrams.

82. Strawberries

Its delicate package belies this berry's aggressive nutritional defenses. Starting with the more conventional heart disease and cancer fighters, 1 cup of strawberries covers 136 percent of the DV for vitamin C and contributes 3 grams of fiber. Moving on to the more exotic, strawberries are one of the richest sources of ellagic acid, a hot commodity in research labs that is proving to be a potent anti-cancer agent. Ellagic acid destroys the enzymes that turn chemicals into carcinogens, and it stimulates the production of enzymes that destroy carcinogens. It's also an antioxidant, which means it offers both cancer and heart disease protection. One of the pigments that gives strawberries their color—anthocyanin—is also a powerful antioxidant.

How much/how often: Count ¾ cup of strawberries toward your one or more daily servings of citrus/berries.

83. Sunflower Seeds

They may be little, but sunflower seeds are a mighty source of fiber, minerals, B vitamins, and hard-to-get vitamin E. Sunflower seeds are particularly rich in folate, giving you 19 percent of the DV in a ¼-cup handful. This B vitamin helps prevent neural tube defects and is linked to a lower risk of heart disease. Sunflower seeds are also high in phytosterols, compounds that help keep cholesterol down.

How much/how often: Count 1 ounce toward your 5 ounces of nuts or seeds per week.

84. Sweet Peppers

Green, red, and yellow bell peppers are fantastic sources of vitamin C, covering two to three times the DV in one pepper. Red peppers offer an antioxidant bonus over the others with both higher C levels and more beta-carotene per pepper, covering over 100 percent of the DV for vitamin A. (The body converts beta-carotene to A as needed.) Also, red peppers are loaded with another antioxidant carotenoid, beta-cryptoxanthin.

How much/how often: Count 1 cup of sliced red, orange, or yellow pepper toward your one or more daily servings of deep yellow, orange, or red vegetables. Count 1 cup of green pepper slices toward your one or more daily servings of greens.

85. Sweet Potatoes

Sweet potatoes are a comfort food that's actually great for you. They are stuffed with beta-carotene. And a Japanese study also showed that sweet potatoes, especially the darker red-purple varieties, contain another class of antioxidant compounds: anthocyanins. They work similarly to beta-carotene to disable cancer-causing substances and prevent heart disease. Sweet potatoes have off-the-chart numbers for a few other prime protectors. One cup of mashed sweet potatoes has 82 percent of the DV for vitamin C and 6 grams of fiber, plus a healthy sprinkling of minerals and B vitamins.

How much/how often: Count ½ cup of mashed sweet potatoes or one medium (5 inches long, 2 inches in diameter) baked sweet potato toward your one or more daily servings of deep yellow, orange, or red vegetables.

86. Tahini

You can thank the Arabs for this one. Their delicious imports— chickpea-based hummus and eggplant-based baba ghannouj—are made with tahini, which is simply ground sesame seeds. Tahini is a nutritionally impressive food: Just 1 tablespoon has 1.4 grams of fiber and provides 12 percent of the DV for copper and thiamin (a B vitamin that helps convert food into energy), plus a sprinkling of other minerals and B vitamins (11 percent of the DV for manganese and phosphorus; 4 percent of the DV for riboflavin, niacin, and folate). It also sports antioxidants unique to sesame called sesaminol, sesamonlinol, and pinoresinol—all of which fight heart disease and cancer.

How much/how often: Count 2 tablespoons of tahini as one of your five weekly servings of nuts or seeds.

87. Tangerines

Tangerines are usually lumped in with oranges as far as nutrition goes. But they have a unique phytonutrient claim to fame: tangeretin. Test-tube studies show that this compound helps prevent breast cancer. And a Chinese study found that people who ate the most tangerines were at lower risk of lung cancer than those who ate the least. Tangerines are also exceptionally rich in another protective compound, beta-cryptoxanthin. It's an antioxidant that the body converts to vitamin A.

Like all citrus, tangerines are a great source of vitamin C. There's 122 percent of the DV in a cup of tangerine juice, 43 percent in a medium tangerine.

One warning: Although test-tube experiments show that tangeretin helps prevent breast cancer, a Belgian animal experiment showed that taking it in conjunction with tamoxifen (the breast cancer prevention drug) weakens the drug's effectiveness. The researchers warn against taking tangeretin supplements when on tamoxifen.

How much/how often: Count one large or two small tangerines or ¾ cup tangerine juice toward your one or more daily servings of citrus/berries.

88. Tea

Whether you're sipping green, oolong, or black tea, you can feel pretty good about a beverage that's been around for 4,000 years. That's because dozens of studies link tea to decreased risk for disease. In fact, in some parts of the world, people drink 10 cups of tea a day, and it only seems to improve their health. A study published in the *Archives of Internal Medicine* tracked the eating habits of 3,454 Dutch men and women for 2 to 3 years. In general, those who drank the most tea (5 cups a day) decreased their risk of developing severe atherosclerosis (clogged arteries) by 70 percent over those who didn't drink tea at all. Drinking 3 to 4 cups daily cut risk by 53 percent; 1 to 2 cups, 46 percent.

These remarkable risk reductions are less surprising when you take a look at what's in tea. There are three major types of tea: green (dried *Camellia sinensis* leaves), oolong (partially fermented green tea), and black (fermented green tea). All are loaded with antioxidants. One powerful antioxidant, epigallocatechin gallate (EGCG), makes up 30 percent of the weight of dried green tea leaves. When green tea gets oxidized into oolong and black tea, EGCG forms other compounds called polyphenols, which are also strong antioxidants.

These compounds account for the four main protective effects of tea that researchers have uncovered thus far.

- Tea contains antioxidants that disarm chemicals that cause cancer and initiate heart disease before they can work their mischief.

- Tea spurs the production of your body's own enzymes that detoxify carcinogens.

- Tea slows down the rate of growth of new cancer cells.

- Tea brings down the level of unfriendly bacteria in the gut (such as *E. coli*) and encourages the growth of protective bacteria like lactobacillus.

Decaffeinated tea is also protective, but bottled and powdered iced teas usually contain other ingredients, like sugar and corn syrup, and very little tea, so they aren't as protective. If you want tea's protective compounds, make your own iced tea. Use five tea bags for every 2 cups of boiled water and let it steep for 5 minutes. Drink it up within a day to get the most of the beneficial compounds. Herb teas don't contain these compounds at all. The only known risk of tea-drinking is an increased likelihood of throat cancer for those who drink their tea hot enough to burn the throat.

How much/how often: Have 1 to 5 cups of tea daily. If the caffeine makes you jittery or if you have a medical condition that prevents you from taking in caffeine, switch to decaffeinated.

89. Tempeh

This ancient Indonesian food is a combination of soy and grains incubated with an edible mold. Although an acquired taste, it has many fans. Use it in sandwiches and spreads.

How much/how often: One-half cup of tempeh has 36 milligrams of isoflavones; you need one serving daily of 30 to 50 milligrams.

90. Textured Vegetable Protein (TVP)

Available in granular form or chunks, it's a great substitute for ground beef in dishes like chili, sloppy joes, and tacos. It's made from defatted soy flour that has been compressed to the point where it changes form. Before cooking, rehydrate it by mixing 1 cup of TVP with a scant cup of boiling water.

How much/how often: One-quarter cup of dry coarse TVP has 47 milligrams of isoflavones; you need one serving daily of 30 to 50 milligrams.

91. Tofu

This familiar Asian staple is made by curdling hot soy milk with a coagulant. Tofu's blandness is its strength, because it blends well with both sweet and savory foods. If you think you don't like tofu, go to a good Japanese or Chinese restaurant; the creamy, rich tofu used in these restaurants will win you over. Then try it at home in stir-fries, casseroles, and shakes as a great vegetarian protein source. Many types are processed with calcium, giving you a bonus of 45 percent of the DV for this mineral.

How much/how often: One-half cup of tofu has 24 to 27 milligrams of isoflavones; you need one serving daily of 30 to 50 milligrams.

92. Tomatoes

File this in the too-good-to-be-true drawer: Pizza and ketchup can actually help ward off heart disease and cancer. The credit goes to tomatoes, which contain an array of disease-fighting compounds.

What better place to study the effects of tomatoes than Italy, where tomatoes are a dietary staple? An Italian study compared the eating habits of 2,709 people with various types of cancer with those of 2,879 cancer-free men and women. The conclusion: People who ate the most tomatoes cut their risk of stomach and colon cancer by more than half and were about a third less likely to develop cancer of the mouth and esophagus. And a well-publicized Harvard study tracking the eating habits of nearly 48,000 men found that eating at least 10 servings of tomatoes a week cut prostate cancer risk by 53 percent over those eating less than 1½ servings.

Those are just two of the 70-plus published research papers on the connection between tomatoes and cancer. Taking all the research into account, a *Journal of the National Cancer Institute* review concluded that eating lots of tomatoes can lower cancer risk by 40 percent. In studies, tomato sauce, ketchup, pizza, other tomato-intense foods, and raw tomatoes counted.

The compound giving the cancer protection is lycopene, a plant pigment of the carotenoid family that gives tomatoes their red color. Lycopene is considered a more powerful antioxidant than its more famous cousin, beta-carotene.

Lycopene appears to protect the heart as well. In a European study, men who suffered heart attacks had lower body stores of lycopene compared to healthy men. Based on these findings, researchers concluded that the higher your lycopene levels, the lower the risk for having a heart attack. Tomatoes were the real star of this study, since they are the main source of lycopene in the diet.

Processed tomato products such as spaghetti sauce are even more concentrated sources of lycopene than fresh tomatoes. The lycopene is absorbed better if the tomatoes have been cooked or if they are eaten with a little fat, such as olive oil.

Tomato-wise, lycopene gets some help from vitamin C. An average-size tomato has nearly 40 percent of the DV for this antioxidant vitamin. In addition, tomatoes contain coumaric acid and chlorogenic acid, compounds that help block the action of cancer-causing substances called nitrosamines (found in cigarette smoke and formed naturally in the body from nitrates in cured meats and in other foods). Chlorogenic acid is also linked to a reduced risk of colon cancer.

How much/how often: Count one tomato, 1 cup of sliced tomatoes or cherry tomatoes, or ½ cup of tomato sauce toward your one or more daily servings of deep yellow, orange, or red vegetables.

93. Turmeric

The pigment that gives this curry spice its yellow color—curcumin—is a potent disease fighter and the subject of many studies. It reverses liver damage caused by toxins, lowers the levels of cancer-causing compounds in smokers, and raises levels of enzymes that destroy carcinogens. It helps prevent skin, colon, and stomach cancers in mice. And it is anti-inflammatory, which means it helps reduce the risk of heart disease, asthma, and other diseases. A Japanese study of rats exposed to a carcinogen found that those on a diet of 1 percent curcumin developed 28 percent fewer breast cancer tumors than those not getting curcumin.

How much/how often: Use as much turmeric as often as you like as one of your one or more daily servings of herbs and spices.

94. Turnips

Turnips, which are cruciferous vegetables, get their pungency partly from cancer-fighting compounds called isothiocyanates. These compounds help disable cancer-causing substances before they trigger the disease. Turnips also have a sprinkling of vitamin C and 3 grams of fiber per cup.

How much/how often: Consider ½ cup of cooked turnips as one of your five or more crucifers per week.

95. Vegetable Juice

Drink up! Three-quarters cup of tomato-based vegetable juice (like V8) has more than twice as much of the powerful antioxidant lycopene as a cup of chopped fresh tomatoes. Add 77 percent of the DV of vitamin C and an array of carotenoids donated by the other vegetables in the juice, and you're drinking liquid nutrition.

How much/how often: Three-quarters cup of vegetable juice covers one of your one or more daily servings of deep yellow, orange, or red vegetables. Since juice doesn't contain a lot of fiber, have it only once a day.

96. Walnuts

Knowing how much walnuts have going for them in terms of heart protection, researchers at Loma Linda University in California gave 18 men without high cholesterol either a standard low-fat diet or a low-fat diet that derived 20 percent of its calories from walnuts. Four weeks later, the average blood cholesterol of the walnut eaters was 12 percent lower than that of those on the standard low-fat diet. LDL cholesterol was 16 percent lower. This study ties in nicely with surveys that link higher nut consumption with lower risk of heart disease.

Among nuts, walnuts are uniquely rich in a type of omega-3 fatty acid called alpha-linolenic acid, which has been shown to lower heart disease risk.

Another compound in walnuts—ellagic acid—also fights heart disease by reducing the formation of artery-clogging plaque. And ellagic acid can help prevent cancer.

How much/how often: Count 1 ounce (14 halves) as one of your 5 ounces of nuts or seeds per week.

97. Watercress

As soon as scientists isolate a disease-fighting compound in a food, they give it—instead of the food—to their subjects. But a compound plentiful in watercress that's been found to render a noxious tobacco carcinogen harmless—PEITC—wasn't approved for human use, so American Health Foundation researchers gave 11 smokers 2 ounces of watercress three times a day for 3 days and tested their urine for up to 2 weeks. On the watercress-enriched diet, the smokers excreted 34 percent more of a breakdown product of the tobacco carcinogen, which meant that the watercress was actually disabling the carcinogen. (Don't take this as a license to smoke. PEITC disabled only a fraction of the carcinogen, and there are plenty of others in tobacco.) Lab animal research shows that PEITC is also protective against breast cancer. On a more familiar note, watercress is a decent source of other cancer fighters: vitamin C and carotenoids.

How much/how often: Count 2 cups of chopped watercress as one of your five or more cruciferous vegetables per week or toward your one or more daily servings of greens.

98. Wheat Bran Cereal

It's amazing how much a morning bowl of bran cereal can do for you. The benefits begin—but don't end—with fiber. Bran cereal, especially the highest fiber types (such as All-Bran and Fiber One), is one of the most concentrated sources of insoluble fiber. Piles of research papers show that high-fiber diets help combat heart disease and cancer. And in many of these studies, wheat bran emerges as particularly protective.

On the heart disease front, even the traditionally cautious American Heart Association concluded: "Diets high in complex carbohydrate and fiber are associated with reduced mortality rates from coronary heart disease and other chronic diseases."

Two large-scale Harvard University studies attest to this. The first, the ongoing Health Professionals' Study of 43,757 male health professionals, found that those who ate the most fiber per day (29 grams) over a 6-year period were 40 percent less likely to have a heart attack as men eating the least fiber (12.4 grams). Cereal fiber (including wheat bran) stood out as especially effective. The other ongoing Harvard study, tracking 68,782 nurses, found that women who ate the most fiber from all sources (23 grams daily) over a 10-year period had a 23 percent lower risk of heart disease than those eating less than 12 grams.

Oddly, that same study did not show that fiber helps prevent colon cancer, a finding that perplexed many in the research community. Dozens of animal studies show that adding wheat bran to the diet does help prevent colon cancer. The difference may be that colon cancer takes only weeks to develop in rats but decades in humans, so the definitive human study hasn't been done. There are, however, promising studies showing that a high-fiber diet including wheat bran reduces polyps, a major risk factor for colon cancer.

Bran cereals prevent constipation by drawing water into the stools, which makes them easier—and quicker—to pass. This process also may reduce colon cancer risk by diluting stools and reducing the concentration of carcinogens that come into contact with the colon. (The same process is responsible for lowering cholesterol and reducing heart disease risk.) Fat, cholesterol, and your body's own bile acids (made from cholesterol) move out of the bowels more quickly on a high-fiber diet. Speedier transit time may also play a role in the reduction of hormone-triggered cancers, because estrogen and other hormones are whisked out of the body before they can be absorbed back by the intestines.

Studies indicate that wheat bran may reduce the risk for breast cancer. One possible reason is that wheat bran has been shown to lower estrogen levels in some, but not all, studies. Breast cancer—as well as endometrial cancer—is triggered by estrogen and testosterone; lower levels mean lower risk. In one of the studies showing a positive effect, American Health Foundation researchers gave 22 women enough wheat bran to raise their fiber intake from 15 grams a day to 30. Two months later, their estrogen levels declined by 15 to 20 percent.

Cereal fiber may protect against diabetes, a disease that afflicts 16 million Americans. The Harvard study of nurses found that women who ate the most fiber from cereal (7.5 grams daily) were 28 percent less likely to develop diabetes than those eating only 2 grams. The theory on the diabetes protection is that fiber slows the release of glucose into the blood, making fewer demands on the hormone insulin and thus keeping blood sugar under better control.

Besides fiber, wheat bran stashes away other weapons against disease. It's a rich source of lignans, which help fend off hormone-dependent cancers such as breast cancer. Cereals made from wheat bran are naturally loaded with health-promoting minerals like magnesium (which protects the heart). Add to that all of the vitamins and minerals that cereal manufacturers throw in, and you can see why a single bowl of cereal is such a valuable ally in your fight against chronic disease.

How much/how often: Check labels for the cup measure of cold or hot wheat bran cereal that is 70 to 90 calories' worth. That counts as one of your 5 to 10 daily whole grain servings.

99. Wheat Germ

The germ of a grain is its food warehouse, which is why wheat germ is such a concentrated source of so many vitamins and minerals. One-quarter cup mixed into your daily bowl of cereal or incorporated into recipes provides between 8 and 32 percent of the DV of most vitamins and minerals. Wheat germ boasts particularly high levels of these health-promoting heavyweights: vitamin E (shown to reduce incidence of heart attacks), zinc (linked to decreased cancer risk and better wound healing), and folate (prevents birth defects and is linked to lower risk of colon cancer and heart disease).

How much/how often: Count ¼ cup of wheat germ as one of your 5 to 10 servings of whole grain foods. Eat it as often as you like. You don't need to eat the full serving at one time. Try mixing a little into your cereal, yogurt, or fruit at breakfast. Add some more to recipes or other foods throughout the day.

100. Whole Wheat Foods

Every time you eat white bread or white pasta, you're missing out on a great nutrition opportunity. You get three times more fiber in a slice of whole wheat bread than in a slice of white. Whole wheat pasta also gives you three times the fiber of white (6 grams per cup versus 2). Clearly, making the switch to whole wheat puts a serious dent in the 20 to 35 grams of fiber you need daily.

Don't stop with bread and pasta, however. Try whole wheat waffles, pancakes, couscous, graham crackers, and crackers. Since whole wheat retains the bran part of wheat, you get, in smaller doses, all of the disease-fighting compounds of wheat. And you may even lose some weight, because whole wheat foods make you feel fuller on fewer calories. Since blood sugar levels don't rise as high as with white flour foods, you're also less likely experience the hunger that comes after a blood sugar spike.

How much/how often: One slice of bread, ½ to 1 cup of cold cereal (equal to 70 to 90 calories), ½ cup of hot cereal, ½ cup of cooked pasta, or ½ cup of cooked grains counts as one of your 5 to 10 daily servings of whole grain foods.

101. Yogurt

Scientists are just starting to catch up with natural healers, who have been using yogurt for centuries. Yogurt is milk that's been coagulated by certain bacteria, usually *Lactobacillus bulgaricus* and *Streptococcus thermophilus*, and it's these guys that help us out in many ways. The active live cultures in yogurt survive harsh stomach acids and wind up in the gut, where they have many benefits.

Lessened lactose intolerance. Yogurt makes dairy a lot more pleasant for people with lactose intolerance. This condition is caused by low levels of the enzyme that splits lactose—milk sugar—into two simple sugars that get absorbed in the intestines. With diminished levels of the enzyme, lactose winds up unabsorbed in the gut and causes gas and discomfort. Yogurt contains only about a third of the lactose of milk because its bacteria predigest the milk sugar for you.

Freedom from diarrhea. A Danish review of the research on yogurt and traveler's diarrhea, infant diarrhea, and the diarrhea that comes from antibiotic use concluded that most of the studies show that yogurt helps alleviate these conditions.

Fewer vaginal infections. Vaginal yeast infections plague most women at one time or another; for some, the condition is chronic. In an Israeli study of 46 women, 60 percent started the study with a yeast infection, and 60 percent had bacterial vaginitis, another common vaginal infection. (Some women had both types of infections.) After 4 months of eating ½ cup of yogurt daily, the proportion of women with either infection fell to about 25 percent.

Enhanced immunity. Both animal and human studies show that eating yogurt stimulates the immune system—both the local immune defense system in the intestines and immunity throughout the whole body. To see just what this means in terms of day-to-day symptoms, researchers from the University of California, Davis, gave people either 8 ounces of regular live-culture yogurt daily, 8 ounces of yogurt in which the bacteria were destroyed by heating, or no yogurt at all. Over the course of a year, those who ate the live-culture yogurt cut back on allergies and itching by about 90 percent.

If you like your yogurt with fruit, do your waistline and your blood sugar a favor: Make it yourself. A cup of fat-free yogurt mixed with a teaspoon of honey and ¼ cup of sliced peaches comes to 166 calories—store-bought fat-free peach yogurt would cost you 213 calories.

It is important to note that, unlike milk, yogurt is not fortified with vitamin D. If yogurt is your only source of dairy, make sure to take a multivitamin and mineral supplement providing 400 IU of vitamin D.

How much/how often: One cup of plain low-fat or fat-free yogurt covers one of your daily two to three dairy servings. With 415 milligrams of calcium per cup of low-fat plain yogurt and 452 milligrams per cup of fat-free plain yogurt, it is an even better source of calcium than milk. For men and women over 50, even with three dairy servings daily, you may need to take a calcium supplement to meet the 1,500-milligram recommendation.

Your Day-to-Day Power-Eating Plan

BY JANIS JIBRIN, M.S., R.D. Now that you have a virtual shopping list of 101 Power Foods from which to stock your pantry and plan menus, you're probably wondering, "Just how do I eat 35 servings of fruits and vegetables a week—plus get all the grains, beans, and other nutrient-packed foods I need to build health?"

Get ready for a nutritious eating frenzy. This chapter breaks through two of the biggest barriers to power eating: prep time and boredom. You'll find all sorts of quick and easy ways to put together healthful meals without spending all your free time slaving over a cutting board. And don't worry about having to live on skinless chicken and steamed vegetables. With this plan, it's easy to go for variety.

Power eating is easy and efficient. With these strategies and shortcuts, your diet will improve overnight—guaranteed.

Must-Have Foods for the Power Cook

You're on a coming-home-late streak, missed your weekly supermarket trip days ago, and find yourself in your kitchen scrounging for food. The difference is that this time you calmly reach into the freezer, open the cupboard, and presto! Your family has a supernutritious dinner in 20 minutes flat. The trick behind this sleight of hand is staples from the "new" food groups: greens,

POWER FOOD GROUPS: YOUR DAILY QUOTA

To help you take research on Power Foods out of the lab and onto your dinner plate, use this handy chart, developed by Paul Lachance, Ph.D., director of the nutraceuticals program at Rutgers University in New Brunswick, New Jersey, and professor of food science and nutrition. Meeting all of the frequency criteria will provide you with complete daily nutrition.

FOOD	SERVING SIZE	SERVINGS	FREQUENCY
Vegetables	1 to 2 cups raw; ½ cup cooked	4 or more	Daily
Greens	2 cups raw; ½ cup cooked	1 or more	Daily
Cruciferous vegetables	1 cup raw; ½ cup cooked	1 or more	5 days a week or more
Deep yellow, orange, or red vegetables, including tomatoes	1 cup raw; ½ cup cooked; 6 oz vegetable juice (tomato- or carrot-based juices are best)	1 or more	Daily
Fruits	1 fruit; 1 cup sliced fruit; 6 oz fruit juice	2 or more (have juice no more than once a day)	Daily
Citrus/berries	¾ cup berries; ½ grapefruit; 1 orange; 1 to 2 tangerines; 6 oz citrus juice	1 or more	Daily
Onions, garlic, leeks, shallots, or chives	¼ cup raw; 2 Tbsp cooked; except garlic: ½ or 1 clove	1 or more	At least every other day

cruciferous vegetables, tomatoes and other yellow and orange vegetables, fruits, whole grains, beans and soy foods, onions and garlic, nuts or seeds, dairy, meat, herbs, and healthful oils.

You can customize this list with your personal favorites. But if you keep these backups in stock, you'll be able to make most of the Power Recipes in this book. And you'll never be caught nutritionally short.

FOOD	SERVING SIZE	SERVINGS	FREQUENCY
Beans (pinto, black, lentils) or soy foods	½ cup cooked or canned beans; 1 serving of soy (2 Tbsp miso; 3 Tbsp dry-roasted soybeans or soy protein; ½ cup cooked fresh soybeans, tempeh, or tofu; 1 cup soy milk; ¼ cup textured vegetable protein)	1 or more; vegetarians: 3–4 servings (only 1 soy) daily	3–7 days a week
Whole grain foods	½–1 cup cold cereal (70–90 calories); ½ cup hot cereal; 1 slice bread; ½ cup pasta or cooked grains	5–10	Daily
Nuts or seeds	1 oz	1	Five times a week
Dairy	1 cup fat-free or 1% milk or yogurt; 1 cup calcium-fortified soy milk; 1 oz reduced-fat cheese	2–3	Daily
Fish, poultry, meat, or a vegetarian equivalent	2–3 oz fish, skinless poultry, shellfish, or lean meat (no more than 6 oz daily); ½ cup tofu or cooked beans	2–3 (only 1 tofu)	Daily; 2 vegetarian days per week and fish twice a week or more
Healthful oils (olive, canola, sesame, flaxseed, rice bran)	1 tsp	5–10	Daily
Herbs and spices	1 tsp or more fresh; ¼ tsp or more dried	1 or more	Daily
Hot or homemade iced tea	1 cup	1–5	Daily

Freezer Finds

Frozen vegetables. Keep broccoli florets, cauliflower florets, asparagus, chopped spinach, and other greens (like kale) on hand for stir-fries, pasta dishes, quickly sautéed or microwaved side dishes, toppings for baked potatoes (with melted reduced-fat cheese), vegetable mashed potatoes, additions to casseroles and soups, and mixed Mediterranean dishes like ratatouille.

Boneless chicken breast. Grill it, bake it, or use it in stir-fries or pasta dishes.

Veggie burgers. Keep an assortment of soy or other bean-based patties on hand for variety.

Whole grain pita, sliced bread, and rolls. Keep a supply for sandwiches and veggie burgers.

Gingerroot. Store it in the freezer. Take it out and grate what you need, then refreeze the rest. Use it in stir-fries, bean dishes, and marinades. You can also buy grated ginger in a jar.

Refrigerator Fixes

Whole wheat tortilla or lavash bread. Make burritos, fajitas, or wraps. Fill the wraps with chicken, fish, tofu, imitation soy sausage, vegetables, beans, tofu, salsa, peanut butter and jelly, or leftovers.

Prewashed baby carrots. Serve them as no-fuss crudités with dip as lunchbox snacks, layered in casseroles, in wraps, sautéed with black beans as a side dish, shredded into pasta sauce, or added to a ready-made soup.

Sturdy greens. A bag of spinach or a head of romaine lettuce makes a great salad base. But it also doubles as a fresh-cooked vegetable, an addition to soups or stir-fries, or filler for tacos and wraps.

Reduced-fat cheeses. Buy mozzarella and Swiss, American, or Cheddar. Experiment with different brands until you find one you like.

Low-fat or fat-free plain yogurt. Use it as a staple for making "cream" sauces for pasta (a little holds together one-dish pastas containing vegetables and chicken), topping for fruit (mix it with a little honey), dip (for thicker dip, put yogurt in a sieve lined with a coffee filter and refrigerate it for 3 or more hours, then combine it with your favorite seasonings), soup base, salad dressing base, topping for baked potatoes, or fruit smoothies.

Fresh or jarred salsa. Use it to top low-fat nachos made with melted reduced-fat Cheddar and chopped jalapeños (add chicken and chopped fresh tomatoes for a complete meal), in lasagna (layered with beans and tortillas instead of lasagna noodles), as a topping for baked potatoes, as a seasoning for wraps or burritos, or as an accompaniment for grilled meat, poultry, or seafood.

Reduced-sodium soy sauce and sesame oil. They add instant Asian flavor to steamed vegetables and stir-fries and marinades. Refrigerating

POWER-SHOPPING STRATEGIES

The worst time to shop for food is on weekdays between 5:00 and 8:00 P.M. or on busy weekends, when you're fighting the crowds. If you work all day, go after 9:00 P.M. If you have a more flexible schedule, go in the morning. Here are some other tips to take the headache out of grocery shopping.

- Do one big trip for staples, then fill in with fresh produce midweek.
- Shop with an older child or your husband, then divide up the list and meet at the cash register.
- If you hate grocery shopping, period, find a supermarket that will shop for you. Simply call or fax in your order, and pick it up or have them deliver it to your home. Other options are home food delivery services and Internet shopping.

these items will help them preserve their flavor if you don't use them up quickly.

The Well-Stocked Pantry

Beans, beans, beans. Be sure that you have no less than one can each of black beans (great in beans and rice), white beans (wonderful in bean salads and mashed with garlic and oil on crusty bread), and refried beans (to go into a burrito with salsa). Supplement these with kidney beans (for chili and tacos), chickpeas (for bean salads and hummus), and canned soybeans.

Canned soups and broth. Unless you're highly sodium sensitive, canned soups like minestrone, black bean, split pea, or lentil are a handy way to work beans and vegetables into your daily diet.

Pastas. Keep a variety of shapes on hand—elbow macaroni, shells, ziti, penne, fusilli, orzo, or others—for bean salads; baked ziti (use reduced-fat cheese); one-dish meals combining vegetables, seafood, or chicken with pasta of any shape; lasagna; spaghetti with red sauce; thicker soups (throw in orzo); cold pasta salads with parsley and vegetables (any short pasta works well); and noodle casseroles.

Tomato sauce. Keep it handy for pasta with red sauce; chicken, veal, or fish cacciatore; lasagna; pizza; and vegetable stews.

Brown rice. You don't want to run out. Like pasta, rice is the perfect anchor for vegetables, fish, chicken, and soy foods.

Countertop Caddies

Olive and canola oils. For the best-tasting salad dressings, light sautéing, pasta dishes, dips for bread, or dressing for steamed vegetables, buy extra-virgin olive oil. Canola oil is good for stir-fries.

10 CURES FOR VEGETABLE BOREDOM

Peas and carrots. Or steamed broccoli. Or green beans. Again.

Here are 10 ways to break out of a vegetable rut. Some use oil—and that's good: Studies show that carotenoids—antioxidants in dark green, orange, and red vegetables—are better absorbed with a little oil.

1. AU NATUREL. Crudités (raw vegetables) are real time-savers, especially if your supermarket carries good-quality, prechopped raw vegetables. Serve them with your favorite dip; hummus or yogurt-based dips are supernutritious choices.

2. BEYOND TOSSED SALAD. In the late summer, when tomatoes and cukes are at their peak, try a Middle Eastern–style chopped salad. That's diced tomatoes, cucumbers, green peppers, parsley, and mint with a little lemon juice and oil. And keep green salads interesting by adding combos like tangerines and almonds or beets and walnuts.

3. VEGETABLE SALSA. Chop some carrots, avocados, tomatoes, or other vegetables with cilantro, onion, and garlic, and your kids will forget they're eating vegetables.

4. GRILL. Brush sturdy vegetables like zucchini, eggplant, portobello mushrooms, peppers, and onions with your favorite marinade and place them on the outdoor grill or under the oven broiler. Throw in some garlic cloves and tomatoes, too, for a healing dose of garlic's allylic-sulfide compounds and some lycopene.

5. LAYER. Making a lasagna, noodle, or rice casserole? Add a layer of vegetables in the middle: Spinach or frozen chopped vegetables work well.

Balsamic vinegar. It wakes up salads, is a fat-free way to sauté, and is great combined with olive oil in marinades.

Garlic. No well-stocked kitchen is complete without garlic, a staple of Mediterranean cuisine.

Onions. Keep a couple of these on hand—red, yellow, white, shallots, and scallions. Sautéed onion gives prepared foods (such as jarred spaghetti sauce, canned beans, and soups) a homemade aroma and taste.

6. ROAST. Heat the oven to 425°F, and pop in vegetables of your choice (beets, potatoes, onions, sweet potatoes, and carrots stand up particularly well). Brush the vegetables with olive oil. Make sure to throw in whole, unpeeled garlic cloves. Roast them for 20 to 40 minutes, depending on the vegetables. When it's all done, squeeze out the molten garlic to flavor the rest of the vegetables.

7. SAUTÉ. A little olive oil, a little thyme, some chopped shallots, and lots of mushrooms (they shrink), and you have a heavenly side dish or sauce. Vary the herbs, vary the vegetables—it's nearly impossible to go wrong.

8. STEAM. Both microwaving and steaming preserve the most nutrients. For best results, don't overcook. Remove vegetables from the heat when they're still bright and firm. Then dress them with a simple spritz of lemon juice (excellent for asparagus). Also, a sauce made by combining tahini, lemon juice, water, and garlic stands up well to steamed cruciferous vegetables such as cauliflower.

9. PUREE. After boiling, roasting, or steaming vegetables, stick them in the blender or food processor. Add purees to mashed potatoes (for broccoli mashed potatoes) or to other pureed vegetables (butternut squash, carrots, and grated ginger), or pool them at the bottom of the plate for a brilliant splash of color (red pepper puree is a dramatic choice).

10. STIR-FRY. Heat canola oil and toss in ginger, garlic, a splash of soy sauce, a few drops of sesame oil, and your vegetable of choice—all vegetables take to this method.

Also use it when cooking ground white meat turkey, stir-fries, and home-made soups.

Bananas. They are great for topping cereal, as snacks, or dipped in a little chocolate syrup for a dessert.

One-Dish Wonders

If your image of a nutrition-packed meal consists of individually pre-pared items—meat, potatoes or rice, two vegetables, and a salad—think again. A beautifully set table loaded with side dishes is nice, but who has time? These one-dish meals cover all the nutrition bases with ease.

"Kitchen sink" pasta. For every cup of cooked ziti, rigatoni, linguine, or other favorite pasta, add 1½ to 2 cups fresh, steamed, grilled, or lightly sautéed vegetables seasoned with fresh or dried herbs. Then throw in cooked chicken, shrimp, or another high-protein food, or go completely vegetarian with beans (chickpeas and white beans work well). Toss it with 1 to 3 teaspoons of oil per person, and moisten the sauce with a few tablespoons of the pasta cooking liquid or, when available, juicy tomatoes.

Super soup. Bean-based soups topped with a little grated Parmesan cheese and served with a hunk of whole grain bread make an incredibly satisfying meal. If you don't have time to make your own soup from scratch, toss some broccoli, spinach, cherry tomatoes, or any other vegetables into minestrone, pasta and bean, black bean, split pea, or lentil soup.

Pizza party. Throw together homemade pizzas with whole wheat pita rounds topped with tomato sauce, reduced-fat cheese, and veggies.

Lasagna. Use preshredded reduced-fat mozzarella or mozzarella and reduced-fat ricotta, and layer with sliced vegetables. To save time, you don't have to boil the lasagna noodles in advance. Just use 20 percent more sauce than the recipe calls for, and bake the dish covered. Try a Mexican-style version layering tortillas with beans, salsa, and vegetables.

Rice dishes. Start with a layer of quick-cooking brown rice. Use 2 cups of liquid per cup of uncooked rice. From that point on, your imagination's the limit. Here are some ideas: Pour in chicken broth and herb-rubbed chicken pieces or a layer of lentils or canned beans with your favorite seasonings. Or use a thin, nonchunky tomato-based sauce for spicy red beans and rice.

Chicken or fish in foil. Pour barbecue sauce or reduced-fat Italian salad dressing on a piece of aluminum foil, add the chicken and top with

FIVE OR MORE IN THREE EASY STROKES

Ideally, experts recommend eating no fewer than five fruits and vegetables a day. Yet most women barely eat one. According to one survey, on a given day, only half of all Americans eat fruit or drink fruit juice. And while about 80 percent of us have a vegetable, most choose either french fries or another type of potato. Dark leafy greens, cruciferous vegetables, squash, and other vegetables high in superhealing nutrients get short shrift.

Getting more fruits and vegetables—other than french fries and iceberg lettuce—isn't really that difficult. Here's what it takes.

BREAKFAST. Add a glass of juice and a banana to whatever you usually eat. Two down with zero prep time.

LUNCH. Have a carrot with your sandwich. And use romaine lettuce. That's four down, two to go.

DINNER. Serve pasta with chicken and spinach in a tomato sauce. Last two down the hatch.

sliced onions and frozen vegetables. Seal the foil, put the packet into a 350°F oven, and bake for 40 minutes (take a 30-minute power walk and a 10-minute shower, then take dinner out of the oven). You can prepare fish this way, too, and it takes less time, just 25 to 35 minutes.

Meal-size salads. Start with a layer of salad greens (prepared supermarket greens are fine), and top them with just about anything. Try homemade tuna salad with low-fat mayo; grilled strips of meat, poultry, or fish; shellfish; or seasoned lentils or other beans. Throw on potatoes, corn, or any other vegetables. Drizzle on some dressing and you're set. (Preseasoned cooked chicken strips now available in the poultry section save lots of time.)

The 7-Day Food-Power Menu

BY DAYNA WINTER, M.S., R.D. Busy women want to eat well but don't always have the time to plan meals more than a day in advance, if that. Here, we've pulled together a 7-day menu based on the Day-to-Day Power-Eating Plan on page 541, using 28 of the Power Recipes in this book and many of the 101 Power Foods on page 480.

Follow this menu—or a similar scheme, based on your tastes—and you are guaranteed to get your quota of vitamins, minerals, fiber, antioxidants, and the many phytonutrients that scientists say benefit women.

If you don't have time to prepare all the Power Recipes called for, substitute the simpler serving suggestions from the chapters in which they appear.

On this plan, you get three meals plus a snack and dessert every day for an average of 1,800 calories daily, appropriate for sedentary women who get little physical exercise on the job, at home, or in their leisure activities. If you're more active and want to bump up your calorie intake to make up for what you burn exercising, just add another serving of grains, vegetables, fruit, or even a dessert like Chocolate Cheesecake (page 434).

DAY 1

Breakfast

1 cup Power Oatmeal (page 66)

½ pink grapefruit

1 cup fat-free milk (or 1% milk or calcium-fortified soy milk)

Snack

6 ounces vegetable or carrot juice

Lunch

2 servings Power Broccoli Salad (page 170)

2 pieces toasted whole grain bread of your choice, drizzled with 2 teaspoons olive oil and sprinkled with chopped fresh or dried rosemary

Snack

1 apple

1 ounce reduced-fat cheese of your choice

2 rye crisp bread crackers

Dinner

1 serving Power Fish Fillets (page 351)

1 cup brown rice (or choose another grain such as quinoa or bulgur)

1 cup Swiss chard sautéed with 2 teaspoons olive oil

Dessert

1 cup sliced fruit (try a tropical fruit like papaya, mango, or pineapple)

DAY 2

Breakfast

1½ cups Power Milkshake (page 109)

1 piece whole grain bread with 2 teaspoons all-fruit jam preserves

Snack

¾ cup strawberries or other berries

1 ounce sunflower seeds (dry-roasted, unsalted are best)

1 cup fat-free milk (or 1% milk or calcium-fortified soy milk)

Lunch

1 serving Power Tuna Salad (page 90) served over 2 cups fresh spinach and 1 cup cherry tomatoes

1 small whole grain roll

Snack

1 cup sliced raw vegetables (try red and yellow peppers, carrots, broccoli, and summer squash), dipped in ¼ cup fat-free plain yogurt mixed with 1 tablespoon chopped fresh or 1 teaspoon dried herbs, such as cilantro, dill, basil, or any other favorite herb

Dinner

1½ cups cooked pasta (preferably whole wheat) tossed with 2 tablespoons Power Pesto (page 58)

1 grilled or broiled 3-ounce chicken breast, skin removed (To prepare chicken: Mix 1 tablespoon olive oil, 1 tablespoon lemon, and 1 tablespoon fresh basil and use half of this mixture to brush meat before cooking.) Serve separately or slice over pasta and pesto.

1 cup roasted vegetables (You can buy these ready prepared or make them easily on your own. Try zucchini and yellow squash sliced lengthwise and brushed with the olive oil mixture from above. Roast them at 400°F for about 15 minutes.)

Dessert

1 cup frozen purple grapes

DAY 3

Breakfast

¾ cup mixed berries (blueberries, strawberries, or raspberries), topped with 1 cup fat-free plain yogurt, 1 ounce chopped nuts, and 1 cup low-fat granola

Snack

1 ounce reduced-fat Cheddar cheese

¾ cup raw baby or sliced carrots

2 large whole grain crackers

6 ounces unsweetened apple juice

Lunch

3 ounces baked tofu with lettuce, tomato, and mustard on whole grain bread (You can buy premade baked tofu in health food stores or the health food section of some supermarkets. Otherwise, you can just broil firm tofu in an oven or toaster oven.)

1 serving Power Cauliflower Salad (page 212)

Snack

½ mango, 2 to 3 fresh apricots, or 4 to 6 dried apricot halves

Dinner

1 cup Power Chili (page 282)

2 cups mixed salad greens (try premixed), tossed with 1 tablespoon Power Salad Dressing (page 133)

½ to 1 cup steamed vegetables

1 whole grain dinner roll

Dessert

1 Power Cookie (page 376)

DAY 4

Breakfast

2 Power Muffins (page 306)

1 cup fat-free milk (or 1% milk or calcium-fortified soy milk)

½ pink grapefruit

Snack

½ cup 1% cottage cheese

1 cup halved cherry tomatoes with 1 tablespoon chopped fresh herbs (try dill, cilantro, or basil)

Lunch

1 cup brown rice or other grain such as millet or whole wheat couscous

1 cup red and yellow peppers and 1 cup steamed asparagus, tossed with 1 table-spoon Power Salad Dressing (page 133)

Snack

1 cup Power Shake (page 183)

2 tablespoons nut butter of your choice (peanut, cashew, or almond butter) spread on 1 slice whole grain bread or 3 crackers

Dinner

1 Power Burger (page 104)

1 serving Power Potatoes (page 355)

1 cup steamed greens (such as spinach, kale, or Swiss chard), tossed with 2 tea-spoons olive oil

Dessert

1 apple or other fruit

DAY 5

Breakfast

About 1 cup whole grain bran cereal (equal to 70 to 90 calories) served with 1 cup fat-free milk (or 1% milk or calcium-fortified soy milk), ½ sliced banana, and ½ cup blueberries

Snack

1½ cups Power Fruit Slush (page 151)

Lunch

1 serving Power Pizza (page 270)

1 to 2 servings Power Greens (page 73) or 2 cups mixed salad greens (try pre-mixed) with 1 sliced tomato, tossed with 1 tablespoon Power Salad Dressing (page 133)

Snack

1 cup steamed edamame (young, green soybeans) or 3 tablespoons dry-roasted soybeans

6 ounces vegetable or carrot juice

Dinner

1 serving Power Mushrooms (page 344)

1 serving Power Rice (page 167)

1 cup Power Soup (page 207)

Dessert

1 Power Brownie (page 374) or 2 Power Cookies (page 376)

DAY 6

Breakfast

1 serving Power Breakfast (page 451)

1 cup fat-free milk (or 1% milk or calcium-fortified soy milk)

Snack

⅓ cup cranberry raisins

Lunch

2 cups mixed salad greens (try premixed), 1 sliced tomato or 1 cup cherry tomatoes, 2 to 3 ounces sliced turkey breast (without skin), and 1 ounce grated reduced-fat Cheddar cheese, tossed with 1 tablespoon Power Salad Dressing (page
133) or 1 tablespoon olive oil and the juice of half a lemon, with 1 tablespoon
chopped fresh herbs such as basil, cilantro, or fresh mint

2 slices whole wheat baguette (long, thin French loaf), 1 whole wheat pita bread, or
1 whole wheat dinner roll

Snack

1 serving Power Dip (page 32)

Dinner

4 to 5 ounces baked halibut, marinated in 2 teaspoons olive oil and juice of ½
lemon

1 serving Power Veggies (page 410)

1 large baked sweet potato

Dessert

1 baked apple with ½ cup Power Fruit Topping (page 83)

DAY 7

Breakfast

Three whole wheat pancakes (4-inch) or waffles with ½ cup Power Fruit Topping (page 83) and ½ cup fat-free plain yogurt

6 ounces orange or tangerine juice

Snack

1 cup baby or sliced carrots to munch throughout the day

Lunch

1 serving Power Citrus Salad (page 178)

1 small whole wheat or oat bran bagel with 2 tablespoon reduced-fat cream cheese

Dinner

5 ounces grilled lamb chops (fat removed)

1 serving Power Casserole (page 190)

1 whole grain dinner roll

Dessert

1 serving Power Pudding (page 174)

INDEX

Underscored references indicate boxed text.